T0289496

HISTORICAL DICTIONARY

The historical dictionaries present essential information on a broad range of subjects, including American and world history, art, business, cities, countries, cultures, customs, film, global conflicts, international relations, literature, music, philosophy, religion, sports, and theater. Written by experts, all contain highly informative introductory essays on the topic and detailed chronologies that, in some cases, cover vast historical time periods but still manage to heavily feature more recent events.

Brief A–Z entries describe the main people, events, politics, social issues, institutions, and policies that make the topic unique, and entries are cross-referenced for ease of browsing. Extensive bibliographies are divided into several general subject areas, providing excellent access points for students, researchers, and anyone wanting to know more. Additionally, maps, photographs, and appendixes of supplemental information aid high school and college students doing term papers or introductory research projects. In short, the historical dictionaries are the perfect starting point for anyone looking to research in these fields.

HISTORICAL DICTIONARIES OF RELIGIONS, PHILOSOPHIES, AND MOVEMENTS

Jon Woronoff, Series Editor

Orthodox Church, by Michael Prokurat, Alexander Golitzin, and Michael D. Peterson, 1996

Civil Rights Movement, by Ralph E. Luker, 1997

North American Environmentalism, by Edward R. Wells and Alan M. Schwartz, 1997

Taoism, by Julian F. Pas in cooperation with Man Kam Leung, 1998

Gay Liberation Movement, by Ronald J. Hunt, 1999

Islamic Fundamentalist Movements in the Arab World, Iran, and Turkey, by Ahmad S. Moussalli, 1999

Cooperative Movement, by Jack Shaffer, 1999

Kierkegaard's Philosophy, by Julia Watkin, 2001

Prophets in Islam and Judaism, by Scott B. Noegel and Brannon M. Wheeler, 2002

Lesbian Liberation Movement: Still the Rage, by JoAnne Myers, 2003

Unitarian Universalism, by Mark W. Harris, 2004

New Age Movements, by Michael York, 2004

Feminism, Second Edition, by Janet K. Boles and Diane Long Hoeveler, 2004

Jainism, by Kristi L. Wiley, 2004

Methodism, Second Edition, by Charles Yrigoyen Jr. and Susan E. Warrick, 2005

Kant and Kantianism, by Helmut Holzhey and Vilem Mudroch, 2005

Olympic Movement, Third Edition, by Bill Mallon with Ian Buchanan, 2006

Feminist Philosophy, by Catherine Villanueva Gardner, 2006

Logic, by Harry J. Gensler, 2006

Leibniz's Philosophy, by Stuart Brown and Nicholas J. Fox, 2006

Non-Aligned Movement and Third World, by Guy Arnold, 2006

Epistemology, by Ralph Baergen, 2006

Bahá'í Faith, Second Edition, by Hugh C. Adamson, 2006

Aesthetics, by Dabney Townsend, 2006

Medieval Philosophy and Theology, by Stephen F. Brown and Juan Carlos Flores, 2007

Puritans, by Charles Pastoor and Galen K. Johnson, 2007

Green Movement, Second Edition, by Miranda Schreurs and Elim Papadakis, 2007

Husserl's Philosophy, by John J. Drummond, 2008

Existentialism, by Stephen Michelman, 2008

Zionism, Second Edition, by Rafael Medoff and Chaim I. Waxman, 2008

Coptic Church, by Gawdat Gabra, 2008

Jehovah's Witnesses, by George D. Chryssides, 2008

Hume's Philosophy, by Kenneth R. Merrill, 2008

Mormonism, Third Edition, by Davis Bitton and Thomas G. Alexander, 2008

Hegelian Philosophy, Second Edition, by John W. Burbidge, 2008

Ethics, by Harry J. Gensler and Earl W. Spurgin, 2008

Bertrand Russell's Philosophy, by Rosalind Carey and John Ongley, 2009

Baptists, Second Edition, by William H. Brackney, 2009

Homosexuality, by Brent L. Pickett, 2009

Buddhism, by Carl Olson, 2009

Holiness Movement, Second Edition, edited by William Kostlevy, 2009

Reformed Churches, Second Edition, by Robert Benedetto and Donald K. McKim, 2010

The Reformation and Counter-Reformation, by Michael Mullett, 2010

Heidegger's Philosophy, Second Edition, by Frank Schalow and Alfred Denker, 2010

Jesus, by Daniel J. Harrington, S.J., 2010

Metaphysics, by Gary Rosenkrantz and Joshua Hoffman, 2011

Shinto, Second Edition, by Stuart D. B. Picken, 2011

The Friends (Quakers), Second Edition, by Margery Post Abbott, Mary Ellen Chijioke, Pink Dandelion, and John William Oliver Jr., 2011

Lutheranism, Second Edition, by Günther Gassmann with Duane H. Larson, and Mark W. Oldenburg, 2011

Hinduism, New Edition, by Jeffery D. Long, 2011

Calvinism, by Stuart D. B. Picken, 2012

Hobbes's Philosophy, by Juhana Lemetti, 2012

Chinese Communist Party, by Lawrence R. Sullivan, 2012

New Religious Movements, Second Edition, by George D. Chryssides, 2012

Catholicism, Second Edition, by William J. Collinge, 2012

Radical Christianity, by William H. Brackney, 2012

Organized Labor, Third Edition, by James C. Docherty and Sjaak van der Velden, 2012

Witchcraft, Second Edition, by Jonathan Durrant and Michael D. Bailey, 2013

Lesbian and Gay Liberation Movements, by JoAnne Myers, 2013

Nietzscheanism, Third Edition, by Carol Diethe, 2014

Human Rights, by Jacques Fomerand, 2014

Welfare State, Third Edition, by Bent Greve, 2014

Wittgenstein's Philosophy, Second Edition, by Duncan Richter, 2014

Civil Rights Movement, Second Edition, by Christopher M. Richardson and Ralph E. Luker, 2014

Sikhism, Third Edition, by Louis E. Fenech and W. H. McLeod, 2014

Marxism, Second Edition, by Elliott Johnson, David Walker, and Daniel Gray, 2014

Slavery and Abolition, Second Edition, by Martin A. Klein, 2014

Seventh-Day Adventists, Second Edition, by Gary Land, 2015

Judaism, Third Edition, by Norman Solomon, 2015

Ancient Greek Philosophy, Second Edition, by Anthony Preus, 2015

Descartes and Cartesian Philosophy, Second Edition, by Roger Ariew, Dennis Des Chene, Douglas M. Jesseph, Tad M. Schmaltz, and Theo Verbeek, 2015

Anglicanism, Second Edition, by Colin Buchanan, 2015

Sufism, Second Edition, by John Renard, 2016

Shamanism, Second Edition, by Graham Harvey and Robert Wallis, 2016

Socialism, Third Edition, by Peter Lamb, 2016

Schopenhauer's Philosophy, by David E. Cartwright, 2016

Native American Movements, Second Edition, by Todd Leahy and Nathan Wilson, 2016

Environmentalism, Second Edition, by Peter Dauvergne, 2016

Islam, Third Edition, by Ludwig W. Adamec, 2017

Shakers, Second Edition, by Stephen J. Paterwic, 2017

Utopianism, Second Edition, by Toby Widdicombe, James M. Morris, and Andrea L. Kross, 2017

Chan Buddhism, by Youru Wang, 2017

Islamic Fundamentalism, Second Edition, by Mathieu Guidère, 2017

Salvation Army, Second Edition, by John G. Merritt and Allen Satterlee, 2017

Medical Ethics, by Laurence B. McCullough, 2018

Historical Dictionary
of Medical Ethics

Laurence B. McCullough

ROWMAN & LITTLEFIELD
Lanham • Boulder • New York • London

Published by Rowman & Littlefield
A wholly owned subsidiary of The Rowman & Littlefield Publishing Group, Inc.
4501 Forbes Boulevard, Suite 200, Lanham, Maryland 20706
www.rowman.com

Unit A, Whitacre Mews, 26-34 Stannary Street, London SE11 4AB

British Library Cataloguing in Publication Information Available

Library of Congress Cataloging-in-Publication Data

Name: McCullough, Laurence B., author.
Title: Historical dictionary of medical ethics / Laurence B. McCullough.
Description: Lanham : Rowman & Littlefield, [2018] | Series: Historical dictionaries of religions,
    philosophies, and movements | Includes bibliographical references.
Identifiers: LCCN 2017053094 (print) | LCCN 2017053496 (ebook) | ISBN 9781538114292 (elec-
    tronic) | ISBN 9781538114285 (hardcover : alk. paper)
Subjects: | MESH: Ethics, Medical—history | Dictionary
Classification: LCC R724 (ebook) | LCC R724 (print) | NLM W 13 | DDC 174.2—dc23
LC record available at https://lccn.loc.gov/2017053094

Printed in the United States of America

For four friends and mentors:

My Doktorvater, Ignacio Angelelli, who taught me the history of philosophy at the University of Texas by showing me how to live in and for old books.

H. Tristram Engelhardt Jr., who launched me on and sustained me in my academic career as a philosopher–medical educator.

Warren T. Reich, who asked me to write an entry for his encyclopedia, which launched my scholarship in the history of medical ethics, and who then brought me to Georgetown University.

Baruch A. Brody, who brought me to Baylor College of Medicine and Houston and taught me by example and precept to dedicate myself to medical education and scholarship in medical ethics.

Contents

Editor's Foreword

Although the subject of medical ethics has been around for well over two millennia, since before the Hippocratic Oath in the fifth century BCE, only in the past half century or so has it become central to human society. Its significance keeps increasing, with the activities of not only medical associations and civil society but also the international community, which agreed on the *Declaration of Helsinki* in 2013. It is hard to read the news without being reminded of the importance of medical ethics, with current debates on abortion, eugenics, gene splicing, human cloning, and the need for death with dignity, so it is past time that we added this *Historical Dictionary of Medical Ethics* to the Rowman & Littlefield series Historical Dictionaries of Religions, Philosophies, and Movements.

This book approaches the topic in two basic ways. The chronology and introduction provide a chronological review, reviewing how medical ethics has been a global phenomenon since ancient times. An alphabetical review is then provided in the dictionary section, with entries on people from John Gregory and Thomas Percival to present-day scientists and researchers and organizations including the American Medical Association, the World Medical Association, and the United Nations. Other entries deal with core concepts of medical ethics and the tools of ethical reasoning. The detailed bibliography then provides a wealth of additional sources of information.

The author, Laurence B. McCullough, is a philosopher and medical educator, one of the leading authorities on medical ethics and its history, and adjunct professor of ethics in obstetrics and gynecology at the Weill Medical College of Cornell University, New York City, as well as distinguished emeritus professor at the Center for Medical Ethics and Health Policy of the Baylor College of Medicine in Houston, Texas (where he was honored with the institution's highest teaching award in 2013). During his 40 years in the field, he has taught and mentored numerous students and engaged actively in research on topics such as the conflict of interest in scientific research. He has written extensively, with more than 600 papers and chapters and 14 other books, such as *The Professional Responsibility Model of Perinatal Ethics*. This *Historical Dictionary of Medical Ethics* is quite different in approach and form from the work Dr. McCullough has done before, but his many years of experience as a medical educator made him the ideal author. The book will benefit numerous readers already active in the field as well as others who know relatively little and want to learn more.

Jon Woronoff
Series Editor

Preface

Effective and reliable patient care relies on effective and reliable communication among all members of the care team. Effective and reliable communication relies on precision in thought and speech. This includes communication about the ethical dimensions of patient care. Philosophers understand well the demand for precision in thought and speech: we learned it when we first read, and now teach it to first readers of, Plato's *Dialogues*, starting with Socrates's exchange with the hapless Euthyphro in the eponymous dialogue about piety and continuing with *Republic*'s sustained analysis of justice. The classroom study of medical ethics, like all areas of philosophical inquiry, depends vitally on precision of thought and speech.

Precision of thought and speech is achieved by undertaking and completing the tasks of ethical reasoning: achieving clarity about the meaning of concepts relevant to a case or topic and then identifying the implications of those concepts for a case or topic. These are the skills of ethical analysis and argument, or ethical reasoning, by which students and professors of medical ethics read the literature critically and then communicate with each other effectively and reliably about what they have read and thought. Mastery of these two skills results in the intellectual discipline of ethical reasoning. Precision of thought and speech is also essential in clinical medical ethics, research ethics, organizational ethics, and the ethics of health policy. In all four domains, the lives and health of patients are at stake, lending urgency to precision of thought and speech in clinical ethical reasoning.

I wrote the *Historical Dictionary of Medical Ethics* to support sustained precision of thought and speech about medical ethics by its users, just as I have endeavored to teach precision of thought and speech for the past four decades. Readers of the medical ethics and bioethics literatures—from high school students to college and university students; to medical students, residents, and fellows; to clinical faculty and practicing physicians and health policy makers; and to professors of medical ethics, both new and seasoned—will encounter words, phrases, names, and document and book titles, the meanings of which may be uncertain or even unknown. Teachers and students may use or hear these words and phrases. Care teams and trainees in the clinical and research settings may have similar experiences. I have written the definitions for these diverse communities, who participate in the multiple levels and settings of the discourses of medical ethics and should do so to standards of intellectual excellence.

My teachers and mentors set me on the decades-long path that has led to this book. Patients, students and trainees, and superb clinical and philosophical colleagues, especially those with whom I have been privileged to collaborate in teaching and scholarship, have sustained me. All that is philosophically sound and clinically useful in this book I owe to them, especially the four friends and mentors to whom this *Historical Dictionary of Medical Ethics* is dedicated.

Reader's Notes

Medical educators and philosophy teachers know well the task of teaching the basics, without which one can quickly become lost in the thickets of unfamiliar words and phrases and their complex relations. This book has been designed as an antidote to this outcome, by including definitions of words and phrases that play central roles in medical ethics and therefore appear in many other definitions. These basics include the definitions of medical ethics, professional medical ethics, and bioethics and how they differ; ethical reasoning and its tools of ethical analysis and argument; ethical principles of beneficence, justice, nonmaleficence, respect for autonomy, and respect for people; the professional virtues of compassion, integrity, self-effacement, self-sacrifice, and patience—the grist for the mill of ethical reasoning. Readers who start with these basics will be well prepared to undertake exploring the book, to learn the meaning of the words and phrases, along with their histories and interconnections, that constitute the discourses of medical ethics, professional medical ethics, and bioethics.

The defining feature of this book is that these definitions are placed in the context of the history of medical ethics. These definitions are complemented with definitions for texts and figures from the history of medical ethics.

The users of this book will discover the prominent place of two physician-ethicists in it: John Gregory (1724–1773) of Scotland and Thomas Percival (1740–1804) of England. In my reading of it, the history of medical ethics pivots on these two extraordinary figures. Before them there may have been gestures in the direction of professional medical ethics, but these two physicians invented professional medical ethics. The history of Western, indeed global, medical ethics turns on their accomplishment.

To facilitate the rapid and efficient location of information and to make this book as useful a reference tool as possible, extensive cross-references appear in the dictionary section. Within individual entries, terms that have their own entries are **boldface** the first time they appear. Related terms that do not appear in the text are indicated in *See also* references at the end of an entry. *See* entries refer to other entries that deal with the topic.

Acronyms and Abbreviations

ADA	Americans with Disabilities Act
AIDS	acquired immune deficiency syndrome
AMA	American Medical Association
CCU	critical care unit
CIOMS	Council of International Organizations of Medical Sciences
CPR	cardiopulmonary resuscitation
CVICU	cardiovascular intensive care unit
DHHS	U.S. Department of Health and Human Services
DSD	disorders of sexual development
DSMB	Data Safety and Monitoring Board
ECMO	extracorporeal membrane oxygenation
ECT	electroconvulsive therapy
ELSI	Ethical, Legal, and Social Implications research program of the National Human Genome Research Institute
EMTALA	Emergency Treatment and Active Labor Act
ESRD	end-stage renal disease
GINA	Genetic Information Nondiscrimination Act
HIPAA	Health Insurance Portability and Accountability Act
HIV	human immunodeficiency virus
IACUC	Institutional Animal Care and Use Committee
ICH	International Council on Harmonisation
ICSI	intracytoplasmic sperm injection
ICU	intensive care unit
IRB	Institutional Review Board
IVF	in vitro fertilization
MRI	magnetic resonance imaging
NICU	neonatal intensive care unit

NIPT	noninvasive prenatal testing
NMA	National Medical Association
OHRP	Office for Human Research Protection
OOH-DNR	Out-of-Hospital Do-Not-Resuscitate Order
OPRR	Office for the Protection from Research Risks
PGD	prenatal genetic diagnosis or preimplantation genetic diagnosis
PICU	pediatric intensive care unit
RCT	randomized clinical trial
REC	Research Ethics Committee
ROSC	restoration of spontaneous circulation
SACHRP	Secretary's Advisory Committee on Human Research Protections
TTTS	twin-twin transfusion syndrome
UNAIDS	United Nations Programme on HIV/AIDS
UNESCO	United Nations Educational, Scientific and Cultural Organization
UNOS	United Network for Organ Sharing
WHO	World Health Organization
WMA	World Medical Association

Chronology

Tenth to sixth centuries Compilation of the books of the Torah, the sacred texts of Judaism, traditionally thought to have been given to Moses at Mt. Sinai, the major resources for Jewish moral theology and medical ethics.

551–479 Confucius: Chinese philosopher and sage who based his moral philosophy on the concept of *ren*, or humanity, and filial piety, the obedience to the decisions of one's parents. Confucian medical ethics is based on medicine as "the art of *ren*," emphasizing the physician's virtues.

ca. 460–ca. 370 Hippocrates: Greek physician and ethicist to whom is attributed Hippocratic Corpus, including the *Hippocratic Oath*, *The Art*, and *Epidemics*.

Fifth century Theravāda Buddhist medical ethics, precepts for physicians and the sick, based on prohibitions against taking life, stealing, adultery, lying, and consuming spirit beverages. These texts are included in the Pali Canon, a major resource for Buddhist moral theology and medical ethics.

Late fifth and early fourth centuries Hippocratic Corpus, a collection of texts on clinical and ethical topics in medicine produced by multiple authors, attributed to Hippocrates. *Hippocratic Oath*, attributed to Hippocrates, a "written covenant" of loyalty to teachers and to preserving the "art" (*techné*) of medicine with prescriptions and proscriptions but no supporting ethical reasoning. *The Art*, a text in the Hippocratic Corpus. The text is notable for its admonition not to continue treatment when disease has "overmastered" the sick individual, to avoid the "madness" of such treatment. *Epidemics*, a text in the Hippocratic Corpus. Mistakenly cited as the origin of the dictum "First do no harm" (later Latinized as *Primum non nocere*). The text reads: "Declare the past, diagnose the present, foretell the future; practice these acts. As to diseases, make a habit of two things—to help or at least to do no harm."

Third century *Caraka Samhitā* and *Suśruta-Samhitā*, texts of Hindu moral theology and Hindu medical ethics, presenting a comprehensive medical ethics, focusing on Āyurveda or knowledge of long life and happiness, are major resources for Hindu moral theology and medical ethics.

ca. 427–ca. 347 Plato: Greek philosopher, author of the *Dialogues*, in which he elaborates on metaphysics and moral philosophy. His quest for certainty has intellectual descendants such as Immanuel Kant (1724–1804), who influenced medical ethics in the 19th century and bioethics in the 20th century.

384–322 Aristotle: Greek physician, scientist, and philosopher who wrote on metaphysics, logic, and moral philosophy. His quest for reliability has intellectual descendants such as David Hume (1711–1776) and Richard Price (1723–1791), who influenced medical ethics in the 18th and 19th centuries.

Second to first centuries Author unknown: *Yellow Emperor's Classic of Medicine* (*Huangdi Neijing*) has the status in the history of Chinese medicine that the Hippocratic Corpus has in the history of Western medicine. This text calls for physicians to follow the *Dao*, or way, of medicine and describes medicine as the ultimate virtue.

134 Chinese government adopts Confucian medical ethics.

106–43 Marcus Tullius **Cicero:** Roman politician, lawyer, and Stoic philosopher. His *De Officiis* appeals to role-related obligations, which influences the medical ethics of Thomas Gisborne (1758–1846) and Thomas Percival (1740–1804).

14 BCE–50 CE Aulus Cornelius Celsus: Roman encyclopedist. Like Scribonius Largus (ca. 1–ca. 50 CE), he emphasizes the virtue of compassion, which, for the surgeon, must be managed carefully, so that the surgeon does not lose control and remains focused on benefiting the sick individual upon whom the surgeon is operating.

THE COMMON ERA

First century The New Testament, including the four Gospels about Jesus, the Son of God, and other books, is a major resource for Christian moral theology and medical ethics.

ca. 1–ca. 50 Scibonius Largus: Roman court physician and ethicist. His *Compositiones*, a text on pharmacy, includes text on medical ethics, based on *humanitas* or love of humanity and the virtue of compassion, which creates the physician's obligation to care for all who present for care.

ca. 47 Scribonius Largus's *Compositiones*.

130–210 Galen: Greek physician and philosopher. His medical texts influenced the history of medicine for centuries. He wrote commentaries on ethics in the Hippocratic Corpus and *That the Best Physician Is Also a Philosopher*.

Early Christian era *The Oath according to Hippocrates, in So Far as a Christian May Swear It.* It is sometimes presented in cruciform format and is distinctive for prohibiting inducing abortion from "above" or "below."

329–379 Saint Basil the Great: Orthodox Christian theologian whose moral theology of medicine treats medicine as a gift from God, to use to relieve human suffering.

354–430 Saint Augustine of Hippo, in Roman Africa: Roman Catholic theologian and philosopher, Latin Father, and Doctor of the Church who urged physicians to make cure of the sick their main goal.

Sixth century Buddhism is developed in Japan, appealing to concepts of *sho* (coming into existence, life), *ro* (aging), *byo* (becoming sick), and *shi* (dying and death) to explain the life cycle. The concepts continue to influence Buddhist medical ethics in Japan.

Eighth and ninth centuries The *Qur'an*, the revealed word of God to the prophet Mohammed, and *Hadiths*, the collection of the sayings of the prophet Mohammed, become major resources for Islamic moral theology and medical ethics.

Ninth century Ishāq bin Ali al-Ruhāwī, known as al-Ruhāwī: Arab physician and philosopher, author of the first text in Islamic medical ethics in Arabic medicine, *Practical Ethics of the Physician*. He is known for the quote "The philosopher can only improve the soul, but the virtuous physician can improve both body and soul."

845–925 Mohammad ibn Zakariya al-Razi, known as Rhazes: Persian physician and philosopher whose medical ethics emphasized obligations to both friends and enemies.

1058–1111 Abu Hamid al-Ghazālī, known as al-Ghazālī: Persian theologian and philosopher whose medical ethics includes trust in God and acceptance of medical treatment, understood to be invested with power to heal by God.

1135–1204 Moses ben Maimon, known as Maimonides: Spanish Talmudist and physician whose medical ethics emphasizes the primacy of the care of the sick even on the Sabbath. "Oath of Maimonides" and "The Daily Prayer of a Physician" are attributed to him but were probably written by Marcus Hertz (1747–1803).

1194–1250 Frederick II: Holy Roman Emperor (1212–1250). He called for experienced physicians to protect the sick from incompetent physicians.

13th to 15th centuries An ethics for traditional healers among the Kukutu, developed in what is now Kenya, that emphasizes confidentiality and acknowledges limits on therapy in hopeless cases.

1220–1274 Guglielmo da Saliceto: Italian physician. His surgical ethics describes the good physician, based on the concept of solemnity or solidity of character, especially when sharing bad news with the sick.

1225–1274 Saint Thomas Aquinas: Italian Roman Catholic Dominican priest and Doctor of the Church, theologian and philosopher. His writings address topics in medical ethics, for example, ensoulment of the fetus after 40 days gestation, with important implications for the ethics of induced abortion.

ca. 1240–1311 Arnald of Villanova (Arnaldus de Villa Nova): Spanish physician and ethicist in the *de cautelelis* tradition of providing cautions to physicians, *De Cautelis Medicorum* (*On the Cautions of a Physician*). He provides admonitions implicitly based on the virtue of prudence.

n.d. Arnald de Villanova's *De Cautelis Medicorum* (*On the Cautions of a Physician*).

1260–1316 Henri de Mondeville: French surgeon and ethicist. He wrote one of the first texts on surgical ethics, included in his *Chirugia*, using intellectual and moral standards based on the concept of the conscientious, competent surgeon who helps the sick by providing surgical management only when it is needed.

1290–1370 Guy de Chauliac: French physician. He wrote medical ethics based on the requirement that the physician be competent, which benefits the sick.

1306 Henri de Mondeville's *Chirugia* (*The Surgery of Master Henry de Mondeville*), unfinished upon his death.

1352 al-Ghazālī's *Ihya 'ulum ad-dīn* (Kairo: Matba'a al-'Utmaniya, 1933).

1445–1505 Gabriele Zerbi: Italian physician and ethicist. In the *de cautelis* tradition, he wrote *De Cautelis Medicorum*, emphasizing the fidelity of the physician to the sick.

1478–1535 Saint Thomas More: English lawyer, philosopher, statesman, and Roman Catholic. He opposed King Henry VIII's separation from the Roman Catholic Church and was executed for treason. In his *Utopia* (1516), he considered the permissibility of suicide and euthanasia (in the sense of a death with minimized pain).

1495 Gabriele Zerbi's *Opus perutile de cautelis medicorum*.

1528 Gabriele Zerbi's *De Cautelis Medicorum*.

1547–1628 Giovanni Condronchus: Italian physician and ethicist. He wrote *De Christiana ac Tuta Medendi Ratione* (*Christian and Careful Method of Medicine*), based on virtues, the most fundamental of which is justice.

fl. 1550–1580 John Securis: English physician. He argued that only learned physicians have the capability to heal and warned against commercialization of clinical practice.

1550–1627 Rodrigo de Castro: Portuguese Jewish physician and ethicist in the *medicus politicus*, or politic physician, tradition, which is based on the virtue of prudence of the physician who was subordinate to the power of the rich, royalty, and cities hiring municipal physicians.

1640s Medical curriculum in Spanish colonies in America is mandated to include medical ethics.

1572–1631 John Donne: English poet and cleric of the Church of England. His work on ethics included an argument against regarding suicide as an "irremissible" sin.

1584–1659 Paulus Zacchias: Italian physician, medical educator, and papal physician who wrote a comprehensive medical ethics that also incorporated legal reasoning.

1561–1626 Francis Bacon: English philosopher, statesman, scientist, and jurist. He developed scientific method for clinical investigation and practice based on "experience" (the carefully observed and reported results of natural and controlled experiments, for example, effects of medication), a nascent form of evidence-based medicine, and an ethics of the offices (*officiis*) or role-related obligations of physicians.

1591 Giovanni Condronchus's *De Christiana ac Tuta Medendi Ratione*.

1614 Rodrigo de Castro's *Medicus Politicus* (*The Politic Physician*).

1620 Francis Bacon's *Novum Organum* (*The New Organon*).

1621–1625 Paolo Zachia's *Questiones Medico-Legales* (*Medical-Legal Questions*).

1623 Francis Bacon's *De Augmentis Scientiarum* (*On the Dignity and Advancement of Learning*).

1630–1714 Ekiken Kaibara: Japanese physician and Confucian scholar who wrote *Yojokun* (*Teaching and Care of Life*), which emphasizes a multi-faceted concept of health that physicians should support and restore when lost.

1660–1738 Friedrich Hoffmann: German physician and ethicist in the *"medicus politicus,"* or the "politic physician," tradition, which provides an account of the ethics of the physician who is subordinate to the power of those who employed him, based on the virtue of prudence. Hoffmann's distinctive contribution was to interpret prudence as enlightened self-interest.

1662 Rodrigo de Castro's *Medicus Politicus (The Politic Physician).*

1663–1728 Cotton Mather: New England Puritan minister whose teachings include that being a physician and a cleric is an "angelic conjunction."

1696–1787 Alphonsus Liguori: Italian Roman Catholic bishop. His moral theology addresses both the obligations and sins of physicians. He systematized casuistry, or analogical reasoning, from paradigm cases of right or wrong behavior or good or bad character to new cases.

1711–1776 David Hume: Scottish moral scientist, philosopher, historian, and diplomat. In his *Treatise on Human Nature*, he reports the scientific discovery and mechanism of the principle of sympathy, the natural capacity of all human beings to enter into the affective life of others that motivates us to respond to the pain, distress, and suffering of others, which influenced John Gregory's (1724–1773) and Thomas Percival's (1740–1804) medical ethics.

1713 Ekiken Kaibara's *Yojokun (Teaching and Care of Life).*

1723–1791 Richard Price: Welsh Dissenter and philosopher, a founder of moral realism, the view that moral judgments are based on moral properties of things in the world that can be discovered reliably using the methods of observation elaborated by Francis Bacon (1561–1626), which influenced Thomas Percival's (1740–1804) medical ethics. He wrote *A Review of the Principal Questions of Morals.*

1724–1773 John Gregory: Scottish physician and ethicist, professor of medicine at the University of Edinburgh, and first physician to His Majesty the King in Scotland. He is the author of the first modern text on professional medical ethics, based on Baconian scientific method and the principle of sympathy from David Hume's (1711–1776) moral science.

1738 Friedrich Hoffmann's *Medicus Politicus (The Politic Doctor).*

1740–1804 Thomas Percival: English physician and ethicist. His is the author of probably the first text titled "Medical Ethics" in the global history of medical ethics, *Medical Ethics*, based on Baconian scientific medicine, the moral science of Richard Price (1723–1791), and the moral theology of Dissenters and an influence on the 1847 *Code of Medical Ethics* of the American Medical Association.

1742–1821 Samuel Bard: American physician and ethicist, a founder of what is now the College of Physicians and Surgeons of Columbia University. He is the author of *A Discourse upon the Duties of a Physician*, based on Scottish moral science, which he learned as a medical student at the University of Edinburgh.

1745–1821 Johann Peter Frank: German physician and hygienist. He wrote *System einer vollständigen medicinischen Polizei* (*A System of Complete Medical Police*), based on the concept that the physician's primary obligation is to the state or monarch, which influenced medical ethics in the Soviet Union (1917–1989).

1746–1813 Benjamin Rush: Physician and American patriot who signed the Declaration of Independence for Pennsylvania and served as surgeon general of the Continental Army. Rush studied medicine at the University of Edinburgh and brought John Gregory's medical ethics to North America in his *Observations on the Duties of a Physician, and the Methods of Improving Medicine: Accommodated to the Present State of Society and Manners in the United States.*

1747–1803 Marcus Hertz: German physician and philosopher. He is the probable author of "Oath of Maimonides" and "The Daily Prayer of a Physician," attributed to Maimonides (1135–1204).

1748–1832 Jeremy Bentham: English philosopher and jurist, and utilitarian. He wrote a moral science of duties, which influenced the French *Déontologie médicale* approach to medical ethics in the 19th century.

1753–1821 James Gregory: Physician and son of John Gregory (1724–1773). His critiques of the management of the Royal Infirmary of Edinburgh emphasized that the physician's primary commitment should be to patients and not to the self. He also argued that the managers of the Royal Infirmary have an ethical obligation to see to it that every patient receives clinical management supported by the scientific judgments of physicians and surgeons.

1758–1846 Thomas Gisborne: English Anglican priest and moral theologian. His moral philosophy of role-related ethical obligations ("offices") influenced Thomas Percival's medical ethics. He wrote *An Enquiry into the Duties of Men in the Higher and Middle Classes of Society in Great Britain Resulting from Their Respective Stations, Professions and Employment.*

1762–1836 Christian Hufeland: German physician and ethicist. He wrote a medical ethics influenced by the German philosopher, Immanuel Kant (1724–1804), emphasizing treating the patient as an end in himself or herself and not a mere object of experiments. Wrote *Enchiridion Medicum* (*Manual of the Practice of Medicine*), which influenced the development of Japanese medical ethics in the 19th century.

1766–1842 Baron Dominique-Jean Larrey: French surgeon who introduced and applied the concept of rapid evacuation of wounded soldiers to field hospitals. This resulted sometimes in the number of patients exceeding available resources, leading Larrey to invent the concept of triage, or prioritizing patients by medical need and urgency.

1769 Samuel Bard's *A Discourse upon the Duties of a Physician*.

1770 Anonymous (John Gregory): *Observations on the Duties and Offices of a Physician.* As was then common, Gregory published his text on professional medical ethics anonymously to test public reception of his ideas. The book was well received, and he followed it with a revised and retitled book in 1772.

1771–1865 Félix Janer: Spanish physician and ethicist. He wrote *Elementos de Moral Médica* (*Treatise on Moral Medicine*), in which he acknowledges the influence of John Gregory's (1724–1773) medical ethics.

1772 John Gregory's *Lectures on the Duties and Qualifications of a Physician.* Upon positive reception of *Observations*, Gregory revised and retitled the text and published it under his own name. The text introduces professional medical ethics that replaced the contractual ethics that had dominated the previous history of medical ethics. Gregory's medical ethics becomes an acknowledged source of influence of the 1847 *Code of Medical Ethics* of the American Medical Association.

1778 Anonymous German translation of Gregory's *Lectures*.

1779 Johann Peter Frank's *System einer vollständigen medicinischen Polizei* (*A System of Complete Medical Police*).

1785–1863 William Beaumont: U.S. Army surgeon. He made contributions to gastric physiology based on the research carried out, starting in the 1820s, on Alexis St. Martin (1794–1880), who suffered a gunshot wound to the abdomen that did not close, allowing for direct observation of gastric function. St. Martin consented to become a research subject.

1787 Richard Price's *A Review of the Principal Questions of Morals*.

1790s Baron Dominique-Jean Larrey's concept of triage is introduced to manage the challenge of the number of wounded soldiers in a field hospital exceeding available resources to treat them.

1791–1855 Theodoric Romeyn Beck: American physician and medical educator who wrote the first major work on medical jurisprudence in the United States, *Elements of Medical Jurisprudence.*

1794 Thomas Gisborne's *An Enquiry into the Duties of Men in the Higher and Middle Classes of Society in Great Britain Resulting from Their Respective Stations, Professions and Employment.* Thomas Percival's *Medical Jurisprudence; or, A Code of Ethics and Institutes, Adapted to the Professions of Physic and Surgery* is privately published in Manchester, England, and circulated to acquaintances and scholars for comment. In response to comments, Percival revised and retitled the text and published it in 1804 as *Medical Ethics; or, A Code of Institutes and Precepts, Adapted to the Professional Conduct of Physicians and Surgeons.*

1796–1872 John Bell: American physician and ethicist who played a leading role in creating the 1847 *Code of Medical Ethics* of the American Medical Association.

1796–1877 Karl Friedrich Heinrich Marx: German physician who took the view that "medicine is a part of ethics" and that physicians were justified in sometimes not accepting some wishes of patients.

1796–1879 Isaac Hays: American physician and ethicist who played a leading role in creating the 1847 *Code of Medical Ethics* of the American Medical Association.

1789 Italian translation by F. F. Padovano of Gregory's *Lectures.*

1797 French translation by B. Verlac of Gregory's *Lectures.*

19th to 20th centuries Influence of medical ethics of colonial European and trading powers on medical ethics in African and Asian countries.

1800–1840 Michael Ryan: Irish physician and author of a text on medical jurisprudence that included what is regarded as the first history of medical ethics, *A Manual of Medical Jurisprudence, Compiled from the Best Medical and Legal Works.*

1803 Thomas Percival's *Medical Ethics; or, A Code of Institutes and Precepts, Adapted to the Professional Conduct of Physicians and Surgeons.* Spanish translation of Gregory's *Lectures*, titled *Discurso sobre los deberes, qualidades y conocimientos del medico, con el método des sus estudios.*

1805 Benjamin Rush's *Observations on the Duties of a Physician, and the Methods of Improving Medicine: Accommodated to the Present State of Society and Manners in the United States.*

1806–1872 Worthington Hooker: American physician, educator, and ethicist. He wrote *Physician and Patient; or, A Practical View of the Mutual Duties, Relations and Interests of the Medical Profession and Community*, emphasizing the scientific practice of medicine combined with professional virtues. The Latinate version of "First, do no harm," or "*Primum non Nocere*," is sometimes attributed to Hooker.

1807, fl. 1845–1865 Maximilien Isidore Amand Simon: French physician. He wrote on the duties of physicians in his Déontologie médicale, in which he applies the "science of duties" of Jeremy Bentham (1748–1832) to the obligations and rights of physicians.

1812–1886 Austin Flint: American physician and ethicist who defended the 1847 *Code of Medical Ethics* of the American Medical Association from its critics. He wrote *Medical Ethics and Medical Etiquette: The Code of Ethics Adopted by the American Medical Association with Commentaries by Austin Flint, M.D.*

1813–1878 Claude Bernard: French physiologist and experimental biomedical scientist. He wrote on the ethics of research with animal subjects and with human subjects in his *Introduction à l'étude de la medicine expérimentale* (*Introduction to the Study of Experimental Medicine*).

1813–1884 J. Marion Sims: American physician. He is noted for his development of the surgical procedure to repair vesico-vaginal fistulas, developed using unanesthetized slaves. He was a vocal opponent of the American Medical Association's *Code of Medical Ethics* of 1847.

1817 First American edition of John Gregory's *Lectures on the Duties and Qualifications of a Physician.*

1819 The Kappa Lambda Society of Hippocrates is founded by Dr. Samuel Brown (1796–1830), a professor at the University of Transylvania medical school in Lexington, Kentucky. The society privately published "extracts" of *Medical Ethics* of Thomas Percival (1740–1804) that became the conduit through which passages from *Medical Ethics* were included in the 1847 *Code of Medical Ethics* of the American Medical Association.

1820s Statements on ethics of the medical societies of the various states in the United States, known as "Medical Police" or "System of Medical Ethics," are developed.

1823 Theodoric Romeyn Beck's *Elements of Medical Jurisprudence.*

1831 Michael Ryan's *A Manual of Medical Jurisprudence, Compiled from the Best Medical and Legal Works*. Félix Janer's *Elementos de Moral Médica* [*Treatise on Moral Medicine*].

1835–1920 Father Charles Coppens, SJ: American Jesuit priest of the Roman Catholic Church. He wrote a Roman Catholic moral theology of medicine titled *Moral Principles and Medical Practice: The Basis of Medical Jurisprudence.*

1836 Christian Hufeland's *Enchiridion medicum order Anleitung zur medizinische Praxis* (*Manual of the Practice of Medicine*).

1841–1920 Karl Binding: German lawyer and advocate. He and Alfred Hoche (1865–1943) wrote of voluntary and involuntary euthanasia in their *Die Freigabe der Vernichtung lebensunwerten Lebens* (*The Release and Destruction of Life Devoid of Value*), which became part of the justificatory framework for the crimes against humanity carried out by physicians in Nazi Germany during World War II.

1845 Maximilien Isidore Amand Simon's *Déontologie médicale* (Medical Deontology).

1845–1934 Lewis Pilcher: American physician and ethicist. In his essay "Code of Medical Ethics," he fiercely criticized the 1847 *Code of Medical Ethics* of the American Medical Association because requiring adherence to it violated the sovereignty of individual conscience.

1846–1847 American Medical Association is founded. All members are required to accept its *Code of Medical Ethics*. Later in the 19th century, physicians challenge this requirement on the grounds that it violates the sovereignty of individual conscience. This results in shortening the *Code* into *Principles of Medical Ethics.*

1847 American Medical Association's *Code of Medical Ethics* addresses obligations of physicians to patients and society, of patients to physicians, and of society to physicians. The latter two obligations are based on an argument for reciprocity: physicians have the professional obligation to patients to provide effective medical care; physicians therefore have a right to expect patients to cooperate in, and society to support, this undertaking; this right creates the obligations of patients and society to cooperate with and support the provision of effective medical care.

1849 Worthington Hooker's *Physician and Patient; or, A Practical View of the Mutual Duties, Relations and Interests of the Medical Profession and Community.*

1849–1919 William Osler: Canadian physician and cofounder of the Johns Hopkins University medical school in Baltimore, Maryland. He wrote on *aequanimitas*, or equanimity, of physicians in patient care: the physician should in all circumstances appear "imperturbable."

1851–1902 Walter Reed: U.S. Army physician. He supported the hypothesis that yellow fever, epidemics of which were common and incapacitated soldiers in camp and in the field, is an infectious disease transmitted by mosquitos. His research to test this hypothesis was based on good science and required the informed consent of soldiers in writing to become research subjects, creating what is considered a model for the conduct of research in military medicine and military medical ethics.

1856 The British Medical Association is founded. Attempts to adopt a code of medical ethics were not successful, a reliance on good moral character having been thought to be sufficient.

1860s Zemskaya medicine is first developed in Russia; it is a prototype of socialized healthcare based on an ethics of access to free medical care, including preventive medical care.

1862–1939 Albert Moll: German physician whose *Ärtzliche Ethik* (*Doctor's Ethics*) is comprehensive. The text includes ethics of research with human subjects, arguing that written consent is required for research with significant risks. Translated into Russian in the late 19th century, the text provoked a critical response.

1865 Claude Bernard's *Introduction à l'étude de la médecine expérimentale* (*Introduction to the Study of Experimental Medicine*).

1865–1943 Alfred Hoche: German physician and advocate. He and Karl Binding (1841–1920) wrote of voluntary active euthanasia and involuntary active euthanasia in their *Die Freigabe der Vernichtung lebensunwerten Lebens* (*The Release and Destruction of Life Devoid of Value*), which became part of the justificatory framework for the crimes against humanity carried out by physicians in Nazi Germany during World War II.

1868–1939 Richard C. Cabot: American physician and ethicist. His medical ethics emphasized cooperation among healthcare professionals caring for a patient, an ethics of cooperation that anticipated the now standard hospital practice of team care.

1876 Karl Friedrich Heinrich Marx's *Ärtzlicher Katechismus: Über die Anforderungen an die Ärtze.*

1876–1958 Pope Pius XII: Head of the Roman Catholic Church (1939–1958). In an address, he stated that Roman Catholic moral theology supports aggressive palliation for a dying patient, provided that the physician does not intend to cause the patient's death.

1882 Austin Flint's *Medical Ethics and Medical Etiquette.*

1882–1954 Willard Sperry: American Protestant theologian and dean of Harvard Divinity School. He wrote *The Ethical Basis for Medical Practice*, which emphasizes the importance of codes of ethics.

1883 Lewis Pilcher's "Codes of Medical Ethics."

1893–1956 Guobin Song: Chinese physician and ethicist. He wrote *Professional Ethics in Medicine*, the first professional medical ethics in China in the 20th century, integrating Western medical ethics into Chinese clinical practice.

1889 William Osler's *Aequanimitas*.

1893–1978 Andrew C. Ivy: American physician and physiologist. He served as representative of the American Medical Association and gave testimony in *United States of America v. Karl Brandt et al.*

1895 The National Medical Association for African American physicians is founded in the United States for African American physicians who were at that time excluded from membership in the American Medical Association.

1896–1978 Chauncey Leake: American biomedical scientist and leader in academic medicine. His 1927 edition of Thomas Percival's (1740–1804) *Medical Ethics* (1803) made this landmark text in the history of medical ethics readily available for physicians, medical educators, scholars, and students.

1897 Father Charles Coppens's *Moral Principles and Medical Practice: The Basis of Medical Jurisprudence*.

1902 Albert Moll's *Ärtzliche Ethik* (*Doctor's Ethics*).

1902–1964 Father Gerald Kelly, SJ: American Jesuit priest of the Roman Catholic Church who wrote a Roman Catholic moral theology of medicine, titled *Medico-Moral Problems*.

1903 *Principles of Medical Ethics* of the American Medical Association replaces *Code of Medical Ethics*.

1905–1991 Joseph Fletcher: Protestant theologian and advocate of "situational ethics" (a version of act utilitarianism). A founder of the field of bioethics, he wrote *Morals and Medicine*, which emphasizes the patient's rights.

1908–2001 Pedro Laín Entralgo. Spanish medical scientist and historian of medicine, a major source of influence on bioethics and medical ethics in Spain and Latin America and their emphasis on the medical humanities.

1912 A revised version of *Principles of Medical Ethics* of the American Medical Association is published.

1920 Karl Binding and Alfred Hoche's *Die Freigabe der Vernichtung lebensunwerten Lebens: Ihr Mass und ihre Form* (*The Release and Destruction of Life Devoid of Value: Its Measure and Form*).

1920–2013 Edmund D. Pellegrino: American physician, medical educator, and ethicist. He is a founder of the field of bioethics and the founding editor of the *Journal of Medicine and Philosophy*.

1921–1999 Immanuel Jacobovitz: Jewish rabbi and scholar. He is the author of *A Comparative and Historical Study of the Jewish Religious Attitude to Medicine and Its Practice*, a broad examination of topics in medical ethics from the perspective of Jewish moral theology.

1927 Chauncey Leake's edition of *Percival's Medical Ethics*.

1930–1931 Germany's Reich Health Council promulgates "Regulations Concerning New Therapy and Human Experimentation," providing comprehensive guidance for research with human subjects, which were violated by Nazi physicians.

1931–1972 The United States Public Health Service in Macon County, Georgia, conducts a study of the natural history of syphilis among African American men. The study's name is taken from the Tuskegee Institute, the hospital that collaborated in the study. The enrollment process involved deception, and the study continued after penicillin, a cure for syphilis, became available in 1947. The study was kept secret until it became public in 1972 and was shut down later that year.

1931–2004 John C. Fletcher: American Episcopal priest and one of the founders of the field of bioethics. He was the first chief of bioethics at the Clinical Center of the National Institutes of Health in Bethesda, Maryland, in which position he developed clinical ethics consultation.

1932–1945 Imperial Japanese Army establishes biological warfare programs, such as Unit 731, that conducted unethical experiments using human subjects, comparable to the crimes against humanity of the Nazi doctors. However, no prosecution by Allied countries occurred after the end of World War II in the Pacific.

1933 Guobin Song's *Yiye Lunlixue* (*Professional Ethics in Medicine*).

1945–1991 Era of communist medical ethics in totalitarian states of Eastern Europe under domination by the Union of Soviet Socialist Republics.

1946–1947 *United States of America v. Karl Brandt et al.*, the trial conducted under the auspices of the War Tribunal in Nuremberg, West Germany, to prosecute Nazi physicians for war crimes and crimes against humanity, including unethical experimentation and mass murder. Seven were executed, including Karl Brandt (1904–1948), Adolf Hitler's (1889–1945) personal physician.

1947 *The Nuremberg Code* is promulgated by the War Tribunal in Nuremberg, West Germany. The first international code of research ethics, it includes requirements that consent always be obtained from human subjects of research and that standards of intellectual excellence in scientific investigation must be followed without exception.

1948 The World Medical Association's *Declaration of Geneva: The Physician's Oath* is published, intending to be a modern version of the *Hippocratic Oath*. The text has been revised in 1968, 1983, 1994, 2005, and 2006. The United Nations Universal Declaration of Human Rights is adopted by the United Nations General Assembly. It is a transnational, transcultural, and transreligious statement of rights that all human beings may claim, including the right to health. The United Kingdom's National Health Service is created, implementing healthcare as a right as a matter of public policy.

1949–1954 Gerald Kelly's *Medico-Moral Problems*.

1950 Willard Sperry's *The Ethical Basis for Medical Practice*.

1952 United States Armed Forces Medical Policy Council proposes adoption of the Nuremberg Code of Ethics to guide research with human subjects; it is approved by Department of Defense in 1953.

1953 23 April: The journal *Nature* publishes an article by James D. Watson and Francis H. Crick describing the structure of deoxyribonucleic acid (DNA), launching the era of molecular genetics and genomics in biological sciences and in clinical practice and research.

1954 Joseph Fletcher's *Morals and Medicine*. **23 December:** The first renal (kidney) transplantation, from a living donor, is conducted at Peter Bent Brigham Hospital in Boston, Massachusetts, launching the era of organ transplantation.

1957 *Principles of Medical Ethics* of the American Medical Association is revised to comprise a concise statement of ethical principles, which remains the format of the *Principles*. Pius XII's "Address of 21 November 1957" (*Der Anesthetist* 7: 242–243) endorses aggressive palliation of the dying patient.

1959 Immanuel Jacobovitz's *A Comparative and Historical Study of the Jewish Religious Attitude to Medicine and Its Practice.*

1960 The United States Food and Drug Administration approves the first oral contraceptive, launching the era of the increased control by women over becoming pregnant and detaching sexual intercourse from reproduction. **9 March:** The first placement of a shunt in a patient dying of renal failure is conducted, allowing for attachment to mechanical continuous hemodialysis. It is a scarce resource until federal funding for end-stage renal disease is instituted by Medicare in 1975.

1964 The World Medical Association's *Declaration of Helsinki: Ethical Principles for Medical Research Involving Human Subjects* (revised 1973, 1983, 1986, 1996, 2000, 2002, 2004, 2008, and 2013) provides a statement of principles for comprehensive ethical guidance for research with human subjects.

1965 The London Medical Group, organized around lectures and conferences on a wide range of topics in medical ethics, is founded in England. Medicare (providing limited coverage of medical care for the elderly [over the age of 65] and the disabled) and Medicaid (a state-federal program of limited coverage of medical care and long-term care for the medically indigent) are enacted in the United States.

1966 Henry K. Beecher (1904–1976), an American physician, writes an article for the *New England Journal of Medicine*, reporting on cases of ethically questionable research with human subjects.

1967 3 December: The first heart transplantation is performed at Groote Schur Hospital in Cape Town, South Africa. The donor heart was beating in a patient admitted with "irreversibly fatal brain damage." This inaugurated the era of heart transplantation and the clinical, ethical, and legal challenges of determining when death has occurred for patients on mechanical respiratory support.

1968 25 July: *Humanae Vitae (Of Human Life)* is issued by Pope Paul VI of the Roman Catholic Church, upholding the traditional prohibition of artificial contraception as contrary to natural law. **5 August:** The *New England Journal of Medicine* publishes a report from an ad hoc committee of the Harvard Medical School in Boston, Massachusetts, proposing the use of brain function criteria to determine that death has occurred in a patient on mechanical respiratory support, which precludes the application of cardiopulmonary criteria to determine that death has occurred.

1969 The Institute of Society, Ethics, and the Life Sciences, now the Hastings Center, is founded by the philosopher Daniel Callahan and the physician Willard Gaylin. This private, nonsectarian, independent research center supported and promoted interdisciplinary study in what became the field of bioethics. The institute publishes the journals titled the *Hastings Center Report* and *IRB*. The Ibero-American Bioethics Program at the Institute for the Medical Humanities of the José María Mainetti Foundation in La Plata, Argentina, is founded by Dr. José Alberto Mainetti.

1970 The word "bioethics" is used by the scientist Van Rensselaer Potter (1911–2001), perhaps for the first time, to include study of ethical issues in biomedicine and the environment. Bioethics becomes a multidisciplinary, global field of research, education, and practice.

1971 The Kennedy Institute of Ethics at Georgetown University in Washington, DC, is founded by the Dutch physician and ethicist André Hellegers (1926–1979), with the support of the Joseph P. Kennedy Jr. Foundation. The institute publishes the *Kennedy Institute of Ethics Journal*. Adopted by the Presidium of the Supreme Soviet, the *Oath of the Soviet Physician* is to be taken by all graduates and physicians in the Union of Soviet Socialist Republics, which was dissolved 26 December 1991.

1972 26 July: The *New York Times* reports on the Tuskegee Study of the natural history of syphilis in a population of approximately 600 African American men, funded and conducted by the United States Public Health Service in Tuskegee, Alabama, which was determined by a review panel to be unethical.

1973 22 January: The United States Supreme Court, in majority opinions in two cases that had been joined, struck down laws restricting access to induced abortion. One case was from Texas, *Roe v. Wade*, and the other from Georgia, *Doe v. Bolton*. **25 October:** The *New England Journal of Medicine* publishes an article by Drs. Raymond Duff and Alastair Campbell describing cases in which life-sustaining treatment had been discontinued from neonatal patients with an ethical justification.

1974–1978 The United States' National Commission for the Protection of Human Subjects of Biomedical and Behavioral Research produced the *Belmont Report* that set out an ethical framework based on the principles of beneficence, respect for persons, and justice.

1975 The *Journal of Medicine and Philosophy* is founded by the physician and ethicist Edmund Pellegrino (1920–2013). The *Journal of Medical Ethics* in England is founded by the ethicist Alastair V. Campbell. The Kennedy-Corman Bill becomes law in the United States, adding to Medicare the mandate to provide coverage of treatment for end-stage renal disease (ESRD).

1976 Quinlan Case: The New Jersey Supreme Court supports as legally permissible the discontinuation of life-sustaining treatment in a patient with a "persistent chronic vegetative state" (now known as a "permanent vegetative state") and surrogate decision making for patients who cannot make their own decisions.

1978 The first edition of the comprehensive reference work titled *The Encyclopedia of Bioethics*, edited by Warren T. Reich of the Kennedy Institute of Ethics at Georgetown University, Washington, DC, is published. The text is distinctive for including a large section on the history of medical ethics. **25 July:** The first child conceived by in vitro fertilization is born in England, inaugurating the era of assisted reproductive medicine.

1981 The first cases among homosexual men in the United States of what came to be known as acquired immune deficiency syndrome (AIDS), then a life-taking infectious disease, are reported. The resulting epidemic made urgent the development of ethics for clinical practice, research, and public health of contagious, potentially life-taking diseases.

1982 Baby Doe Case: An infant with Down syndrome (trisomy 21), esophageal atresia, and esophageal-tracheal fistula was not treated, at the request of its parents, and subsequently died, which became public and prompted the administration of President Ronald Reagan (1911–2004; term of office: 1981–1989) to issue federal regulations prohibiting withholding treatment from neonatal patients based on disability.

1982, 1993 The Council of International Organizations of Medical Sciences (CIOMS) and the World Health Organization (WHO) produce guidelines for research with human subjects.

1982 3 December: The implantation of an artificial heart in a human patient at the University of Utah inaugurates the era of mechanical circulation devices.

1983 The first cases of acquired immune deficiency syndrome (AIDS) are reported in sub-Saharan Africa, raising ethical issues of access to treatment and prevention of discrimination of socially and politically vulnerable individuals and groups. The Bioethics Programme of UNESCO (United Nations Educational, Scientific and Cultural Organization), in Geneva, Switzerland, is founded to study ethical and policy dimensions of progress in the life sciences.

1984 In the United States, amendments to the federal law on child abuse are enacted, preventing discontinuation of life-sustaining treatment from neonatal patients, except when continuing such treatment would "merely prolong dying, not be effective in ameliorating or correcting all of the infant's life-threatening conditions, or otherwise be futile in terms of the survival of the infant." **Alkmaar Case:** The Supreme Court of the Netherlands permits euthanasia, in the sense of killing the patient by the physician, provided that the patient has the capacity to make decisions, that the paramount goal is to relieve suffering, and that cases are reported to legal authorities.

1990 In the Netherlands, the Remmlink Report documents cases of euthanasia, in the sense of killing the patient by the physician, of patients who did not have decision-making capacity. In the United Kingdom, the Human Fertilisation and Embryology Authority is created to regulate research and practice in assisted reproduction. The International Conference on Harmonisation (ICH) Guidelines for Good Clinical Practice unifies standards for the approval process of new drugs and devices that aim to protect the rights and interests of human subjects of research and the responsibilities of both investigators and sponsoring organizations.

1991 The Nuffield Council on Bioethics in London, England, is founded by the Nuffield Foundation, a leading center for informing public debate and policy formation on ethical issues in biomedicine.

1992 The International Association of Bioethics is founded.

1994 The *Dakar Declaration* is a statement of legal rights, human rights, and ethical principles for the treatment of individuals infected with human immunodeficiency virus (HIV) and prevention of HIV infection and acquired immune deficiency syndrome (AIDS) with a focus on sub-Saharan Africa. The Regional Program on Bioethics of the Pan American Health Organization, in Santiago, Chile, is created. The Oregon Death with Dignity Act permits physician-assisted suicide for terminally ill patients with decision-making capacity, in the sense of the physician prescribing a life-taking medication that the patient then self-administers.

1995 25 March: *Evangelium Vitae* (*Gospel of Life*), issued by Pope John Paul II of the Roman Catholic Church, affirms the sanctity of human life and its implications for abortion, euthanasia, murder, and capital punishment, providing a broad moral theological context for Roman Catholic medical ethics.

1996 5 July: Dolly, the cloned sheep, is born in Scotland; the sheep dies in 2003.

1999 The *American Journal of Bioethics* is founded by the philosopher Glenn McGee.

2005 United Nations Educational, Scientific and Cultural Organization's Universal Declaration of Human Rights and Bioethics.

2007, 2012 The United Nations Programme on HIV/AIDS (UNAIDS)/World Health Organization (WHO) Guidance Document titled *Ethical Considerations in Biomedical HIV Prevention Trials* provides comprehensive ethical guidance for such clinical trials.

2013 The World Medical Association's *Declaration of Helsinki: Ethical Principles for Medical Research Involving Human Subjects* is a major revision of the statement that provides principles for comprehensive ethical guidance for research with human subjects.

2014 The American Society for Bioethics and Humanities adopts a code of professional ethics for clinical ethics consultants, titled *Code of Ethics and Professional Responsibilities for Healthcare Ethics Consultations*.

Introduction

Medical ethics is the disciplined study of medical morality, with two goals: critically appraising current medical morality and identifying how it should be improved. Medical morality has three components. Physicians, patients, communities, and policy makers have beliefs about what is good and bad character, and right and wrong behavior, in patient care, biomedical research, medical education, and health policy. On the basis of these beliefs, physicians, patients, communities, and policy makers make judgments about how physicians ought to conduct themselves in patient care, research, education, and the formation and implementation of health policy. They then act on their judgments.

These ethical judgments put matters of physicians' character and behavior into one of five categories: ethically impermissible (prohibited character formation and behavior), ethically permissible (allowed character formation and behavior), ethically obligatory (required character formation and behavior), ethically controversial (competing accounts of the impermissible, permissible, or obligatory), or ethically uncertain (no reasoned account has been achieved). Physicians ought never to engage in ethically impermissible character formation (e.g., becoming systematically dishonest), or behavior (e.g., sharing protected health information with the state without proper legal authorization). Physicians may engage in ethically permissible character formation or behavior, but do nothing ethically impermissible if they do not do so. Physicians should engage in character formation that is ethically obligatory (e.g., being honest with patients), and ethically obligatory behavior (e.g., conducting an appropriate informed consent process for the performance of invasive, risky procedures such as coronary artery bypass grafting surgery). Character formation and behavior become ethically controversial when reasoned judgments about its ethical permissibility conflict, for example, selective termination (feticide) of a multifetal pregnancy from a twin to singleton pregnancy for a pregnancy that was initiated using assisted reproductive technology. Character formation and behavior become ethically uncertain when the clinically beneficial harmful outcomes of a new biotechnological development (e.g., gene editing to prevent inherited disorders) are not well enough understood to permit reasoned judgments about them.

The task of ethical reasoning in critical appraisal begins with ethical analysis, which focuses on the concepts that shape moral beliefs. Concepts that are vague or confused will result in highly variable and thus unreliable moral judgments. To prevent this unacceptable outcome in ethical reasoning, ethi-

1

cal analysis seeks the clearest possible expression of concepts. The definitions of words and phrases in this dictionary play an essential role in this task
(Landau 2001). Concepts that are used with shifting meaning in subsequent
judgments will result in highly variable conclusions and, therefore, preventable ethical controversy and uncertainty. To prevent this outcome, once a
concept has been clarified it should be used consistently (i.e., with that meaning and not another). Achieving both clarity and consistency in ethical reasoning requires sustained, close attention.

The task of critical appraisal continues with assessing the quality of reasoning using concepts that have been clarified and then used consistently in
ethical argument. Ethical judgments are based on the implications of clearly
expressed concepts. Ethical judgments should follow these implications to
the conclusions that the implications support and nowhere else. The goal of
routinely doing so is the formation of reliable moral judgments, where "reliable" means that physicians, patients, healthcare organizations, society, and
policy makers can act on them with confidence that their action is ethically
justified.

Ethical judgments about patient care, research, education, and health policy should provide practical guidance about current ethical challenges. Judgments that are expressed in abstract or purely theoretical terms will not meet
the test of applicability, especially clinical applicability. Ethical judgments
should also be adequate: they should provide at least initial guidance to
reflection when new, unexpected ethical challenges arise. Meeting the test of
adequacy serves as a powerful antidote to the view, frequently found in the
ethics literature about new and emerging biomedical technologies, that such
scientific and technologic advancement poses new and unprecedented ethical
challenges that threaten to outstrip our capacity for reliable moral judgments.
The problem for this view is that, from a historical perspective, it is very hard
to do something that is indeed new and unprecedented. Historians, including
historians of medicine and medical ethics, consider the failure to recognize
this reality to be a naive view, at best, and a self-serving view, at worst.

Completing the tasks of ethical analysis and argument results in the disciplined study of medical morality (i.e., medical ethics) expressed in reasoned
ethical judgments about physicians' character formation and behavior. Reasoned ethical judgments are based on clearly expressed concepts, the identification of their implications for the ethical challenge at hand, and following
those implications to the conclusion that they support. The discipline of
medical ethics means that reasoned ethical judgments—and only reasoned
ethical judgments—should guide character formation and behavior of physicians. The discipline of medical ethics also means that reasoned ethical judgments—and only reasoned ethical judgments—should then guide the evaluation of character formation and behavior of physicians and their improve-

ment based on such evaluation. When character formation or behavior is supported by reasoned ethical judgment, then that character formation or behavior is said to be ethically justified.

Achieving and adhering to the intellectual and practical discipline of medical ethics prevents errors in reasoning that can make moral judgments unreliable and jeopardize the quality of patient care, research, education, and health policy. One such error is starting with conclusions about character formation and behavior and then going in search of friendly premises. This error is often made in informal conversation about controversial topics in medical ethics, for example, physician-assisted suicide. Another such error is what Plato (c. 427–347 BCE) at many places in his *Dialogues* has Socrates (c. 470–399 BCE) call "mere opinion," the expression of a conclusion about what character formation or behavior should be without any supporting premises and, in the worst cases, no interest in such premises. Physicians in positions of power over others in clinical or research settings sometimes commit this error, which is a corrupting influence on trainees and the research team. Such behavior is also a source of ethically significant moral distress (Thomas and McCullough 2015). A third error is the attempt to stop ethical reasoning. For example, on rounds in a critical care unit more than two decades ago, I asked whether the limits of treatment might have been reached for a young patient in end-stage multi-organ failure, based on the reasoned ethical judgment of the Society for Critical Care Medicine ("Consensus Statement of the Society of Critical Care Medicine's Ethics Committee," 1997). The attending physician responded to this question with a question: "What do you want us to do? Kill our patient?" This is the exercise of raw power, in other words, the exercise of power detached altogether from ethical reasoning. The response to raw power is to insist that the discipline of medical ethics be followed, not arbitrarily disrupted.

Another important error is to equate law and medical ethics, whether explicitly or, more often, implicitly. An international research group has published a number of papers that analyze the U.S. Centers for Disease Control database to examine the absolute and relative risk of planned home birth compared to hospital birth. This research group has identified increased absolute and relative risk of planned home birth, which can be responsibly reduced by planned hospital birth (Grünebaum et al. 2013). On the basis of these data, this research group argued that planned home birth is inconsistent with the best interests of the child standard in pediatric ethics. Physicians should therefore recommend against planned home birth and explain the evidence base for doing so, in response to women who express an interest in planned home birth (Chervenak et al. 2013). One of the critics of this ethical judgment has written:

> For example, one way to express the difference in neonatal mortality is that in-hospital birth appears to improve neonatal survival over home birth from ~99.85% to 99.95%. This difference does not meet the high threshold generally set for overriding parental decisions for their children suggested by the AAP Committee on Bioethics and others. (Watterberg 2013, 924)

"Overriding" parental decisions is shorthand for seeking court orders for clinical management supported by the best interests of the child standard, a core concept of pediatric ethics, but refused by parents. The error committed here is to assume that, if ethically justified criteria for the use of state power are not satisfied, the evidence-based recommendation against planned home birth and for planned hospital birth is not ethically justified.

This line of reasoning succeeds only if one implicitly equates health law and medical ethics. This equation runs deeply counter to the view advanced by the English Enlightenment physician-ethicist Thomas Percival (1740–1804) in his pivotal *Medical Ethics* (Percival 1803), probably the first book titled "Medical Ethics" in the global history of medical ethics. Percival's view, which he sets out in his chapter on medicine and the law, was that professional medical ethics is autonomous from the law. For example, while Percival agreed that abortion was an egregious moral wrong and that the state was therefore justified in making abortion a criminal offense, the punishment meted out to women was far too harsh. Percival reasoned in an evidence-based way: given the well-known clinical dangers to the pregnant woman of an induced abortion (at that time), no woman who procured for herself, or performed on herself, an induced abortion could be considered to be in her right mind and was therefore considered to have had criminal intent. Then-current English law recognized not being in one's right mind (mens rea) as a factor that should mitigate punishment. If Percival had accepted the equation of medical ethics and law, he could not have made this argument.

THREE HISTORICAL GENRES

The discourses of medical ethics begin in the ancient worlds of China, Greece, and India (Baker and McCullough 2009a). Albert Jonsen characterizes this history as "the long tradition of moral discourse about medicine" (Jonsen 2000, ix), which long predates the "birth of bioethics" (Jonsen 1998) in the 1960s and 1970s. In the ensuing centuries, this "long tradition" of medical ethics developed in every region of the world (Baker and McCullough 2009a). National codes of medical ethics date from the 19th century, for example, the Code of Medical Ethics of the American Medical Association (AMA) (American Medical Association [1847] 1999; Bell [1847] 1999; Baker et al. 1999).

Especially since the end of World War II in 1945, medical ethics has also become international. International associations of physicians in the different specialties have produced codes of medical ethics and ethics statements on clinical practice, research, education, and health policy, for example, the International Federation of Gynaecologists and Obstetricians, headquartered in London, United Kingdom. The major multispecialty international association of physicians, the World Medical Association, headquartered in Ferney-Voltaire, France, near Geneva, Switzerland, has made major contributions to medical ethics, notably its "International Code of Medical Ethics" (World Medical Association [1949] 2006a), "Declaration of Geneva: Physician's Oath" (World Medical Association [1946] 2006b), and its widely influential "Declaration of Helsinki: Ethical Principles for Research with Human Subjects" (World Medical Association [1964] 2013) on research ethics.

There are different ways in which one might seek to organize the vast global literature of the history of medical ethics (Baker and McCullough 2009b). A simple way—I hope not deceptively simple—in which to organize the vast historical and contemporary literature of medical ethics is on the basis of three distinctively different conceptual sources of medical ethics. The first is theological or religious medical ethics, based on moral concepts adopted by and, indeed, definitive of, the various faith communities of the world. The result is a moral theology of medicine. The second is philosophical medical ethics, based on moral concepts of philosophy. The result is a moral philosophy of medicine. Theological or religious medical ethics and philosophical ethics have very long histories, as can be seen in the chronology. The third genre of medical ethics, professional medical ethics, dates from the 18th-century national enlightenments (Porter and Teich 1981) of Scotland and England and not from the *Hippocratic Oath*, as commonly (Veatch 2012) but mistakenly believed, as explained below. Professional medical ethics is based on the ethical concept of medicine as a profession, a secular concept that is transreligious, transcultural, and transnational.

Theological or Religious

Theological or religious medical ethics deploys ethical analysis and argument using concepts that are accessible to, and authoritative for, members of a faith community to reach judgments about medical morality and its improvement that are reliable for all members of that faith community. Theological or religious medical ethics is perhaps the oldest genre of medical ethics. The early textual history of Hindu medical ethics dates to the middle of the second millennium BCE (Young 2009a, 2009c), while the textual history of Buddhist medical ethics and Jewish medical ethics date from middle of the first millennium BCE (Young 2009a, 2009b). Oral and written preservation of beliefs long predated the preparation of these texts.

Religions comprise faith communities defined by a shared commitment (a) to beliefs about reality, including nature and human nature, and the relationship between nature and human beings, on the one hand, and transcendent or divine reality, on the other, and (b) to practices and social orders, including government (e.g., the divine right of kings in Western Europe), based on these beliefs. The transcendent reality may be deities or a deity, as in Christianity, Hinduism, Islam, and Judaism. The transcendent reality, however, need not be deities or a deity, as in Buddhism (Young 2009a, 2009b). Like all moral beliefs, religious beliefs invoke ethical concepts. These concepts have implications for how human beings should form their characters—the virtues that should be cultivated and the vices that should be shunned—and how human beings should behave—right and wrong conduct.

When members of a faith community publicly formulate and share their beliefs—orally or in written form—they create a theology. When a theology of a faith community addresses morality, it becomes a moral theology of that faith community. The close reader of this text will have taken note of the use of indefinite article in the preceding two sentences. This choice is deliberate and is meant as a caution against simplifying religious experience and theology that seeks to give an account of religious experience. The longer that a religion has been in existence, the less likely will it be to speak of *the* theology of that faith community, because that religion will have developed a tradition of faithful but competing interpretations of its sacred texts, experiences, and practices. Indeed, with exceptions such as Roman Catholicism, there is typically no single authority on theology and moral theology in faith communities, especially in Protestant faith communities that emphasize the autonomy of conscience. Yet, even in Roman Catholicism there is faithful disagreement with authority.

Two cautions about moral theology are in order. First, no faith community is as monolithic or homogeneous as it may appear to outsiders. Faith communities, viewed up close by scholars, display marked variation, for example, the diverse legal schools—Hanafites, Malikites, Shafiites, Hanbalites—in Islam (Ilkilic 2009, 171), the striking range of accounts in Christian moral theology on the morality of induced abortion, or the Theravāda, Mahāyāna, and Vajrayāna branches of Buddhism (Young 2009b). This variation is especially marked in faith communities that take themselves to be "living in the question" and not always to have final answers. Second, one should not be surprised—because one should expect—to encounter differences, including sometimes irreconcilable differences, among moral theologies of different faith communities about topics in medical ethics. For example, Roman Catholic moral theology centuries ago introduced the distinction between ordinary medical treatment, which is judged obligatory in all cases, and extraordinary medical treatment, which is not obligatory but also not forbidden and therefore permissible not to initiate or to discontinue. In contrast, Islam takes the view that only Allah gives life and therefore can take life, a core tenet of Islam. Orthodox Judaism permits discontinuation of life-sustaining treatment when a patient is *gosses* or three days from death. Setting limits on life-sustaining treatment becomes very difficult for faithful Muslims and Orthodox Jews. Some Islamic authorities permit induced abortion in the early stages of pregnancy because Allah does not breathe a soul into the developing human being until 120 days, whereas Roman Catholicism prohibits induced abortion because God has infused the soul into gestational life at conception (which occurs before pregnancy, which is defined in obstetrics as the implantation of the embryo into the uterine wall).

One very important function of religions, in all their internal and comparative diversity, is to explain the meaning of reality. Meaning is created when human beings use concepts to discover or create connections among entities and events that otherwise may seem unconnected and therefore meaningless. The sources of these concepts are remarkably diverse and include revelation of the Divine to human being, ways or paths (*Dao*) of life, or deep reflection. These diverse resources result in powerful oral and written traditions, in some cases created and commented on over millennia. These concepts are also conveyed by historical figures—Jesus, the Incarnate God of Christianity, the prophets of Islam and Judaism, or revered teachers such as Buddha or Confucius.

Some religions give meaning to human existence and its relationship to the divine through an account of creation. God made the world and everything in it, as in Christianity, Islam, and Judaism. All living things, including human beings, are thereby and therefore creatures of the Creator. The Creator's extraordinary creative act gives all creatures dependent moral status, in other words, moral status that originates, not in each individual (which is known as independent moral status), but in a social role created by others or, in this case, the Creator. Some religions give meaning to human existence through deep reflection. Consider Buddhism:

> Buddhism denies a Supreme Being or Absolute. It also denies revelation. Its concept of enlightenment is based on insight in the very nature of reality framed by the law of karma (the law of reaping what one sows) and cosmic and individual cycles of existence (*samsārsa*). (Young 2009b, 185)

The task of giving meaning to human existence typically focuses on the life cycle, because the human life cycle characterizes the existence of every human being. All human beings are conceived, gestated, and born. Liveborn human beings become infants, children, adolescents, and then adults, a passage often marked by diverse rituals across religions. Adults age and often become infirm as they age. Children and adults die. In high-income, developed countries, maternal, infant, and childhood mortality have become very low, as has morbidity from disability, disease, disorders, and injury. In low-income, less-developed countries, this is not the case. It was certainly not the case globally before the advances of biomedical science and its clinical application in the 20th century reduced frightful mortality rates. In the past, death was common, a constant companion. In 18th-century Britain, for example, young women feared marriage, because of the very high probability that they would die in childbirth. Women also feared being unmarried because spinsterhood often meant poverty (McCullough 1998). Women in Britain no longer face such a stark choice.

In the past, the perils of pregnancy and childhood; the constancy of war and its aftermath of death and also of disability, disease, and injury; the constant loss of spouses, children, other family members, friends, and neighbors; and the finality, commonality, and imminence of death for individuals and for those who survive them challenged all human beings to make sense of death and all that precedes it in the human life cycle. All the world's religions have responded over the centuries to this enduring transreligious and transcultural challenge. Acquaintance with the world's religions leads to awareness of the strikingly diverse ways in which they give meaning to the human life cycle (Amundsen 2009a, 2009b; Engelhardt 2009; Fan 2009; Ferngren 2009; Ilkilic 2009; Young 2009b, 2009c; Zohar 2009). The resulting differences shaped cultures and contributed to their striking diversity.

Medicine engages the human lifecycle directly, on a daily basis. Physicians (and other practitioners) have, for millennia, attended birth; treated the diseases of infants, children, and adults; attempted to ameliorate disabilities, disorders, and injuries; and sought to prolong life, in Francis Bacon's (1561–1626) meaning of progressively reducing mortality rates and not as an unlimited ethical obligation to prevent death (McCullough 1998). Medicine and the world's religions thus intersect in the human life cycle, making medicine of great concern for the world's religions and moral theologies. Religions provide accounts of the meaning of health, disability, disease, disorders, injuries, and death; moral theologies provide accounts of what is ethically impermissible, permissible, obligatory, uncertain, and controversial in the character formation and behavior of physicians, the behavior of patients, the education of physicians, the conduct of research, and health policy.

For physicians and patients who are members of a faith community, guidance from religion and moral theology about the meaning of health, disability, disease, disorder, and death and about proper character and behavior becomes essential. Limitations, however, should be acknowledged; not all of the world's religions agree on the meaning of life-cycle events or on the meaning of the life cycle itself.

When there are significant differences within a faith community, especially differences that manifest as controversies, these differences should be acknowledged and respected. Attempts to manage pluralism in moral theology in a faith community should be managed by ongoing discussion and not attempts to shut down discussion by asserting that one's own view is *the* view of the faith community. Similarly, differences between or among the moral theologies of different religions should be acknowledged and respected. This becomes an especially important consideration when diverse moral theologies take incompatible positions. When this occurs, no one religion can claim to have *the correct* moral theological position. This is because there is no, as it were, super-religious perspective to reconcile controversy.

The task becomes one of deciding how to live with irreconcilable moral differences among religions, as is currently the case among faith communities for a number of topics in medical ethics, including not just induced abortion, but also human embryologic stem cell research, organ procurement for transplantation, justified limits on life-sustaining treatment, and physician-assisted suicide. One of the great motivations—and, subsequently, achievements—of the national enlightenments of the 18th century was the recognition that resort to violence does not resolve such irreconcilable moral differences (McCullough 1998). The task became, and remains, how faith communities should live in peace with profound moral pluralism (Engelhardt 1996).

It is also important to responsibly manage friction between religion and medicine. A religion can create friction with medicine when that religion proffers an account of the nature and cause of diseases and disorders that does not pass intellectual muster, as occurred in ancient Greece in the case of what are now known clinically as grand mal seizures. The Hippocratic text, "The Sacred Disease," mounts a sustained and devastating critique of the view that the signs and symptoms of this condition result from the gods seizing an individual in punishment for transgression against the gods (Hippocrates 1923b). The author of this remarkable text, who is unknown, shows that the religious account fails because it is hopelessly riddled with confusion and contradiction. The author goes on to show that the disease originates in the human body, in the brain, to be precise. The seizures are not seizures (the word is still used clinically) at all; the convulsions and other signs and symptoms originate in an imbalance in the brain among the four humors.

From the perspective of contemporary neuroscience, the author of "The Sacred Disease" got the anatomy of seizures correct, but not the physiology. The implication for responsibly managing the boundary between religion and medicine is that the methods of reasoning in religion do not apply to the causal explanation of disease; the empirical methods of scientific medicine apply.

Medicine became increasingly scientific in the 17th and 18th centuries in Europe, especially as physicians began to adhere to Bacon's philosophy of medicine. Medicine should be based on what Bacon called experience, the carefully observed, recorded, analyzed, and reported results of natural and well-designed experiments. Many in Christian faith communities saw the increasingly powerful Baconian science of medicine as putting physicians at risk of becoming atheists. This suspicion was expressed in the commonly used Latin phrase, *"Ubi tres medici, ibi duo atheii"* or "Wherever there are three physicians, there are two atheists." John Gregory (1724–1773), who wrote the first text of modern professional medical ethics, devotes more words to the boundary between medicine and religion than any other topic. The boundary today may perhaps be less fraught, but can still prompt ethical challenges. For example, how should a physician respond when a patient asks the physician, who does not share the patient's religion, to pray with the patient? Is it ethically permissible for a physician ever to offer, unbidden, to pray with a patient who is from the same faith community? From a different faith community?

Finally, it is worth noting the major role played by moral theologians and scholars of religious ethics (the nondenominational study of ethical reasoning in religions) in the development of bioethics in the 1950s and 1960s in the United States. In his landmark account of this remarkable historical development, Jonsen (1998) documents that the first ethicists to respond to emerging ethical challenges in medicine and to work with physicians to fashion reasoned responses to those ethical challenges were moral theologians and religious ethicists. The philosophers came later.

Philosophical

Philosophical medical ethics deploys ethical analysis and argument using concepts that are accessible to anyone committed to reasoned discourse to reach judgments about medical morality and its improvement that are reliable for anyone, regardless of his or her religion, culture, nationality, race, or ethnicity. The goal is to create and sustain transreligious, transcultural, and transnational medical ethics.

Like religious or theological ethics, philosophical medical ethics has ancient roots. In the sixth and fifth centuries BCE in China, Confucius (551–479 BCE) based his philosophy on the concept of *ren*, or humanity, and on the virtue of filial piety, the habitual obedience to the decisions of one's parents, once their decision has been made. His influence on subsequent Chinese medical ethics was profound, especially with the adoption of Confucian medical ethics by the Chinese government in 134 BCE (Fan 2009, 196). Medical ethics was to be based on medicine as "the art of *ren*" with a strong emphasis on the physician's virtues (Fan 2009, 196).

In fourth-century BCE Athens (in present-day Greece), Plato addresses medical morality in his *Dialogues*. Readers of *Republic* know well the passage in which Socrates points out that, in the fevered state of democracy, there will be many physicians. Recent scholarship has noted what can be called a dark side of Platonic medical ethics: the view that the physically infirm should not be treated. Indeed, they should be abandoned, a view that, via Friedrich Nietzsche's (1844–1900) philosophy, influenced the architects of the Nazi medical war crimes in Germany during World War II (Baker and McCullough 2009c).

Jonsen (2009) provides a useful and concise account of the subsequent history of philosophical medical ethics. The conception of philosophical medical ethics presented at the beginning of this section became the self-conscious understanding of philosophical medical ethics during the national enlightenments of the 18th century (Porter and Teich 1981), especially in Great Britain (McCullough 1998; Baker and McCullough 2009c). Some readers may respond to the claim that philosophical medical ethics seeks to be transreligious, transcultural, and transnational with skepticism. Two responses are in order.

As noted above, one of the major motivations for the national enlightenments of the 18th century, including especially in Great Britain and in the nations on the European continent, was a profound weariness with the chronic, destructive religious wars dating to the Protestant reformations of the 16th and 17th centuries. The battlefields of these religious wars had become heaped with the bodies of the dead and wounded, as late as the Scottish civil war between Roman Catholics and Protestants in 1745–1746. Religious differences between Roman Catholics and Protestants and among Protestants could not be reconciled for the reason explained above: the acceptance of a single religion and single moral theology was beyond the realms of both possibility and imagination and therefore utterly unrealistic. This remains the case.

The discourse of peace in medical ethics required a discourse not rooted in, and therefore limited by, a particular religion and its moral theologies. Philosophical medical ethics is equipped to take on the task of a discourse of moral reasoning open to all who are committed to the intellectual and practical discipline of philosophical ethics. This also remains the case. Skeptics bear a burden of proof: to justify abandoning this discourse of peace and to plan for responsibly managing the risks of doing so, risks that will be very difficult to manage in the absence of a discourse of peace.

Philosophical medical ethics, as a subdiscipline of moral philosophy, should not be expected to result in final judgments about medical morality. Rather, philosophical medical ethics aims for reliable judgments. "Reliable" means that we can act on such judgments with confidence that they are ethically justified (i.e., well supported in ethical reasoning). In some cases, those judgments may become settled in the sense that revisiting them is not urgent, for example, the consensus view that informed consent is required for all invasive procedures that incur risk of clinical harm, especially when the probability for clinical harm is high and the clinical harm is serious, far-reaching, and irreversible (e.g., disabling injury from neurosurgical repair to injury to the spinal cord or damage to the brain from micro embolisms generated by mechanical circulation devices). Even for such settled judgments, there are challenges at their limits, in hard cases such as the role of informed consent for patients with progressive mild to moderate cognitive impairments or for older adolescent patients who are legal minors, especially older adolescent patients with chronic disease such as cancers or cystic fibrosis. Then, too, controversies exist in philosophical medical ethics, for example, about euthanasia (in the sense of direct killing by the physician) for patients who are capable of informed consent and even more so for patients who are not capable of consent. In short, there are important limitations to the results of philosophical reasoning in medical ethics, and these limitations should be kept constantly in mind, to prevent overweening confidence that one's reasoned judgment is the only reliable reasoned judgment.

Religious or theological medical ethics has the serious limitation that judgments about medical morality emanate from a specific set of concepts that may have no or only little currency outside the faith community of their origin. This is not to gainsay that religious or theological medical ethics may invoke concepts of wide currency, such as moral status. But the concept of moral status is a philosophical concept. The judgments of religious or theological medical ethics, however reliable they may be in clarity of their concepts and the rigor of argument based on the implications of those concepts, will almost always be of limited applicability in other religious or theological contexts, as well as in nonreligious contexts.

Philosophical medical ethics does not have this limitation. In pluralistic societies and across pluralistic societies—in a pluralistic world—philosophical medical ethics is the preferred approach to medical ethics, if one aims to maximize the opportunity for a transreligious, transcultural, and transnational discourse of medical ethics. Philosophical medical ethics makes such a discourse possible because the concepts of philosophy are secular. Secular concepts have two characteristics: (1) they are the product of a reasoned discourse that makes no reference to divinity, revelation, or spiritual insight and need not do so; and (2) there is no necessary hostility between philosophical and religious or theological concepts.

Professional

Professional medical ethics deploys ethical analysis and argument using concepts that are accessible to anyone committed to reasoned discourse to reach judgments about medical morality and its improvement that are reliable for all physicians, regardless of an individual physician's religion, culture, nationality, race, or ethnicity. To achieve this goal, professional medical ethics invokes the ethical concept of medicine as a profession, which is a philosophical, secular concept.

Many physicians, as well as scholars and teachers of medical ethics and bioethics (more on the relationship between medical ethics and bioethics in the next section), hold the view that professional medical ethics has ancient roots, specifically in the Hippocratic Corpus and even more so in the *Hippocratic Oath*. Steven Miles, for example, understands the *Hippocratic Oath* to provide an ethical basis for a "new profession" (Miles 2004, 18). One also commonly encounters the claim that there is a Hippocratic tradition in professional medical ethics of paternalism, the bête noire of bioethics.

Both readings are at best dubious. Jacques Jouanna (1999), in his masterful book on Hippocrates, makes a convincing case that the *Oath* was created to address an acute problem: the physicians of the Koan school of medicine did not have enough sons to perpetuate their merchant guild and its secrets that, without hesitation, sons could be trusted to protect and preserve. Strangers needed to be formally inducted into what had been a family guild, sworn to loyalty and to preserving the secrets of the guild, all themes that appear in the *Oath*. The *Oath* announces itself in the opening section as a "written covenant" (von Staden 1996, 2009) of loyalty from the nonfamily initiates to the family guild. There then follow a series of moral proscriptions and prescriptions, none accompanied by any ethical reasoning.

To claim for the *Oath* the status of a document for medicine as a profession is to read into this text what is not in it, an egregious presentism. We do know that, at that time (fifth to fourth centuries BCE) in the various city states of what later becomes Greece, medical practitioners were not licensed and there was no uniform theory of health and disease and education based on that theory. Physicians were itinerants and struggled for market share of those who could afford their fees—a very small market, to be sure—in fierce competition with other physicians, surgeons, and all manner of other practitioners. Gaining the reputation for high mortality among the sick whom one had treated was a recipe for market failure followed rapidly by poverty. Preventing such an unwelcome reputation became a priority. It is no surprise, therefore, that preserving reputation is a central focus of the *Oath* (von Staden 1996, 2009).

Protecting a reputation for being a good physician is accomplished by not performing invasive procedures, such as the placement of a pessary to induce abortion, because the pessary was destructive—of the pregnant woman's life. The life of the fetus was not of moral significance, because in ancient Greece the fetus had no moral status. Surgery to remove bladder stones is prohibited in the *Oath*, because it is a high mortality procedure. In *The Art*, the author (again unknown) urges physicians to leave off "desperate cases" (Hippocrates 1923a), in other words, the dying, or the sick individual the gravity of whose disease or injury had outstripped the capacity of medicine to alter its course, so that the disease or injury and not the physician would be blamed for the death soon to follow. The timing of both the announcement that the case has become desperate and the physician's departure become crucial to maintaining one's reputation as a successful physician. These components of the *Oath* explain why reputation looms so large in the *Hippocratic Oath* (von Staden 1996, 2009). Abandoning the dying remained the ethical standard until reversed by Gregory (1770, 1772). Finally, there is no word that can be translated as "patient" in the *Oath*. Instead, the word in Greek for "the sick" is used. Words express and track concepts: the use of "the sick" signals a contractual relationship for services between the sick individual and the physician. This is a patient-physician relationship, not a physician-patient relationship.

Grant, for the sake of argument only, that the *Oath* was a statement of professional medical ethics. There is no unbroken practice of physicians taking the *Oath*, which falls out of favor not too many centuries later (Nutton 2009). Vivian Nutton has shown that the *Oath* was brought back into use early in the 20th century in the United States in an attempt to shore up medicine at a time in which its social status was weak. This was still the era before widespread health insurance and government payment for medical care, medical education, and biomedical research created what historians of medicine call the "social success" of medicine, which came after World War II (Nutton 2009). Hippocrates, a revered figure, was invoked to support a position—professionalism in medicine—that he did not take and would not recognize, a role to which the Father of Medicine has often been recruited (Gâlvao-Sobrinho 1996). There is no Hippocratic tradition and therefore no unbroken history of professional medical ethics that originates in the Hippocratic Corpus.

In the subsequent practice of medicine in the fiefdoms and principalities of Europe, entrepreneurialism dominated the private practice of medicine and medicine provided by physicians employed by cities and princes. The relationship between the sick (*aegrotus* in the Latin texts) and the physician was contractual. The sick individual had power, deriving either from wealth or political position. In both cases, the payer had the power of the purse and the physician was subordinate to this power.

In response, there emerged a genre of medical ethics known as *medicus politicus*, the politic physician (Castro 1614; Hoffmann 1738). "Politic" should not be equated to "political." The political physician seeks power in a healthcare organization or in governmental processes for making and implementing health policy. The politic physician, relative to the payer for his (no women were physicians during the Renaissance and late Renaissance period in Europe when the literature of the politic physician was created) services, has no or very little power. Physicians did not enjoy the social and political status that they currently do in the United States and other developed countries, including the high degree of sustained economic security that came after World War II. Medicine in the late 17th and early 18th centuries in Europe was not yet a profession and so its social status was fragile. Princes, royal leaders of cities, and wealthy private citizens had the power of the purse and also political power over physicians. Failure to acknowledge and work successfully within the bounds of this considerable power imbalance meant loss of income and even the dire outcome of poverty.

In situations of asymmetrical power, the individual who is subordinate to power, when that individual has no, or few, means to limit another's power and who wishes to survive economically, puts a premium on self-interest and therefore the virtue of prudence. This virtue schools one in the discipline of identifying one's legitimate interests and then acting to protect and promote those legitimate self-interests. Friedrich Hoffmann's (1660–1742) *Medicus Politicus* was written for his medical students at the University of Halle, some of whom would seek employment by the princes of the German states (Hoffmann 1738). The full title of this work, which can be read as the culmination of the *medicus politicus* literature, is *Medicus Politicus; sive, Regulae Prudentiae secundum quas Medicus Juvenis Studia sua & Vitae Rationem Dirigere Debet*, which translates from the Latin as *The Politic Doctor; or, Rules of Prudence according to which a Young Physician Should Direct His Studies and Reason of Life*. Hoffmann made the distinctive contribution to the history of medical ethics of explicating the virtue of prudence by invoking the concept of enlightened self-interest. An individual subordinate to the economic and political power of another needs to consider the interests of this other powerful individual. Failure to do so could result in serious, far-reaching, and irreversible harm to one's economic and reputational interests. Hoffmann knew whereof he spoke; he interrupted his work as a professor at Halle to serve as the royal physician in Berlin (1708–1712).

Consider Hoffmann's advice on how the male physician (his students were all men) should comport himself with females under his care (what are now known as obstetricians were then known as "man-midwives"): "The midwife above all should be pious, chaste, sober, not timid, taciturn, and experienced." Pious meant that the "physician should be a Christian." Sobriety was required because, given the paucity of potable water, the sick offered guests cordials (spirit beverages) to slake thirst. The physician should not be so timid as to be unable to act, including touching the woman when clinically necessary. Taciturnity is the virtue of keeping secrets, now known as the professional ethical obligation of confidentiality. To be experienced, in Baconian discourse, means that one knows what one is doing clinically because one is basing clinical practice on experience, the results of natural and controlled experiments and therefore not personal bias. Fulfilling all these requirements will protect and promote the physician's self-interests. Hoffmann recognized two key points. First, fulfilling these requirements will also protect and promote the woman's interests. Second, thus protecting and promoting the interests of the woman becomes a very effective means to protecting and promoting the physician's self-interest, especially in remaining employed.

As in the Latin literature before him, Hoffmann uses *aegrotus*, which translates as the sick one or sick individual. He does not use "patient." The word "patient," which is core to the discourse of professional medical ethics, appears later in the 18th century, in the professional medical ethics of Gregory, in Scotland, and Percival, in England. Gregory and Percival wrote their professional medical ethics in response to two challenges.

The first challenge was the loss of intellectual trust (that physicians knew what they were doing, "experienced" in Hoffmann's text above) and of moral trust (that physicians were primarily concerned with the health and life of the sick and not with their own wealth, power, and reputation) (Porter and Porter 1989; McCullough 1998). At this time, the first response to illness was to self-diagnose and self-treat (there was no government regulation of medicinals that were then readily available, such as laudanum, a form of liquid opium taken for relief of pain). This was known as "self-physicking." (It is still practiced under such names as "self-care.") The sick turned to a physician or surgeon only when self-physicking failed, but the rampant distrust only compounded the anxiety and fear of the sick.

The second challenge derived from the advent of the era of hospital practice, for Gregory the Royal Infirmary of Edinburgh and for Percival the Royal Infirmary of Manchester, both of which continue to serve patients to this day. The royal infirmaries were established in British cities starting in the middle of the 18th century. They were created by landed aristocrats and industrial leaders of such enterprises as coal mines, mills, and shipyards, to provide free medical and surgical care for the men, women, and children who worked for them. These wealthy individuals paid an annual "subscription" that funded the costs of operating an infirmary. The sick came from a lower social class than physicians, resulting in an imbalance of social power. Physicians also gained power over the sick, by reason of the organizational hierarchy that anyone who has been hospitalized or visited a loved one in a hospital appreciates.

Medical ethics provided no guidance for how to wield this new power over the sick. The major resource, the literature of *medicus politicus*, with which Gregory and Percival would have become acquainted during their medical studies in Leiden in the Netherlands, provided prudence-based guidance for the physician over whom power is wielded by others. Prudence-based guidance is inadequate for circumstances in which the physician has gained power over the sick, rupturing the connection between the physician and the sick upon which the concept of enlightened self-interest vitally depends.

The response of Gregory and Percival to these two challenges was to invent the ethical concept of medicine as a profession. This concept requires three commitments of physicians: (1) become and remain scientifically and clinically competent; (2) make the protection and promotion of the patient's health-related interests the physician's primary concern and motivation, keeping self-interest systematically secondary; and (3) sustain medicine as a public trust (the phrase is Percival's) that exists for the benefit of current and future patients, physicians, healthcare organizations, and society, rather than a guild, which medicine had been for centuries, that protects the economic, social, and political status and power of physicians as its primary concern and motivation (McCullough 2006; Chervenak and McCullough 2014). That medicine is a profession is made true by physicians making and sustaining these three commitments. In this sense, the ethical concept of medicine as a profession is a pragmatic concept.

This concept has three significant implications for professional medical ethics. First, physicians and surgeons become one profession and professionals who are worthy of intellectual and moral trust, especially in the use of their power over others in the clinical setting, as well as in research and education. In 18th-century Britain, physicians used the word "professional" at a time when there was no standard medical curriculum and, indeed, one could purchase an M.D. degree from an impecunious university. But physicians used "professional" in a self-interested way, to differentiate themselves as university educated practitioners superior to apprentice-trained surgeons, apothecaries, midwives, and the host of "irregular" medical practitioners crowding the fiercely competitive marketplace of medical care. Gregory and Percival gave "professional" substantive ethical content for the first time in the history of medical ethics.

Second, coming under the care of a professional physician transformed the sick into patients, individuals cared for by a physician committed to knowing what he was doing and to protecting life and health as his primary concern and motivation. This includes protecting patients from abuse of the physician's power (i.e., the self-interested or clinically harmful use of power). Adhering to the obligations of a professional physician becomes the antidote to intellectual and moral distrust and to abuse of the physician or surgeon of his power in the hospital setting.

Third, Gregory and Percival wrote their medical ethics for a secular profession, in the sense explained above. The University of Edinburgh, where Gregory served as professor of medicine (1766–1773), defined itself as a center of *lehrenfreiheit* or the freedom to teach unrestrained by theological dogma or political position. As a result, the University of Edinburgh drew a remarkably pluralistic group of faculty and students. Percival was a Rational Dissenter from the Church of England and, as a matter of conscience, would not sign the articles of faith then required for admission to Oxford and Cambridge universities. He went to Edinburgh, leaving in 1765 for the completion of his medical studies at Leiden. Both Gregory and Percival took religious pluralism seriously and created a professional ethics intended to become transreligious, transcultural, and transnational.

They succeeded. Gregory's books (1770, 1772) on professional medical ethics were translated into French (1797), German (1778), Italian (1789), and Spanish (1803) (McCullough 1998). Scholarship on the history of the influence of Gregory's professional medical ethics through these translations has begun (Gracia 2009), but there remains much scholarly work to be completed. Gregory's (1770, 1772) and Percival's (1803) books were brought to the English colonies in North America (in Gregory's case) and the new United States of America (in Percival's case) (Baker 2013). In 1847, the framers of the first modern national professional code of ethics, the "Code of Medical Ethics" of the then-new AMA, explicitly cite Gregory and Percival as sources of influence (American Medical Association [1847] 1999; Bell [1847] 1999; Baker et al. 1999). In an era innocent of plagiarism concerns, whole passages from Percival's *Medical Ethics* (1803) appear in the Code without attribution, via the work of the marvelously named Kappa Lambda Society of Hippocrates, whose members helped write the Code (Baker 2013).

The 1847 Code has evolved into the *Principles of Medical Ethics* of the AMA (American Medical Association 2001), which is self-consciously a statement of professional medical ethics. It has been joined in the United States by professional codes of medical ethics of specialty organizations of physicians. As noted above, many national and international specialty and multispecialty organizations of physicians have produced codes of ethics.

BIOETHICS AND MEDICAL ETHICS

Bioethics (or biomedical ethics) deploys ethical analysis and argument using theological concepts that are usually limited to the faith community in which they originate or philosophical concepts that are accessible to anyone committed to reasoned discourse to reach judgments about the morality of the healthcare professions, patients, healthcare organizations, and health policy that are reliable for all individuals, organizations, and states, regardless of religion, culture, nationality, race, or ethnicity. Some take the view that bioethics originated in the United States (Jonsen 2000, 2009), while others claim this accomplishment for Great Britain (Campbell 2000; Baker 2013). No one would disagree that bioethics has become global, reflected in the *International Association for Bioethics* and the international scope of authorship and subject matter in the academic journals of the field of bioethics.

Typically, in the bioethics literature, medical ethics is understood to be a subfield of bioethics with nothing distinctive about its methods or content. In the first edition of the landmark reference work *The Encyclopedia of Bioethics* (Reich 1978)—now in its fourth edition (Jennings 2014)—K. Danner Clouser, a philosopher–medical educator and one of the founders of the field of bioethics, wrote the entry "Bioethics" (Clouser 1978). He described the new field of bioethics as "not a new set of principles of maneuvers, but the same old ethics being applied to a particular realm of concerns" (Clouser 1978, 116). Medical ethics is to be understood as "a first approximation" of bioethics:

> Medical ethics is a special kind of ethics only insofar as it relates to a particular realm of facts and concerns and not because it embodies or appeals to some special moral principles or methodology. It is applied ethics. It consists of the same moral principles and rules that we would appeal to, and argue for, in ordinary circumstances. It is just that in medical ethics these familiar moral rules are being applied to situations peculiar to the medical world. We have only to scratch the surface of medical ethics and we break through to the issues of "standard" ethics as we have always known them. (Clouser 1978, 116)

The burning "issues" that bioethicists addressed may be new, unprecedented, and special, but the methods of ethics for their study was not. In Clouser's conception, widely shared at the time and to this day, professional medical ethics differed from bioethics perhaps only for its subject matter—medical practice, research, education, and health policy—but not for its ethical methods and the core concepts deployed to address this subject matter. The history of medical ethics, including the history of professional medical ethics, was not pertinent to bioethics, relegated to the category of antiquarian interests of scholars and therefore of no importance for bioethics. The notion that philosophical concepts are timeless and therefore not shaped by history was taken for granted at that time (Strawson 1963) and still is by many bioethicists and philosophers.

BIOETHICS AND PROFESSIONAL MEDICAL ETHICS

The ahistorical character of bioethics has resulted, according to at least one critic, in the deprofessionalization of medical ethics (McCullough 2011). From the perspective of professional medical ethics as described previously, bioethics as explained by Clouser and the many bioethicists who embrace this self-understanding of bioethics should not be equated with professional medical ethics.

There is another reason why this equation should not be made: the moral pluralism of bioethics that defines it but does not define professional medical ethics. Bioethics is a distinctively interdisciplinary field of study, to which many disciplines contribute, including the creative and literary studies, the healthcare professions, law, philosophy, the qualitative and quantitative social sciences, religious ethics, and moral theology. Works in normative bioethics are thus written from many disciplinary bases, resulting in a marked pluralism of approaches to bioethics. Professional medical ethics is written from a single disciplinary perspective, moral philosophy, and—in order to be transcultural, transnational, and transreligious—does not appeal to moral theology or law. Indeed, professional medical ethics is autonomous from these sources. Professional medical ethics is also based on a single philosophical concept: the ethical concept of medicine as a profession.

Bioethics thrives on moral controversy (Baker 2002); professional medical ethics does not. Professional medical ethics seeks consensus as the outcome of ethical reasoning, so that physicians, physician leaders of healthcare organizations, and health policy makers have reliable guidance for professional character formation and behavior.

The commitment, reflected in this dictionary, to the view that ethical concepts in professional medical ethics and in philosophical medical ethics are not timeless but have a historical origin does not entail a commitment to the view that ethical concepts are time-bound and therefore cannot become transreligious, transcultural, and transnational. Key concepts such as medicine as a profession and becoming a patient, as well as the professional virtues and ethical principles that explicate the implications of these key concepts, now shape the international discourse of professional medical ethics. The international discourse of professional medical ethics as secular and therefore transreligious, transcultural, and transnational owes a considerable intellectual debt to Gregory's and Percival's transformation of the history of medical ethics from religious or theological ethics and philosophical ethics into professional medical ethics. This landmark accomplishment would not have been possible were it the case that ethical concepts cannot transcend the historical context in which they came into intellectual and practical currency. The international discourse of bioethics takes the transcendence of philosophical concepts for granted but for the wrong, ahistorical reason, marking yet another important difference between professional medical ethics and bioethics.

A

ABANDONMENT. Discontinuing **clinical management** of a **patient**. The legal requirements for notification must be met in all cases. Notification is also **ethically obligatory** in **professional medical ethics**.

The abandonment of patients who have become desperately ill and who therefore are at a high risk of **death** was a **norm** in **clinical practice**, articulated as early as the **Hippocratic Corpus**. The main reason appears to be the desire to preserve a good **reputation**, one of the two core concepts of the *Hippocratic Oath*. If a physician stayed with a patient who died, the physician risked being blamed for the death, which would result in a reputation as a physician whose patients die. The result would be loss of market share and income at a time when physicians did not enjoy the economic security they have experienced in the United States in the post–World War II period. Outside the Roman Catholic religious foundations, in which monks provided care for the sick in the infirmary and who cared for patients until death as an **ethical obligation** in **Roman Catholic moral theology**, the Hippocratic norm guided practice. **John Gregory** (1724–1773) appears to have been the first to reject this norm and replace it with an ethical obligation to care for the dying up to the moment of death. *See also THE ART*; END-OF-LIFE CARE; PALLIATIVE CARE.

ABORTIFACIENT. A drug or device that disrupts pregnancy (which commences with implantation of the embryo in the uterine wall), resulting in an **induced abortion**. The ethical challenges of abortifacients are therefore the same as the ethical challenges of induced abortion. This word is also used by some to classify drugs or devices that prevent implantation of the embryo in the uterine wall (i.e., that prevent the initiation of pregnancy). This is an error because it conflates two distinct ethical challenges: induced abortion before viability, which results in **feticide**, and prevention of a pregnancy that results in **embryocide**. Drugs or devices that prevent implantation may be understood to be forms of **contraception** that prevent pregnancy by causing embryocide. For those who believe that the embryo has **independent moral status** or **dependent moral status**, the use of such drugs and devices is at least ethically controversial or **ethically impermissible**. Whether the embryo has such **moral status** is itself ethically controversial. *See also* ABORTION; TERMINATION OF PREGNANCY.

ABORTION. The evacuation of the contents of a pregnancy (which commences with implantation of the embryo in the uterine wall) from a woman's uterus before **fetal viability**. An abortion can occur as either an **induced abortion** or a **spontaneous abortion**. Both induced and spontaneous abortions result in death of the fetus. After viability, evacuation of the uterus is either a spontaneous delivery, an induced delivery, or a cesarean delivery. Delivery results in either a liveborn or stillborn infant. Induced abortion, spontaneous abortion, and delivery all result in **termination of pregnancy**. The use of *abortion* and *termination of pregnancy* interchangeably is a conceptual error, because termination of pregnancy encompasses more than abortion.

The ethics of induced abortion turns on how the **moral status** of the fetus should be understood and the **ethical obligations** of others to protect the fetus's life based on its moral status. These others include the pregnant woman, physicians, and other healthcare professionals; individuals whose behavior affects a pregnancy; and the state. Those who hold that the moral status of the fetus creates an **absolute ethical obligation** to protect its life are committed to the position that induced abortion is always **ethically impermissible**. Those who hold that the moral status of the fetus creates a strong but **prima facie ethical obligation** to protect its life are committed to the position that induced abortion is sometimes but not always ethically permissible. Those who hold that the fetus has very weak or no moral status are committed to the position that induced abortion is (almost) always **ethically permissible**.

In the global histories of **moral philosophy** and **moral theology**, there has been no agreement on the moral status of the fetus and, therefore, no agreement on the ethics of induced abortion. In the global histories of moral philosophy and moral theology, there has also been no agreement on a method that would have the intellectual authority to bridge all philosophies and theologies and thus resolve this millennia-old disagreement. There is, therefore, no likelihood of agreement on the moral status of the fetus and therefore on the ethics of abortion.

How to responsibly manage this irresolvable disagreement becomes a central topic in the ethics of abortion. Any specific **health policy** on induced abortion will be limited in its **authority** when such policy appeals to a specific position on the moral status of the fetus and the ethics of abortion in a particular philosophy or theology.

The **common law** has had a strong influence on whether induced abortion should be considered ethically permissible. The first stage was based on the imputed constitutional **right** to **privacy** applied first to **contraception,** in 1965 in the **Griswold Case** (*Griswold v. Connecticut* (381 U.S. 479), in which the U.S. Supreme Court held that the right to privacy protected the **decision making** of a married couple with their physician from interference by the state, and second to **induced abortion,** in 1973 in *Roe v. Wade* (410 U.S. 113) and *Doe v. Bolton* (410 U.S. 179), in which the Supreme Court held that the **right to privacy** protected a woman's decision making with her physician about the disposition of her pregnancy from interference by the state. The state must establish a **compelling state's interest** to justify such interference and failed to satisfy the **burden of justification** in all three cases.

The second stage was based on a liberty **interest,** which the Supreme Court adopted as the basis for decision making in 1992 in *Casey v. Planned Parenthood of Eastern Pennsylvania* (505 U.S. 833). A liberty interest is clearly based on the 14th Amendment and not imputed as the right to privacy is. A liberty interest, however, is weaker than a constitutional right. The state may interfere with the exercise of a liberty interest so long as doing so is not an undue burden (clarified by subsequent courts to mean blocking access to physicians and clinics providing termination of pregnancy services). *See also* PUBLIC POLICY; RIGHT TO LIFE.

ABORTION CASES. *See* ABORTION.

ABSOLUTE ETHICAL OBLIGATION. An action that one must complete without limitation or exception. In **ethical reasoning,** the **burden of justification** is on the party that asserts that an **ethical obligation** is absolute, and the burden can be steep because absolute ethical obligations are rare. *See also* LEGAL OBLIGATION; PRIMA FACIE ETHICAL OBLIGATION.

ABSOLUTE ETHICAL PRINCIPLE. An **ethical principle** that generates an **absolute ethical obligation.** *See also* PRIMA FACIE ETHICAL PRINCIPLE.

ABSOLUTE NEGATIVE RIGHT. A **negative right** that creates an **ethical obligation** of noninterference that has no justified limits or exceptions. An absolute negative right creates an **absolute ethical obligation.** *See also* PRIMA FACIE NEGATIVE RIGHT.

ABSOLUTE POSITIVE RIGHT. A **positive right** that creates an **ethical obligation** to spend the time, energy, and resources of others, in order to protect and promote that individual's **interests**, that has no ethically justified limits. Because there are always ethically justified limits on one's claim on the resources of others, in **ethical reasoning** it is very difficult, if not impossible, to establish that a positive right is absolute. The **burden of justification** is steep, because rights often conflict with each other or with existing obligations. An absolute positive right is of theoretical interest only. *See also* PRIMA FACIE POSITIVE RIGHT; RIGHT.

ABSOLUTE RIGHT. A **right** that creates an unlimited or exceptionless **ethical obligation**. The **burden of justification** to establish that a right is an absolute right is on the advocate for such a right. The burden of justification is steep, because rights often conflict with each other or with existing obligations. *See also* ABSOLUTE NEGATIVE RIGHT; ABSOLUTE POSITIVE RIGHT; PRIMA FACIE RIGHT.

ACCEPTABLE OPPORTUNITY COST. *See* OPPORTUNITY COST.

ACCESS TO HEALTHCARE. Access to healthcare exists when there are no obstacles that prevent an individual from becoming a **patient** and receiving clinical care required by **deliberative clinical judgment**. These obstacles can be financial (there is no source of payment for the clinical care provided or the individual is underinsured), geographic (the individual is at a great distance from healthcare facilities), psychological (the individual is reluctant, for whatever reason, to seek healthcare), social (**invidious discrimination**), or cultural (health beliefs that support self-care as the first response to changes in one's health).

Underinsurance means that the scope of coverage may not include clinical management that the patient needs or that deductibles (the amount that the individual must spend himself or herself before insurance payment starts) or copayments (the amount that the patient has to pay for clinical management) are so high that the individual cannot afford them. Psychological reasons include an individual's history of bad experiences as a patient (e.g., being disrespected or mistreated). Invidious discrimination occurs when access to healthcare is denied for reasons that are **ethically impermissible** in **justice**-based **ethical reasoning**, including denial of access based on race, religion, color, politics, sex, gender, or other clinically irrelevant reasons. The **right to healthcare** includes access to healthcare. *See also* HEALTH POLICY; PUBLIC POLICY.

ACQUIRED IMMUNE DEFICIENCY SYNDROME (AIDS). Acquired immune deficiency syndrome is an infectious disease caused by **human immunodeficiency virus** (HIV). When this infectious disease was first reported in the United States in the early 1980s, most of the patients were homosexual males. Patients who had received blood transfusions also became infected, as well as those who shared needles while using intravenously injected controlled substances. AIDS was found only very rarely among the general population.

Three features of the early period of AIDS before treatment became available in the 1990s were the following: (1) there was no treatment, and almost all patients died from the infection; (2) there was a stigma attached to infected patients who were gay or sharing needles; (3) it had been almost a half century since physicians and other healthcare professionals had been put at risk for life-threatening infection (tuberculosis). These features combined synergistically to create **invidious discrimination** and to call into question physicians' **duty to treat** when fulfilling that duty risked life. Under the **ethical principle of justice**, invidious discrimination is **ethically impermissible. Consensus** rapidly formed that there was indeed a duty to treat, a duty that was familiar to and accepted by other physicians, for example, military physicians attend the wounded in Mobile Army Surgical Hospitals (MASH units) near combat and can come under direct attack by enemy forces.

In the 1990s, with the advent of treatment that slowed the infectious process and then later achieved remission for many patients, AIDS was transformed from a uniformly fatal condition to a chronic disease for those who had **access to healthcare**. In addition, uniform infection control measures were shown to be effective in minimizing infection to healthcare professionals. As a result, AIDS has become "normalized" in **professional medical ethics**.

One very clinically significant success story of AIDS is the prevention of vertical transmission from a pregnant woman to her infant(s) by a drug treatment regimen that also benefits the woman, to the point that in the United States and other high-income countries the birth of an HIV-infected child is a very rare event. AIDS in low-resource countries, especially sub-Saharan Africa, remains a major public health challenge, to which international health organizations and nongovernmental organizations (NGOs) have responded with the support of high-resource countries, for example, the United States President's Emergency Plan for Aids Research (https://www.pepfar.gov/, accessed 14 September 2017), which continues to provide billions of U.S. dollars to programs of treatment and research. *See also* HEALTH POLICY.

ACTIVE EUTHANASIA. Killing a **patient**. This can be done with the patient's authorization in the **informed consent process**, which is known as **voluntary active euthanasia**. When the patient authorizes the physician to prescribe a life-taking medication and the patient ingests that medication, this is known as **physician-assisted suicide**. This can be done without such authorization, which is known as **involuntary active euthanasia**. *See also* PASSIVE EUTHANASIA.

ACTIVE INVOLUNTARY EUTHANASIA. *See* INVOLUNTARY ACTIVE EUTHANASIA.

ACTIVE VOLUNTARY EUTHANASIA. *See* VOLUNTARY ACTIVE EUTHANASIA.

AD HOC COMMITTEE OF THE HARVARD MEDICAL SCHOOL TO EXAMINE THE DEFINITION OF BRAIN DEATH. A 1968 statement that calls for determination of death of a **patient** by brain function criteria. Patients receiving mechanical ventilation, a form of **life-sustaining treatment**, in a **critical care** unit cannot be determined to have died by cardiopulmonary criteria, because mechanical ventilation supports or supplants cardiopulmonary function, preventing the **determination of death** by cardiopulmonary criteria. This has two clinical consequences that are **ethically impermissible**. First, a scarce resource—a critical care bed and healthcare professionals to staff it—is being used for a dead individual (i.e., to perfuse a cadaver, and not a patient). This can also create an **unacceptable opportunity cost** for other patients in the hospital or the hospital's emergency department. Second, if the patient or the patient's surrogate has provided **informed consent** to **organ procurement**, surgery to remove organs would violate the **dead donor rule**, which is ethically impermissible.

To address these two clinical consequences, the committee proposed criteria to reach a **deliberative clinical judgment** that the patient can be determined to be dead by brain function criteria ("A Definition of Irreversible Coma," 1968). This inaugurated the era of clinical examination of the patient to determine that death has occurred based on the irreversible absence of brain function. This allows for continued perfusion of the cadaver from which organs are to be procured for **transplantation**, followed by discontinuation of mechanical ventilation. This also allows for mechanical ventilation and other physiological interventions to be discontinued immediately for a cadaver from which organs are not to be procured. *See also* BRAIN DEATH; CARDIAC DEATH; CARDIOPULMONARY DEATH; DONATION AFTER CARDIAC DEATH.

ADA. *See* AMERICANS WITH DISABILITIES ACT.

ADDICTION. The diminished ability to resist repeated use of tobacco products, spirit beverages, drugs, and other substances. This diminished ability, like all human traits, displays variation. Historically, addiction was understood as a moral failing. In this view, an individual made **voluntary** choices that were not **prudent** and wound up out of control in his or her use of spirit beverages or drugs like opium. The solution to moral failing is to recover self-mastery and thereby stop the self-destructive behavior as a matter of prudence. Failure to do so resulted in social opprobrium, (e.g., being turned out by one's family or being subject to criminal proceedings).

Modern neuroscience has discredited this account and replaced it with a **biopsychosocial** account of addiction as a brain **disorder** or **disease** in which, after a first exposure, voluntary or **involuntary** (e.g., in response to peer pressure from other adolescents), to a chemical, the brain's demands for reexposure are difficult to resist. Like all biological traits, addiction displays biopsychosocial variation.

As with all disorders and diseases, there is an **ethical obligation** in **professional medical ethics** to provide **clinical management** for **patients** with addiction. Social opprobrium and criminalization become outmoded responses and, therefore, should be abandoned. In many societies, however, the moral failure model retains a hold on the popular imagination, which can impede efforts to seek or to provide access to clinical management of addiction, an example of how scientifically discredited ideas remain socially and politically influential in part because of their long history of acceptance. *See also* ALCOHOL ABUSE.

ADEQUACY. *See* CLINICAL ADEQUACY.

ADMINISTRATIVE LAW. Law that governs the decisions and actions of the executive branch of government, based on **common law** and **statutory law**. Decisions under administrative law by public payers such as **Medicare** and **Medicaid** and state and local government can limit resources available for **patient care**, **innovation**, and **research** and therefore require **ethical justification**. *See also* PUBLIC POLICY; REGULATORY LAW.

ADULT CRITICAL CARE. Critical care of adult patients. *See also* END-OF-LIFE CARE; LIFE-SUSTAINING TREATMENT.

ADVANCE DIRECTIVE. A **decision** by a **patient** made in advance of a **condition** that results in loss of **decision-making capacity** or, when allowed by applicable law, by the patient's **surrogate**, to authorize or refuse to authorize clinical management or to assign an individual to act as the patient's surrogate under applicable **statutory law** and **common law**. The phrase *advanced directive* is not accurate and should not be used. Advance directives include a **Directive to Physicians, Durable Power of Attorney for Healthcare, Living Will, Medical Power of Attorney**, and **Out-of-Hospital Do-Not-Resuscitate Order**. These directives may be in oral or written form, as provided for in applicable statutory and common law.

These statutes began with the enactment in 1976 of the California **Natural Death Act**. Starting in the 1990s, these statutes became known as **Advance Directives Acts**. Statutory law supporting advance directives was spurred by a series of landmark cases, starting with in 1976 with the Quinlan Case, *In re Quinlan*, in which the New Jersey Supreme Court found that, when a patient has been diagnosed with a "persistent chronic vegetative state" (now known as a "**permanent vegetative state**") and there is therefore no probability of returning to a cognitive, sapient state, the state no longer has a **compelling state's interest** in requiring **life-sustaining treatment**, and that when such patients cannot make decisions for themselves to refuse such **clinical management**, a surrogate may do so. The Court called for the creation of ethics committees (prognosis committees) to aid in such decision making (*In re Quinlan* 70 N.J. 10, 355 A.2d 647 [NJ 1976]). *See also* END-OF-LIFE CARE; FUTILITY; HEALTH POLICY; INFORMED REFUSAL; PUBLIC POLICY.

ADVANCE DIRECTIVES ACT. Statutory law that provides for the creation and implementation of a **patient's advance directive**, including a **Directive to Physicians, Medical Power of Attorney**, and **Out-of-Hospital Do-Not-Resuscitate Order**, and for discontinuation of **life-sustaining treatment** for a patient who has lost **decision-making capacity** and who has a terminal or irreversible condition but who has no advance directive. Typically, an Advance Directive Act applies to neonatal, pediatric, and adult patients but does not apply to fetuses. Typically, an Advance Directives Act provides for protection from both civil and criminal liability for clinicians and healthcare organizations when a patient who has lost decision-making capacity and who has a terminal or irreversible condition is allowed to die. *See also* END-OF-LIFE CARE; FUTILITY; HEALTH POLICY; INFORMED REFUSAL; PUBLIC POLICY.

ADVERTISING. The use of media of various kinds (print, electronic) to offer goods or services for sale. Advertising by physicians was very common in the history of medicine but was banned as **ethically impermissible** in the

American Medical Association *Code of Medical Ethics* **of 1847**. The U.S. Federal Trade Commission ruled in 1975 that restricting advertising was a legally impermissible violation of **statutory law** against "restraint of trade."

Advertising by physicians creates a **conflict of interest** between the physician's **professional ethical obligation** to patients and the physician's financial interests from increasing his or her number of patients. To manage this conflict of interest in a professionally responsible way, advertising by physicians should be understood as the initiation of the **informed consent process**, which requires that all statements by a physician be truthful and evidence based. Advertising by physicians that blurs these professional standards is at best **ethically controversial** and at worst ethically impermissible. Advertising by physicians that violates these standards is ethically impermissible. *See also* TRUTH-TELLING.

ADVISORY COMMITTEE ON HUMAN RADIATION EXPERIMENTS. Established in 1994 during the administration of President William Jefferson Clinton (1993–2001) and charged to investigate and report on radiation **experiments** during the Cold War (1947–1991), often without consent or public knowledge. The detailed report was completed in 1994 and led to a public, formal apology by President Clinton to survivors and family members. *See also* PRESIDENTIAL COMMITTEE; PUBLIC POLICY.

AEGROTUS. Latin, past perfect participle of *aegroto* (to be ill, sick), used in the Latin literature in the history of medical ethics to designate a sick individual who is in a **contractual relationship** with a clinical practitioner (physician, surgeon, apothecary, midwife, or irregular) before the **ethical concept of medicine as a profession** was introduced into the history of medical ethics by **John Gregory** (1724–1773) and Thomas Percival (1740–1804).

The **Hippocratic Corpus**, including the *Hippocratic Oath*, uses the Greek word with the same meaning. Both the Greek and Latin terms are often mistranslated as "patient," suggesting that the ethical concept of medicine as a profession dates from the ancient Greek and Roman periods. Words express concepts, and it is an error to mistranslate a word when the result is to suggest the introduction of a concept into the history of thought, including the history of medical ethics, before that introduction occurred. *See also* OATH.

AEQUANIMITAS. A concept set out by **Sir William Osler** in his essay *Aequanimitas* (1899), in which he describes a fundamental character trait or **virtue** of physicians: distancing oneself from the affective dimensions of the **patient**'s condition by achieving an "imperturbability" that allows the physician to focus solely on making a diagnosis and formulating a treatment plan on scientific grounds. In Osler's view, entering into the lived experience of the patient risked inadequate patient care. This view is the opposite of **John Gregory**'s (1724–1773) account of **sympathy** and anticipates the concept of **empathy**.

AGGRESSIVE OBSTETRIC MANAGEMENT. The use of invasive medical or surgical treatment, including fetal monitoring and imaging, maternal-fetal intervention, **maternal-fetal surgery**, and **cesarean delivery** for fetal or maternal benefit. The **ethical justification** for aggressive obstetric management appeals to the **ethical principle of beneficence**. The pregnant woman has the **autonomy**-based **negative right** to authorize or refuse to aggressive obstetric management in the **informed consent process**. There is **ethical controversy** in **obstetric ethics** about whether this negative right is an **absolute negative right** or a **prima facie negative right**. *See also* NON-AGGRESSIVE OBSTETRIC MANAGEMENT.

AGISM. Sometimes spelled *ageism*. A negative set of attitudes and behaviors, which lack an evidence base, about older individuals, including geriatric **patients**. Such attitudes are not acceptable as components of **deliberative clinical judgment**, because they are **biased**, sometimes so biased that behavior based on such attitudes is justifiably **judged** to be **invidious discrimination**. **Geriatric ethics** rejects agism in all its forms, including **rationing** based on age. Geriatrics and gerontology teach that one's age reliably predicts how old one will be on one's next birthday but not much about the clinical condition of a geriatric patient.

AIDS. Acquired immune deficiency syndrome, an infectious disease caused by **human immunodeficiency virus** (HIV).

ALCOHOL ABUSE. In the **biopsychosocial** account of **addiction**, alcohol abuse should be classified as an addiction; its severity displays variation. There is an **ethical obligation** in **professional medical ethics** to provide **clinical management** for **patients** with alcohol abuse.

AL-GHAZĀLĪ (ABU HAMID AL-GHAZĀLĪ, 1058–1111). Persian theologian and philosopher whose **Islamic medical ethics** includes **trust** in God and acceptance of medical treatment, understood to be invested with power to heal by God.

ALKMAAR CASE. The Netherlands Supreme Court (1984) permits **euthanasia**, in the sense of **killing** the patient by the physician, provided that the patient has the capacity to make decisions and the paramount goal is to relieve suffering. Cases of **voluntary active euthanasia** must also be reported to the government. *See also* END-OF-LIFE CARE; REMMLINK REPORT (1990).

ALLOCATION OF ORGANS. *See* ORGAN ALLOCATION.

ALLOCATION OF SCARCE MEDICAL RESOURCES. Ethical reasoning about whether a specific approach to distributing medical resources when they are scarce is ethically justified. Typically, ethical reasoning on this topic appeals to the **ethical principle of justice.** Inasmuch as there is no agreement on how the ethical principle of justice should be understood, there is **ethical controversy** about the allocation of scarce medical resources based on the various **specifications** of this **ethical principle.**

Libertarian justice supports a market approach, in which scarce medical resources are allocated by price. This view assumes that purchasers in the market have access to it and that wealth has been acquired under conditions of **fairness. Egalitarian justice** supports a policy of distribution that ensures equal access and meeting each individual **patient**'s healthcare needs equally insofar as possible. **Utilitarian justice** supports allocation of resources that result in the greatest good for the greatest number. **Rawlsian justice** supports allocation of resources that result in the greatest good for the greatest number provided that the condition of the least well off is improved. **Healthcare justice** supports allocation of medical resources that meet that clinical needs of each patient as these needs are understood in **deliberative clinical judgment.**

Thomas Percival (1740–1804) provides a two-pronged approach to this topic, focusing on the allocation of drugs (Percival 1803, Chap. I, Sect. VIII) in the **Royal Infirmary** of Manchester, a major cost center at that time and to this day. He first invokes a cost-benefit argument that a single but expensive dose of a drug may be more clinically effective than multiple doses of a less expensive drug because the cumulative cost of multiple dosing will be more expensive than the cost of the single-dose drug. This is an important argument because it refutes the claim by many physicians that economic efficiency and **professional medical ethics** are necessarily incompatible.

The second prong of Percival's argument is that, even if economic efficiency is not possible, in cases of the most serious **diseases**, "purest beneficence"—**beneficence**-based clinical judgment uninfluenced by economic considerations—should guide **clinical management.** Percival's ethics of the allocation of scarce medical resources allows for **rationing** in less serious cases, because the patient's life is not at stake. Resource use that results in an **unacceptable opportunity cost** is **ethically impermissible.** *See also* TRIAGE.

ALLOWING TO DIE. *See* LETTING DIE.

AL-RUHĀWĪ (ISHĀQ BIN ALI AL-RUHĀWĪ, NINTH CENTURY CE). Arab physician and philosopher, author of the first text in **Islamic medical ethics** in Arabic medicine, *Practical Ethics of the Physician*, known for the quote "The philosopher can only improve the soul, but the virtuous physician can improve both body and soul."

ALTRUISM. A commitment to an **ethics of care** for others and commensurate **self-sacrifice**, in which one routinely gives priority to the **interests** of others. Altruism, therefore, requires consistent and willing self-sacrifice. *See also* CHARITY CARE.

AMA CODE OF MEDICAL ETHICS. The official **Code of Ethics** of the American Medical Association. The *Code* comprises the **American Medical Association** *Principles of Medical Ethics* and *Opinions* **of the American Medical Association** (American Medical Association 2016). *See also* CODE OF ETHICS; PROFESSIONAL MEDICAL ETHICS.

AMERICAN MEDICAL ASSOCIATION *CODE OF MEDICAL ETHICS* **OF 1847.** A national code of **medical ethics** that is among the first such codes in the modern era. Membership in the American Medical Association (AMA) required acceptance of and adherence to the *Code*. The *Code* addresses **ethical obligations** of physicians to **patients** and society, of patients to physicians, and of society to physicians (Baker et al. 1999). The latter two obligations are based on an argument of reciprocity, an original feature of the *Code*: physicians have the **professional obligation** to patients to provide effective medical care; physicians therefore have a **right** to expect patients to cooperate and society to support this undertaking; this right creates the ethical obligations of patients and society to cooperate with and support the provision of effective medical care.

There was resistance to the requirement to accept the *Code*, led by such physicians as **Lewis Pilcher** (1845–1934). This resistance became strong enough to threaten the existence of the AMA. In response, the AMA divided the *Code* into two components: (1) the *Principles of Medical Ethics*, which, in its current form comprises nine principles, which are "standards of conduct" (American Medical Association 2001); and (2) the *AMA Code of Medical Ethics* (American Medical Association 2016). The *Code* provides guidance to physicians of ethical dimensions of **clinical practice** and **clinical research** on the basis of the *Principles*. The 1847 *Code* is available at https://

www.ama-assn.org/sites/default/files/media-browser/public/ethics/
1847code_0.pdf [accessed 14 September 2017]. *See also* CODE OF ETH-
ICS; PROFESSIONAL MEDICAL ETHICS.

AMERICAN MEDICAL ASSOCIATION *PRINCIPLES OF MEDICAL ETHICS.* After a bitter dispute in the late 19th century about the requirement of members of the American Medical Association (AMA) to accept its **American Medical Association** *Code of Medical Ethics* **of 1847**, the AMA revised the *Code* in 1903. It was renamed the *Principles of Medical Ethics* and characterized as "a suggestive and advisory document" (American Medical Association 1903). Its sections comprise three chapters: "The Duties of Physicians to Their Patients"; "The Duties of Physicians to Each Other and to the Profession at Large"; and "The Duties of Physicians to the Public" (American Medical Association 1903).

The *Principles* were revised in 1912 (American Medical Association 1912), 1957 (in which the document was shortened to a statement of principles, the form it took thereafter to the present) (American Medical Association 1957), and 1980 (American Medical Association 1980). The current form dates from 2001, comprising seven principles, which are "standards of conduct" (American Medical Association 2001) and not advisory as in the 1903 iteration. *See also* CODE OF ETHICS; PROFESSIONAL MEDICAL ETHICS.

AMERICANS WITH DISABILITIES ACT. A federal **statutory law** that protects individuals with a **disability** from **invidious discrimination**, enacted into law in 1990 during the administration of President George H. W. Bush (1989–1993). The definition of *disability* in the statute includes both having a disability and the appearance of having a disability, resulting in a broad scope of application. There is **ethical controversy** about whether an **irreversible condition**, depending on how it is defined in applicable statutory law or **common law**, might also be a disability, creating a potential conflict between the Americans with Disabilities Act and state **Advance Directives Acts**. *See also* PUBLIC POLICY.

AMNIOCENTESIS. The ultrasound-guided passage of a needle into the uterus of a pregnant **patient** to withdraw a sample of amniotic fluid for laboratory, genetic, or genomic analysis. Amniocentesis is a component of **prenatal diagnosis**. The **ethical justification** of amniocentesis is **autonomy**-based: to provide a pregnant woman with information about the **condition** of her fetus(es) so that she can make an informed decision with her physician about the disposition of her pregnancy. When **maternal-fetal surgery** or **maternal-fetal treatment** is a **medically reasonable alternative** or being investigated in either **innovation** or **research**, the ethical justification becomes both **beneficence** based (to provide information for the evaluation of such intervention and to plan for it) and autonomy based (to inform the woman's **decision making** about such clinical management). *See also* CHORION VILLUS SAMPLING.

ANALOGICAL REASONING. Also known as "reasoning by analogy." **Ethical reasoning** about cases, which is conducted in two steps: (1) determining whether the new case is similar in all ethically relevant respects to a **paradigm case**; and (2) applying the ethical reasoning in the paradigm case to the new case. If there is just one ethically relevant respect in which the new case is dissimilar from the paradigm case, then analogical reasoning cannot be used. Analogical reasoning is an essential component of **casuistry**.

Important limits on analogical reasoning are the sources and quality of ethical reasoning in the paradigm. For example, if the resources (**ethical principles** and **virtues**) used in ethical reasoning about a paradigm case are drawn from **moral theology**, they may not be generalizable across faith communities, which limits application of the results of analogical reasoning to the faith community from which the resources were drawn.

ANATOMIC FUTILITY. There is no reasonable expectation in **deliberative clinical judgment** that the patient's anatomy can be restored to a normal or at least clinically manageable acceptable **condition**. The patient's anatomy is incompatible with the successful implementation of a clinical intervention. There are two **ethical justifications** for this **specification** of futility. The first derives from the accepted concept in **ethical reasoning** that *ought* implies *can*. By *modus tolens* (If a, then b; not b; therefore, not a), there no **ethical obligation** to undertake clinical management that is impossible. The second appeals to the **professional virtue of compassion** and the **ethical principle of nonmaleficence**; both prohibit providing clinical management that in deliberative clinical judgment is expected to result in net clinical harm to the patient. *See also* END-OF-LIFE CARE; FUTILITY.

ANENCEPHALY. A rare **condition** in which an infant's brain is severely underdeveloped. This is a neural tube defect in which "higher" brain centers that support cognitive and affective function are missing. There is usually a brainstem, which means that there is cardiopulmonary function. From the perspective of **determination of death** by cardiopulmonary function criteria and by brain function criteria, an infant with anencephaly is alive. Removing vital organs such as the heart would **kill** the **neonatal patient**, which is criminal homicide and would violate the **dead donor rule**. If one waits until the patient has been determined to be dead by cardiopulmonary criteria, the heart and other organs may no longer be clinically acceptable for **transplantation**. Some have argued that such infants are not "brain alive" (i.e., they meet the brain function criteria for the determination of death). This means that procuring vital organs would not violate the dead donor rule, although doing so would remain a homicide. There is **ethical controversy** about this proposal. *See also* DEATH; LIFE; ORGAN PROCUREMENT.

ANIMAL CRUELTY. Causing harm to a sentient being that does not benefit that or any other being and that morally damages the human being causing such harm. This is **ethically impermissible**. *See also* ANIMAL EXPERIMENTATION; VICE; VIVISECTION.

ANIMAL EXPERIMENTATION. Performing **experiments** on animals. When these are not scientifically justified, the experimenter is engaged in **animal cruelty**, which is **ethically impermissible**. When experimentation is scientifically justified, it should be considered **animal subjects research**. *See also* VIVISECTION.

ANIMAL RIGHTS. The **rights** of animals. Many proponents of animal rights assume that the existence and nature of such rights are philosophically settled matters. This is not the case, however, because there is **ethical controversy** about animal rights. There is disagreement among proponents of animal rights about the capacities of animals that provide the basis for an **ethical justification** for alleged rights on the basis of the animal's **moral status**. There is also ethical controversy about whether an animal right can override the right of a human being. Some who hold that this is the case appear to hold that the rights of animals are **absolute rights**. There is ethical controversy about whether such proponents have met the **burden of ethical justification**. *See also* ANIMAL SUBJECTS RESEARCH.

ANIMAL SUBJECTS RESEARCH. Research performed with animals, either to advance science or to improve the care of animal or human **patients**. In the United States and other countries, animal research is **ethically permissible** only when it has received prospective review and approval by an animal research organizational committee, known in the United States as an **Institutional Animal Care and Use Committee**. *See also* ETHICS OF ANIMAL SUBJECTS RESEARCH.

ANIMAL WELFARE ACT. This federal statute, enacted into law in 1966 during the administration of President Lyndon Baines Johnson (1908–1973; term of office: 1963–1969), requires prospective approval and oversight of **animal subjects research** by the **Institutional Animal Care and Use Com-**

mittee (IACUC). An investigator in his or her **research** protocol must provide a scientific justification for the use of animal subjects, including the number needed to test the hypothesis of the **experiments** to be performed. The design of the research must be able to test the hypothesis and thus answer the research question. The kind, level, and duration of expected **pain** and **distress** of the animals must be described and justified. Whether and how the animal will be euthanized at the end of the experiment must be described. If the animal is expected to survive, provision for its care must be described. The IACUC has the **ethical obligation** to evaluate the scientific, clinical, and ethical dimensions of the proposed research for their acceptability. *See also* ETHICS OF ANIMAL SUBJECTS RESEARCH; PUBLIC POLICY.

APPEAL TO AUTHORITY. The assertion of **power** that one has in virtue of being in an institutional role (e.g., chief of service, department chair, dean) in the absence of **ethical reasoning** that provides an **ethical justification** for this appeal and to the use of power that flows from a position of authority. This is one of the informal fallacies of reasoning and is therefore not acceptable in ethical reasoning. *See also* RAW POWER.

APPELLATE COURT. A court of law that provides judicial review of the outcomes in civil and criminal **trial courts** of original jurisdiction. The opinions that result become an essential component of **common law**. In the United States, the first level of appeal in a federal case is to an Appellate Court in one of the circuits and the second and final level of appeal is to the Supreme Court (or its equivalent in the states; some do not use the name *Supreme Court*). The Supreme Court of the United States is the final interpreter of federal law and the United States Constitution. The states have a parallel structure. The opinions of appellate courts at both levels are important sources for the contribution of law to **bioethics, medical ethics,** and **professional medical ethics**. *See also* HEALTH POLICY; PUBLIC POLICY.

APPLICABILITY. *See* CLINICAL APPLICABILITY.

APPRECIATION. *See* DECISION-MAKING CAPACITY.

AQUINAS, SAINT THOMAS (1225–1274). Italian Roman Catholic, Dominican priest, Doctor of the Church, theologian, and philosopher whose writings address topics in **medical ethics** (e.g., **ensoulment** of the fetus after

40 days gestation, creating its **moral status**) have important implications for the ethics of **induced abortion**. *See also* TERMINATION OF PREGNANCY.

ARGUMENT. Identifying the implications of clearly articulated concepts (**ethical analysis**) that are relevant to the clinical case or issue under consideration. Argument is a component of **ethical reasoning**. The intellectual discipline of **ethics** means that one should always go where argument takes one and nowhere else. If one does not accept the conclusion of an argument, one has only two choices: show that there is an error in ethical reasoning and that, when this error is corrected, a different conclusion is supported; or, when such correction does not need to be made, change one's mind by accepting the conclusion.

It is not acceptable in ethical reasoning to start with a conclusion and then go in search of supporting premises. It is also not acceptable to assert a conclusion in the absence of reasons. Plato (427–347 BCE) has Socrates at many places in the *Dialogues* characterize this very bad intellectual habit as "**mere opinion**." Mere opinion has no place in **bioethics, medical ethics**, or **professional medical ethics**. *See also* ARGUMENT-BASED ETHICS.

ARGUMENT-BASED ETHICS. A tool for the critical appraisal of the literature of **normative bioethics** and **normative medical ethics**. Argument-based ethics comprises five questions: "Does the article address a focused ethics question?"; "Are the arguments that support the results of the article valid?"; "What are the results?"; "What are the conclusions of the paper's ethical analysis and argument?"; and "Will the results help me in clinical practice?" (McCullough, Coverdale, and Chervenak 2014). This approach is modeled on tools for the **critical appraisal** of the scientific and clinical literature. *See also* ETHICAL REASONING.

ARISTOTLE (384–322 BCE). Greek physician, scientist, and philosopher who wrote on metaphysics, logic, and **moral philosophy**. His quest for reliability (Gracia 2010) has intellectual descendants such as **David Hume** (1711–1776) and **Richard Price** (1723–1791), who influenced medical ethics in the 18th and 19th centuries.

ARNALD OF VILLANOVA (ARNALDUS DE VILLA NOVA, ca. 1240–1331 CE). Spanish physician and ethicist. In the *de cautelelis* tradition of providing cautions to physicians, *De Cautelis Medicorum* (*On the Cautions of a Physician*, n.d.) is attributed to him. He provides admonitions implicitly based on the virtue of **prudence**. He cautioned against physicians guaranteeing a good outcome, because the power to do so belongs only to God. Physicians should also display **compassion** in **patient care**.

ARS MORIENDI. The art of dying; a body of literature in **Christian moral theology** that provides guidance for **dying** as a member of that faith community. In the ancient western world, the **Stoics** provided such guidance, in some cases, such as **Marcus Aurelius** (121–180), based on philosophy, and **Francis Bacon** (1561–1626), who called for the medicalization of the dying process, especially for effective pain relief, which he called **euthanasia** (Baker and McCullough 2009c). In contemporary **clinical practice**, a **biopsychosocial** approach to **palliative care** can be understood in historical context as *ars moriendi*. *See also* END-OF-LIFE CARE.

THE ART. A text in the **Hippocratic Corpus**. Notable for its admonition not to continue treatment when disease has "overmastered" the sick individual, to avoid the "madness" of such treatment. This became the basis of the **norm** of **abandonment** of **patients** who were seriously ill, a norm that prevailed until the 18th century. This admonition is also invoked in the ethics of **futility**.

ART OF MEDICINE. A phrase used to contrast **clinical practice** as distinct from biomedical and clinical sciences and requiring **judgment** in the application of those sciences to individual **patients**. The *Hippocratic Oath* is often cited as the basis of the distinction, translating *techné* as "art." This, however, is a mistake, because *techné* names the unchanging body of knowledge and skills of the Hippocratic physician. In addition, this distinction is sometimes made to protect the **autonomy** of physicians in clinical practice, without addressing the risk of such autonomy, uncontrolled variation in the processes and outcomes of patient care, which is the definition of poor **quality**. *See also* MEDICAL HUMANITIES.

ARTIFICIAL HEART. A mechanical circulation device or pump that is placed in the **patient**'s body after his or her failing heart has been removed. The first artificial heart was placed in a human patient in 1982, after **animal subjects research**. There has been no success to date of long-term placement of an artificial heart, calling into question whether it is **ethically justified** to implant such devices. The implantation of an artificial heart is **life-sustaining treatment**. This means that a patient has the right to withdraw authorization for continued use of the device, creating an **ethical obligation** to deactivate the device. There is **ethical controversy** about whether the discontinuation of a **mechanical circulatory device** is **letting die** or **killing**. *See also* END-OF-LIFE CARE.

ARTIFICIAL HYDRATION. A **life-sustaining treatment** that provides fluids other than by mouth and swallowing. Some states in their **Advance Directives Acts** have placed limits on discontinuation of artificial hydration. *See also* END-OF-LIFE CARE.

ARTIFICIAL INSEMINATION. The use of **donor sperm** that is placed in the female **patient**'s vagina or uterus or is self-administered ("turkey-baster" baby) with the goal of initiating pregnancy without sexual intercourse. This is a form of **assisted reproduction** used to clinically manage **infertility** and by lesbian individuals or couples to avoid sexual intercourse with a man. The donor may be the woman's partner or spouse, an individual known to her, or an individual not known to her. Ethical challenges of artificial insemination include an adequate **informed consent process** that considers the **biopsychosocial** risks, such as limited access to information about the health status of the donor, informing a future child, and the limited ability of a future child to learn who his or her biological father is. The latter limitations are created by the **professional obligation** of **confidentiality** of physicians to sperm donors, which may be overridden by applicable law. *See also* ASSISTED REPRODUCTIVE TECHNOLOGIES (ART).

ARTIFICIAL NUTRITION. A **life-sustaining treatment** that provides nutrients other than by mouth and swallowing. Some states in their **Advance Directives Acts** have placed limits on discontinuation of artificial nutrition. This is sometimes called "tube feeding," which is a misnomer, inasmuch as food is prepared in the ordinary course of human activities and is taken by mouth, masticated, and swallowed and is therefore not a form of medical treatment. Providing food to those for whose health and life one is responsible is an **ethical obligation**. The Advance Directives Acts in some states place limits on the discontinuation of artificial nutrition and other forms of life-sustaining treatment. *See also* END-OF-LIFE CARE.

ASSENT. Developmentally appropriate decision making by a **patient**. This concept applies to decision making by patients who are pediatric patients and therefore legally excluded from the **informed consent process** because of age, or are adults who have **decision-making capacity** diminished to an extent that warrants **surrogate decision making** but not diminished completely (e.g., geriatric patients with early stages of dementia). Such patients may be able to express their values, which can then be considered by the **surrogate** decision maker. *See also* ASSISTED DECISION MAKING; GERIATRIC ASSENT; PEDIATRIC ASSENT.

ASSISTED DECISION MAKING. Decision making with and by a patient with diminished **decision-making capacity**, who can still express **values** or preferences. The first step in assisted decision making is to assess the impaired components of decision-making capacity to identify reversible impairments and implement **clinical management** to accomplish restoration of the impaired components. Such patients can then exercise their **autonomy** meaningfully in the **informed consent process**. It is **ethically permissible** to ask the patient what is important to him or her and pointing out, if needed, that the patient's values support one or more **medically reasonable alternatives** and asking the patient to authorize one of these medically reasonable alternatives. When decision-making capacity cannot be restored to support the informed consent process, the patient's values should be elicited and considered by the patient's **surrogate** decision maker seeking to implement the **substituted judgment standard** of **surrogate decision making** (Coverdale, Chervenak, and McCullough 2002). *See also* ASSENT; GERIATRIC ASSENT.

ASSISTED REPRODUCTION. The use of various forms of **assisted reproductive technologies** to provide **clinical management** of **infertility** in both female and male **patients**. There are two outcomes sought: (1) the initiation of a pregnancy; and (2) live birth. The **informed consent process** should provide information about the percent occurrence of both of these two outcomes, which are the benefits of assisted reproduction, as well as risks to the patient and the future child, including **biopsychosocial** risks of blurred parenthood when donor zygotes or embryos are used or when a **surrogate pregnancy** occurs. Ethical guidance for physicians specializing in assisted reproduction is provided by the Ethics Committee of the American Society for Reproductive Medicine (http://www.asrm.org/, accessed 14 September 2017) and the American College of Obstetricians and Gynecologists of the American Congress of Obstetricians and Gynecologists (https://www.acog.org/, accessed 14 September 2017). *See also* ARTIFICIAL INSEMINATION; DONOR EMBRYO; INTRACYTOPLASMIC SPERM INJECTION (ICSI); PREIMPLANTATION GENETIC DIAGNOSIS; PRENATAL GENETIC DIAGNOSIS.

ASSISTED REPRODUCTIVE TECHNOLOGIES (ART). Interventions used in **assisted reproduction** to provide **clinical management** of **infertility** in both female **patients** and male patients. These include **intracytoplasmic**

sperm injection (ICSI), **in vitro fertilization**, and **preimplantation genetic diagnosis**. A number of topics have drawn **ethical reasoning** about ART. One is **justice** based: access to ART by patients without a source of third-party payment, given that the out-of-pocket costs can be very considerable. Another is **beneficence** based, concerning the short-term and long-term outcomes (the latter are challenging to study given the difficulties of following **patients** over a long period of time) of ART such as ICSI for the child, with the latter addressed under the **best interests of the child standard** in **pediatric ethics**. With respect to preimplantation genetic diagnosis, ethical challenges include disclosure of **non-paternity** and **risk-assessment** information for genetically related family members.

ASSISTED SUICIDE. The definition is ambiguous between (a) providing an individual with the means to **kill** himself or herself, which means that the individual self-administers, resulting in **suicide**; and (b) killing that individual at his or her request, which is homicide. Assisted suicide in the first meaning by a physician, or **physician-assisted suicide**, is permitted by law in a small number of jurisdictions in the United States and in other countries. Assisted suicide in the second sense is illegal in every jurisdiction in the United States and many other countries. *See also* END-OF-LIFE CARE.

AUGUSTINE OF HIPPO (IN ROMAN AFRICA), SAINT (354–430). Roman Catholic theologian and philosopher, Latin Father, and Doctor of the Church. He urged physicians to make curing the sick their main goal. Consistent with the centrality of the concept of the **sanctity of life** in **Roman Catholic moral theology**, Augustine holds that **suicide** is **ethically impermissible**.

AURELIUS, MARCUS (121–180). Emperor of Rome (161–180) and **Stoic** philosopher. In his *Meditations* (Aurelius 1937 [c. 171–175]), he regards **suicide** as ethically permissible. He distinguishes **mere self-interest**, which arises from our animal nature, from **legitimate self-interest**, which arises from our nature as rational animals. He also addresses *ars moriendi*, or the art of dying (i.e., preparing oneself for **dying** and **death**). This process requires self-mastery, achieved by "[o]ne thing and one alone—Philosophy," which includes "above all waiting for death with a good grace as being but a setting free of the elements of which everything is made up" (Aurelius 1937 [c.171–175 CE], II.17, p. 43). *See also* END-OF-LIFE CARE.

AUTHENTICITY. A concept invoked to characterize a criterion that should be met in order to **judge** a **patient** to have **autonomy**, in addition to having **decision-making capacity**. This concept is used without precision in the literature of **bioethics** and **medical ethics**. In general, the idea behind the concept is that decision-making capacity is abstract and thus separate from actual individuals, who seek to live lives that have coherence over time by developing and adhering to durable **values** and beliefs. An authentic **decision** expresses such values and beliefs. There is **ethical controversy** about this idea, because it appears to demand too much and thus leaves out many patients who should be considered to have autonomy, for example, those who have undergone a significant or even transformative life change, and to whom, therefore, the **ethical principle of respect for autonomy** is clinically applicable.

AUTHORITY. One of the four **virtues** that form the basis for **Thomas Percival**'s (1740–1804) **professional medical ethics**. By *authority* Percival meant the justified claim to superior clinical and moral **judgment** about the health-related **interests** of **patients**. It is important to appreciate that for Percival this concept does not include the **power** to act on this superior judgment. Authority is thus **paternalistic** but not **paternalism**. *See also* CONDESCENSION; MEDICAL PATERNALISM; STEADINESS; TENDERNESS.

AUTOEXPERIMENTATION. Performing **experiments** on oneself. There is a long history of this practice among physicians. Scottish physician James Simpson (1811–1870), seeking an alternative to ether as a form of anesthesia, self-administered chloroform, causing him to become unconscious until he awoke on the floor (Lederer 2009, 560). The willingness of an investigator to experiment on himself or herself is often cited by such investigators to provide an **ethical justification** for conducting the same research on others. This line of reasoning has also been invoked by investigators who performed experiments on their family members. Their line of reasoning presumes that the investigator will hold himself or herself to reasonable limits of sacrificing **legitimate self-interest** imposed by the **virtue** of **prudence**, in the case of autoexperimentation, and the **ethical obligation** not to place children or other family members at unacceptable risk to **health** and **life**. However, there is no one to whom the investigator is accountable, which opens the unwary or reckless investigator to undertaking experiments that are scientifically invalid or unacceptably dangerous. *See also* PARENTAL RESPONSIBILITY; RESEARCH.

AUTONOMY. Self-rule or self-governance in **decision making** and **judgment** and in behavior based on decision making and judgment. There are two prominent **specifications** of this concept. First, an individual has autonomy, or is autonomous, when he or she makes **decisions** and judgments and acts on them without controlling influence by internal factors such as excessive fear, uncontrollable anxiety, or major depression or by external factors such as the actions of others. A stronger view, deriving from the work of philosophers such as Immanuel Kant (1724–1804), holds that an individual is autonomous when he or she is capable of rational, self-conscious decision making and action under the constraints of the moral law (Kant 1964). Autonomy on all accounts of the concept exists in degrees. A threshold concept of autonomy is invoked in the clinical determination that a patient no longer has **decision-making capacity** or is no longer determined in a court of law to be **legally competent**. Autonomy is often contrasted with heteronomy or rule by another, which is usually regarded as unacceptable. *See also* ETHICAL PRINCIPLE OF RESPECT FOR AUTONOMY; ETHICAL PRINCIPLE OF RESPECT FOR PERSONS; PERSON; RIGHT.

B

BABY DOE. *See* BABY DOE CASE.

BABY DOE CASE. A case in which parents refused to authorize life-saving surgical management for an anatomic defect in a newborn with trisomy 21 or Down syndrome, which resulted in the death of the **patient**. Baby Doe was born in 1981 in the state of Indiana with trisomy 21, which results in intellectual **disability** (then called "mental retardation") of varying degrees, and esophageal-tracheal fistula, an opening between the airway and the tube to the stomach. Left unrepaired, this anatomic defect can result in aspiration of fluid or particles into the lungs, which can cause pneumonia and **death**. Repair of the fistula was recommended by the patient's pediatrician and non-repair was recommended by the mother's obstetrician because the developmental outcome for the child would be very poor, which was a false prognosis for trisomy 21. The parents refused to authorize surgical repair of the fistula. The hospital took the case to court, and the court, not appreciating that the obstetrician's reasoning was not evidence based, ruled that, when physicians disagree about the clinical management of a neonatal patient's condition, parents are free to select a plan of **clinical management**. While this decision was being appealed to the United States Supreme Court, the patient died.

There was considerable coverage of this case in the media, which drew the attention of the administration of President Ronald Reagan (1911–2004; term of office 1981–1989). President Reagan instructed the secretary of the Department of Health and Human Services to act to prevent recurrence of nontreatment in such cases. By the mid-1980s, this resulted in a series of regulations issued under **regulatory law** and legislation, known together as the Baby Doe Rule (Placencia and McCullough 2011). A major outcome of the Baby Doe Case is that it has become very difficult to appeal to the presence or prognosis of intellectual or physical disability in the **ethical justification** of nontreatment of neonates with such disabilities. In addition, such patients have had further protection since the enactment of the **Americans with Disabilities Act** in 1990, during President George H. W. Bush's administration (1989–1993). *See also* END-OF-LIFE CARE.

BABY DOE RULE. *See* BABY DOE CASE.

BABY K CASE. A case in which federal courts supported the request for treatment of a baby with anencephaly by her mother. Baby K was born in 1992 in a hospital in northern Virginia. During her mother's pregnancy, **anencephaly** was diagnosed. **Termination of pregnancy** was recommended to Ms. K, which is not compatible with the **professional medical ethics** of obstetrics, which supports offering but not recommending termination of pregnancy for the management of a pregnancy complicated by this catastrophic fetal anomaly. Ms. K refused, and when the baby was born, she refused the recommendation that **life-sustaining treatment** not be initiated and that **palliative care** be provided, on the grounds that anencephaly is a lethal anomaly. She wanted life-sustaining treatment provided.

The hospital sought court review, which upheld the mother's position; the trial court ruling was upheld by the U.S. Fourth Circuit of Appeals (*In re Baby K* 16 F.3d 590 [4th Cir. 1994]) . Baby K spent the next two-and-a-half years in a nursing home with frequent hospital admissions and then died. This case is significant for two reasons. First, the baby's survival meant that anencephaly should be regarded as a condition in which life can be prolonged, but without improvement of brain anatomy or function. The condition is therefore not universally lethal. Second, the **right** of a parent to request **clinical management** that a physician refuses to provide overrides that refusal when it is not based in **deliberative clinical judgment**. *See also* DISABILITY; END-OF-LIFE CARE; FUTILITY.

BACON, FRANCIS (1561–1626). Bacon was a man of many accomplishments in science and politics. In both his **philosophy of science** and **philosophy of medicine**, he insisted that scientific claims and **clinical judgment** should be based on what he called "experience." By this he emphatically did not mean an individual's personal experience. Instead, for Bacon *experience* meant the results of natural and controlled **experiments**. Natural experiments record in an intellectually disciplined way the processes of nature and their outcomes. This intellectual discipline required constant attention to internal and external factors, or **biases**, that can distort the patient observation and precise description of these processes and their outcomes. The goal is to minimize and, ideally, eliminate bias, so that scientific reports will be highly reliable and thus able to be relied upon by other scientists.

An example of a natural experiment in medicine (the phrase *natural experiment* remains in use in clinical discourse) would be to observe the process and outcomes of a currently untreatable **condition, disability,** or **disease** by recording the progression of signs (observable physical or mental changes of what the **patient** is unaware, such as increased heart rate or blood pressure), progression of symptoms (observable physical or mental changes of what the patient is aware, such as increased rate of breathing or pain), results of laboratory analysis or imaging, and outcomes of mortality and morbidity. A controlled experiment is designed to test a hypothesis and should be conducted in the same meticulous manner as natural experiments. An example of a controlled experiment would be to split a compound medication into its components and then test each separately for their effects on the progression and outcomes of a condition, disability, or disease (an example from the lectures on the institutes and practice of medicine of **John Gregory** [1724–1773] at the University of Edinburgh in the 1760s). An example of a controlled clinical experiment in contemporary biomedical science would be a **clinical trial**.

Bacon's philosophies of science and medicine were enormously influential on the development of scientific medicine during the 18th century. They were also enormously influential on the development of **moral science** during the **English** and **Scottish Enlightenments** of the 18th century, especially on the **professional medical ethics** of John Gregory and **Thomas Percival** (1740–1804). Bacon's experience-based philosophy of medicine is a nascent form of what is now known as **evidence-based medicine**, a key component of **deliberative clinical judgment**. Bacon probably coined the term *euthanasia*, by which he meant a "good death" (i.e., a dying process free of pain), thus anticipating **palliative care** by three centuries.

BARD, SAMUEL (1742–1821). American physician and ethicist, a founder of what is now the College of Physicians and Surgeons of Columbia University. He is author of *A Discourse upon the Duties of a Physician*, based on Scottish **moral science** that he learned as a medical student at the University of Edinburgh. There he was exposed to the moral science of the Scottish moralists and their concept of **sympathy**. He was an early champion of this concept. Bard also emphasized the importance of **research** to improve **patient care**, reflecting the Baconian medicine taught and practiced at Edinburgh.

BASIL THE GREAT, SAINT (329–379). Orthodox Christian theologian. His **moral theology** of medicine treats medicine to be a gift from God, to use to relieve human suffering.

BEAUMONT, WILLIAM (1785–1853). U.S. Army surgeon. During the 1920s, he conducted research on gastric function. He used as his **research subject** Alexis St. Martin (1794–1880), who had suffered a gunshot wound to the abdomen that could not be surgically closed. The resulting opening allowed direct observation of gastric function. This research project began in the 1820s. Dr. Beaumont entered into a contract with St. Martin, who thereby gave his **consent**. Contracts are premised on the **ethical principle of respect for patient autonomy**. St. Martin received compensation. This case is an early example of the **human subjects research** with consent and compensation (Lederer 2009). *See also* ETHICS OF HUMAN SUBJECTS RESEARCH; INFORMED CONSENT.

BECK, THEODORIC ROMEYN (1791–1855). American physician and medical educator who wrote the first major work on medical jurisprudence in the United States, *Elements of Medical Jurisprudence* (1823). Beck was concerned about the negative impact on the health of **patients** of unethical and unprofessional behavior of practitioners; he proposed regulating **clinical practice** to prevent such practitioners from harming patients. This concern provides an **ethical justification** for **licensure**. *See also* MEDICAL JURISPRUDENCE.

BEECHER, HENRY K. (1904–1976). American physician. He wrote an article in the *New England Journal of Medicine* (1966), reporting on cases of ethically questionable **human subjects research**. Ignored at first, it later gained considerable influence on the **ethics of human subjects research**.

BEECHER ARTICLE. *See* BEECHER, HENRY K. (1904–1976).

BEHAVIOR CONTROL. The use of medication, physical restraint, **manipulation**, or **coercion** to gain influence over a patient's behavior, including controlling influence, either to protect the **patient** from himself or to protect others from the patient. All these measures are intended to limit the patient's **autonomy** based on the **ethical principle of nonmaleficence**. The **ethical justification** of behavior control must show that implementing the ethical principle of nonmaleficence should be given priority over implementing the **ethical principle of respect for autonomy**. It is very challenging to define clearly the **biopsychosocial** nature of abnormal or pathological behavior. Behavior control was a prominent topic in **bioethics** in the 1970s. It arises currently with respect to the use of physical restraints and the use of medications as chemical restraints of patients who are considered dangerous to themselves or others. *See also* BEHAVIORAL PSYCHOLOGY; NUDGE.

BEHAVIORAL GENETICS. The study of the causal links among the genome, the epigenome, and the environment (everything other than the genome and epigenome), on the one hand, and patterns of human (or animal) behavior, on the other. As there has been throughout the history of human genetics, there is a tendency toward biological reductionism: if we had an adequate science of genomes and the biological pathways to human traits, reductionist thinking asserts, we could understand and influence human behavior biologically. From the perspective of the **biopsychosocial** concept of human traits, including patterns of behavior, biological reductionism is both scientifically and clinically inadequate and, therefore, misleading. There is also the risk of conceptual confusion, for example, in achieving **clarity** about concepts such as violence or cooperation. This lack of clarity precludes establishing causal links between genes and behavior. **Ethical reasoning** about behavioral genetics, therefore, must begin with an appreciation of the complexity of human behavior at the biological, psychological, and social levels. *See also* BEHAVIOR CONTROL; GENETHICS.

BEHAVIORAL PSYCHOLOGY. A field of **research**, teaching, and **clinical practice** that studies psychological processes that affect **decision making** behavior. One important aspect of behavioral psychology for **autonomy** and the **ethical principle of respect for autonomy** is the study of **biases** of decision making. These biases can lead to decisions and behavior based on them that can diminish the exercise of autonomy, calling into question the weight that should be given to the ethical principle of respect for autonomy. This is called further into question by evidence that **manipulation** can affect the biases of decision making, either by blunting or reinforcing their influence. Attempts to blunt the influences of autonomy-reducing biases can be accomplished by the use of strategies under the label **nudge**, which is a kind of **framing effect**. Finally, from the perspective of behavioral psychology, we are creatures of deep habits in our decision making, calling into question whether we are as autonomous as **ethical reasoning** that emphasizes autonomy assumes that we are. *See also* BEHAVIOR CONTROL; BEHAVIORAL GENETICS.

BELL, JOHN (1796–1872). American physician and ethicist who played a leading role in creating the **American Medical Association *Code of Medical Ethics* of 1847**. He was a social contractarian, a political philosophy that influenced the 1847 *Code*'s reasoning that the freely assumed **ethical obligations** of physicians to **patients** and to society created derivative **rights** of physicians to expect that patients and society would do their part to enable physicians to fulfill these freely assumed ethical obligations. These derivative rights create ethical obligations of patients and society to cooperate with physicians in **patient care** and **public health**. *See also* CODE OF ETHICS; HAYS, ISAAC (1796–1879).

THE BELMONT REPORT. A report of the U.S. National Commission for the Protection of Human Subjects of Biomedical and Behavioral Research (1974–1978) published by the U.S. Government Printing Office in 1979 (U.S. National Commission 1979). The report established a framework for the **ethics of human subjects research** that continues to be the basis for the oversight responsibilities of **Institutional Review Boards** in the United States. The framework appeals to the **ethical principle of respect for persons**, the **ethical principle of beneficence**, and the **ethical principle of justice**. The report is distinctive for its treatment of the ethical principle of respect for persons, which includes as a component the **ethical principle of respect for autonomy** but adds the **ethical obligation** "to protect those with diminished autonomy." The latter group includes fetuses, children, **patients** with mental **disorders** and cognitive **disabilities**, and prisoners. *See also* HUMAN SUBJECTS RESEARCH; PRESIDENTIAL COMMITTEE; RESEARCH.

BENEFICENCE. *See* ETHICAL PRINCIPLE OF BENEFICENCE.

BENEVOLENCE. The **virtue** of habitually treating others in accord with the **ethical obligations** generated by the **ethical principle of beneficence** with an attitude of kindness and concern. In **clinical practice** and **human subjects research**, benevolence can also be understood as an expression of the **professional virtue of compassion**. Benevolence also applies in **animal subjects research** in that investigators should prevent **animal cruelty** in the use of animals and how they are confined.

BENTHAM, JEREMY (1748–1832). English philosopher, jurist, and utilitarian. He wrote a moral science of duties, which influenced the French *déontologie médicale* approach to **medical ethics** in the 19th century. He coined the term *deontology*, meaning a science of duty. This is the meaning used by French medical ethicists. This is not the meaning of *deontology* in contemporary **moral philosophy**. *See also* CONSEQUENTIALIST ETHICS; DEONTOLOGICAL ETHICS; UTILITARIAN JUSTICE; UTILITARIANISM.

BERNARD, CLAUDE (1813–1878). French physiologist and experimental biomedical scientist. He wrote on the **ethics of animal subjects research** and the **ethics of human subjects research** in his *Introduction à l'étude de* *la medicine expérimentale* (*Introduction to the Study of Experimental Medicine*, 1865). Bernard called for **research** on animals before undertaking **experiments** on **patients**, both to protect patients and to use the results of research with animals for a plan for research with patients. This established a **norm** for the ethics of human subjects research that assumes that well-designed **animal subjects research** is **ethically permissible** when conducted to benefit **human subjects research**. From the perspective of **animal rights**, making this assumption is an **ethical controversy**.

BEST INTERESTS OF THE CHILD STANDARD. A **beneficence**-based ethical standard that creates an **ethical obligation** of pediatric healthcare professionals, healthcare organizations, and parents or other **surrogates** to make decisions based on **deliberative clinical judgment** about clinical management that will protect the health and life of the **pediatric patient**.

This standard supports the concept of **parental permission (informed permission) in pediatric ethics**. This concept reflects **ethical reasoning** about the **parent-child relationship** as based primarily on **parental responsibility** to protect children and not primarily **parental rights**. The **authority** and strength of parental rights are a function of parents fulfilling parental responsibility. Parents are given some latitude in both pediatric ethics and health law to make decisions with pediatric healthcare professionals about **clinical management** affecting the pediatric patient's health. Parents have an **absolute ethical obligation** to authorize effective life-saving clinical management of a pediatric patient. This ethical obligation is an enforceable **legal obligation** in all jurisdictions in the United States, based on **common law** dating back at least to the middle of the 20th century.

BEST INTERESTS STANDARD. The secondary, **beneficence**-based ethical standard for **surrogate decision making** that requires the **surrogate** to make decisions for an adult patient based on a reliable understanding of what **clinical management** will protect and promote the patient's **interests**, especially the patient's health-related interests. Normally, these health-related interests include prevention of **death** or of serious, far-reaching, and irreversible loss of health resulting from **disease, disability, disorders**, or **injury**. However, when the patient has an **irreversible condition** or terminal **condition** and its outcome cannot be altered by continued treatment, the health-related interests may include limiting or discontinuing **life-sustaining treatment** to prevent **pain, distress**, or **suffering** that result in net clinical harm to the patient. Doing so is therefore **ethically impermissible** because failure to end such pain, distress, or suffering is inconsistent with the ethical principles of beneficence and **nonmaleficence**.

BIAS. Distortion of **decision making, ethical reasoning**, or **judgment** by internal factors such as human psychology or external factors such as **manipulation** or **coercion**. Bias is epistemologically unacceptable because it unnecessarily reduces the reliability of decision making, ethical reasoning, and judgment. Bias was identified as a major epistemological problem by **Francis Bacon** (1561–1626). Bias can also affect decision making by both physicians and **patients**, an area of research in **behavioral psychology**. *See also* EVIDENCE-BASED MEDICINE; NUDGE.

BIG DATA. The use of very large data sets to aid **clinical judgment** about diagnosis and treatment planning. Large data sets on the processes and outcomes of care—specific doses and scheduling of drugs for heart failure and their outcomes, for example—can be analyzed to detect previously unrecognized patterns and develop hypotheses about their causes. This analysis of large data sets has become a component of **precision medicine**. Public data sets are often accessible by patients.

One set of ethical challenges of such data sets is threats to or even violations of **confidentiality** and the **right to privacy**. Large data sets already exist of genome sequences with de-identified sequences (i.e., no identifiers). However, it has been documented that de-identified sequences can be linked to individuals. One response has been to place these data sets behind firewalls, but this is no guarantee against hackers.

Another ethical challenge concerns how to incorporate this information into **decision making** with **patients**. Interpreting large data sets is cognitively demanding for physicians and should be expected to be even more so for patients. There could be information overload in synergy with misinterpretation that could adversely impact the **informed consent process**.

BINDING, KARL (1841–1920). German lawyer and advocate, with **Alfred Hoche** (1865–1943), of **voluntary active euthanasia** and **involuntary active euthanasia** of patients whose lives were considered to have no value to others. Their *Die Freigabe der Vernichtung lebensunwerten Lebens* (*The Release and Destruction of Life Devoid of Value*, 1920) became part of the justificatory framework for the crimes against humanity carried out by Nazi Germany during World War II. *See also* LIFE UNWORTHY OF LIFE; NAZI MEDICAL WAR CRIMES.

BIOBANK. A facility that stores biological materials from **patients** for current and future **research**. The materials are usually de-identified so that investigators will not know from which patient the material came. The facility may keep separate and under limited access a master list that matches the sample identifier (e.g., an alphanumeric sequence) with the name of the patient from whom the sample came. These measures are taken to fulfill the **professional responsibility** of **confidentiality** and to protect the patient's **privacy**. **Consent** is obtained for procurement of materials, either directly or in the course of **clinical management** or **research**.

There is **consensus** that, when clinically significant information comes from results on these biological materials, the facility should make a reasonable effort to contact the patient. The **informed consent process** should describe this policy and its limitations, especially those that derive from patients relocating, a problem that is compounded as time elapses after the original procurement. If data from research become part of databases, the informed consent process should make clear the limitations on the ability to maintain the confidentiality of **big data**. There is **ethical controversy** about whether consent for unlimited research purposes is **ethically permissible** or whether there is an **ethical obligation** to "re-consent" the patient later.

BIOETHICS. The disciplined study of morality—what is **ethically permissible, ethically impermissible**, and **ethically obligatory**—in the practice of the healthcare professions (including allied health, dentistry, medicine, nursing). Bioethics also encompasses the decisions and behavior of **patients**; the policies and practices of healthcare organizations, both public and private (such as private clinics and hospitals, public clinics and hospitals, private and public hospital systems); biomedical **innovation** and **research** with animal and human subjects; and health and environmental policy formulated and implemented by the executive judicial, legislative, and regulatory branches of government at all levels (e.g., in the United States, at the local, regional, state, and federal levels).

The word *bioethics* appears to have first come into use in the United States in the late 1960s and early 1970s and was meant to include both **biomedical ethics** and **environmental ethics**. In subsequent decades in the United States, the focus was almost exclusively on biomedical ethics. In more recent years, the focus has been expanded to once again include environmental ethics.

Bioethics has become a distinctively interdisciplinary field of study, to which many disciplines contribute, including the creative and literary studies, the healthcare professions, law, philosophy, the qualitative and quantitative social sciences, religious ethics, and moral theology. As a rule, works on bioethics can be classified into one of two groups: **descriptive bioethics** and **normative bioethics**. Works in normative bioethics are written from many disciplinary bases, resulting in a marked pluralism of approaches to bioethics. Refer to the introduction and *see also* MEDICAL ETHICS; POTTER, VAN RENSSELAER (1911–2001).

BIOMEDICAL ETHICS. The disciplined study of morality in healthcare and health policy. Bioethics deals with what is **ethically permissible, ethically impermissible,** and **ethically obligatory** in the practice of the healthcare professions; what is ethically permissible, ethically impermissible, and ethically obligatory for patients; the policies and practices of healthcare organizations, both public and private (such as private clinics and hospitals, public clinics and hospitals, private and public hospital systems) as they influence physicians and patients; biomedical **innovation** and **research** with animal and human subjects; and the role of healthcare professionals and **patients** in health and environmental policy formulated and implemented by the executive judicial, legislative, and regulatory branches of government at all levels (e.g., in the United States, at the local, regional, state, and federal levels). *See also* BIOETHICS; MEDICAL ETHICS; PROFESSIONAL MEDICAL ETHICS.

BIOPSYCHOSOCIAL. A concept of health introduced by the American psychiatrist George Engel (1913–1999) to correct the scientific and clinical deficiencies of a concept of health based solely on biological structures and functions, known as biological reductionism or biomedical reductionism. Engel's corrective called for identifying and addresses the biomedical, psychological, and social dimensions of health (Engel 1977).

BIOTERRORISM. The use of biological agents to commit acts of terrorism. These may result in mass casualty events, in which the number of affected individuals may quickly surpass the capacity of an individual hospital or all of the hospitals in the affected area to provide **clinical management**. In **professional medical ethics**, the professionally responsible **allocation of scarce medical resources** will become a major ethical challenge. The ethics of **triage** may not be adequate to the scale of a mass casualty event that quickly overwhelms healthcare organizations and personnel. The response will require an **ethics of cooperation** among multiple healthcare organizations and their professional and lay staffs. The **ethical obligations** of healthcare organizations to protect their staff and family members of staff will become another ethical challenge. To responsibly manage these complex and synergistic ethical challenges will also require guidance from **health policy** and **public policy**.

BIRTH CONTROL. *See* CONTRACEPTION.

BLINDED CLINICAL TRIAL. A method of clinical investigation designed to prevent bias in the **clinical judgment** of investigators and the self-reports of **patients** where the medication being tested against another drug or a **placebo** is not labeled. The **informed consent process** for blinded clinical trials must explain blinding and its purpose to patients who are potential subjects and obtain the patient's **informed consent** to be blinded. *See also* DOUBLE-BLINDED CLINICAL TRIAL; OPEN-LABEL CLINICAL TRIAL; SINGLE-BLINDED CLINICAL TRIAL.

BLINDING. *See* BLINDED CLINICAL TRIAL.

BOUNDARY ISSUES. This phrase is used with two meanings: (1) ethical challenges of maintaining professional boundaries with **patients**, especially regarding romantic or sexual relationships; or (2) intra-professional and interprofessional relationships.

Romantic or sexual relationships can be initiated or accepted by physicians out of **self-interest**, which is incompatible with the **professional virtue of self-effacement** (the attractiveness of a patient is clinically irrelevant and therefore should not be acted upon) and the **professional virtue of self-sacrifice**. In addition, patients can be harmed by such relationships, especially by the imbalance of **power** that transfers from the physician-patient relationship to a romantic or sexual relationship. This outcome is **ethically impermissible** in **beneficence**-based **deliberative clinical judgment**.

There is agreement among professional associations of physicians in the United States that romantic and sexual relationships with current patients are ethically impermissible. This allows as **ethically permissible** ending the professional relationship with a patient before entering into a romantic or sexual relationship. The American Psychiatric Association regards such relationships with past patients as ethically impermissible.

Boundary issues among physicians (intra-professional boundary issues) and between physicians and other healthcare professionals (interprofessional boundary issues), including nurses, physician assistants, dentists, allied healthcare professionals, medical social workers, and chaplains, should be managed based on the first commitment in the **ethical concept of medicine as a profession**, to **competence** in **patient care**. **John Gregory** (1724–1773) addressed this topic in the context of the rivalry between physicians and surgeons, who were then still two separate groups. Gregory asks who should work up a patient who is newly presented for care with a leg fracture and gangrene. The physician has the competence to perform the initial work-up and to make a **clinical judgment** about whether this is a surgical case. If the physician determines that it is a surgical case, he should refer the patient to a surgeon and then not interfere with subsequent **clinical management**. This has general application: intra-professional and interprofessional boundary issues should be managed, first, by recognizing that **professional medical ethics** creates the common ground among those involved and the commitment to clinical competence, and, second, by recognizing that the division of labor among physicians and between physicians and other healthcare professionals should be based on the specialized competence of colleagues.

BRAIN DEATH. The determination that **death** has occurred by brain-function criteria for the irreversible cessation of the brain's integrative functions. This **clinical judgment** that death has occurred is used for patients who are on mechanical life support that prevents a reliable clinical judgment that applies the concept of **cardiac death**. In the United States, the brain-function criteria for the clinical judgment that death has occurred are defined by the American Academy of Neurology (Wijdicks et al. 2010), upon which organizational policy should be based.

There is concern that the use of the term *brain death* can be confusing to the public by suggesting that *brain death* names something different from **cardiopulmonary death**, cardiac death, or circulatory death. All these phrases refer to the death of a patient but determine that death has occurred using different clinically reliable criteria.

Some question the scientific, clinical, and philosophical adequacy of the **determination of death** by brain function criteria. There is also scientific, clinical, and **ethical controversy** about whether current brain-function criteria for death result in determining that patients in a **minimally conscious state**, in which the patient is still alive, are dead. Legally, the determination on the basis of brain function criteria that death has occurred requires that the determination be made by a physician. *See also* AD HOC COMMITTEE OF THE HARVARD MEDICAL SCHOOL TO EXAMINE THE DEFINITION OF BRAIN DEATH.

BUDDHIST BIOETHICS. Bioethics based on Buddhist **moral theology**, drawing on such texts as the Pali Canon, a major resource for Buddhist moral theology and medical ethics, contributing to the pluralism of bioethics (Young 2009a, 2009b). Moral theology, because it is not secular, is not methodologically adequate to serve as the basis of **professional medical ethics**.

BUDDHIST MEDICAL ETHICS. Medical ethics based on Buddhist **moral theology**, drawing on such texts as the Pali Canon, a major resource for Buddhist moral theology and medical ethics (Young 2009a, 2009b). Moral theology, because it is not secular, is not methodologically adequate to serve as the basis of **professional medical ethics**.

BUDDHIST MORAL THEOLOGY. Moral theology drawing on such texts as the Pali Canon, a major resource for Buddhist moral theology and medical ethics, contributing to the pluralism of bioethics (Young 2009a, 2009b). Moral theology, because it is not secular, is not methodologically adequate to serve as the basis of **professional medical ethics.**

BURDEN OF JUSTIFICATION. A requirement in **ethical reasoning** that a **judgment** should not be presumed to be reliable and, therefore, that such a judgment must be shown to be reliable through **ethical justification.** When the judgment runs against very well-established competing judgments, the burden of justification increases. This is referred to as a "steep" burden of justification (or "steep" burden of proof). For example, all adult patients are presumed to have intact **decision-making capacity** and, therefore, decisional capacity. This means that a physician who makes the judgment that a patient lacks such capacity—and therefore should not be considered to have decisional capacity—must provide an ethical justification.

BURDEN OF PROOF. *See* BURDEN OF JUSTIFICATION.

BUSINESS ETHICS. Ethical reasoning about the organization, **organizational culture**, financing, conduct, and regulation of business entities, including healthcare organizations. Adherence to the results of such ethical reasoning and ethical **norms** is an essential component of the business model of physicians' practices and of healthcare organizations. *See also* ORGANIZATIONAL ETHICS.

BYO. One of the four key components in the concept of the life cycle in **medical ethics** in Japan, influenced by **Buddhism** and **Shintoism**. *Byo* means "disease or being sick" (Kimura and Sakai 2009, 132). This concept plays a major role in **Kaibara Ekiken**'s (1630–1714) medical ethics. *See also RO; SHI; SHO.*

C

CABOT, RICHARD C. (1868–1939). American physician and ethicist. His **medical ethics** emphasized competent clinical care and cooperation among healthcare professionals caring for a **patient**, an **ethics of cooperation** that anticipated the now-standard hospital practice of team care. Cabot was also a leader in the development of medical social work in American hospitals.

CADAVER. The dead body of a human being. Medical students learn human anatomy by dissecting a cadaver. Pathologists perform postmortem examinations of cadavers to identify the cause(s) of a **patient**'s death. Inasmuch as no cadaver has any of the intrinsic properties thought to generate **independent moral status**, cadavers do not have independent **moral status**. In addition, because a cadaver is not alive, it cannot benefit from clinical intervention. It follows that no cadaver has the moral status of being a patient. The moral status of a cadaver derives from its social role as the dead body of a former **person** and loved one and as an object of **respect** that should be treated with **dignity**. The dead person's faith community's traditions should be respected. *See also* DEATH.

CANDOR. A **professional virtue** in the **professional medical ethics** of **John Gregory** (1724–1773). Gregory held that all humans have the capacity to be "open to conviction" (i.e., being open to being convinced or to change one's mind based on scientific evidence). Candor is the intellectual **virtue** that creates an **ethical obligation** to be willing to study scientific evidence, from whatever source, about improvements in **clinical practice** and to adopt such improvements when evidence supports them. Individual **self-interest** should never interfere with doing so, especially self-interest in reputation or income (McCullough 1998). Candor has become an essential intellectual virtue for **evidence-based medicine** and for **critical appraisal**, one of the tools of evidence-based medicine. *See also* DELIBERATIVE CLINICAL JUDGMENT.

CAPITAL PUNISHMENT. The implementation of the death penalty by departments of correction in states in the United States and in other countries in which capital punishment is practiced as permitted by law. There is **ethical controversy** about whether physicians should play any role in capital punishment, because of the presumption against killing **patients** in **professional medical ethics**. *See also* KILLING.

CARDIAC DEATH. The **clinical judgment**, following accepted criteria, that **death** is considered to have occurred when there is irreversible cessation of heart function and therefore no expectation of restoration of spontaneous circulation. This clinical judgment is made in settings outside the hospital (e.g., by emergency medical technicians in the field) and in the hospital. The clinical judgment of cardiac death plays a central role in **donation after cardiac death**.

There is concern that the use of the terms *cardiac death*, ***cardiopulmonary death***, and *circulatory death* can be confusing to the public by suggesting that *cardiac death* or *circulatory death* names something different from the term ***brain death***. All these phrases refer to the death of a patient but determine that death has occurred using different clinically reliable criteria. *See also* AD HOC COMMITTEE OF THE HARVARD MEDICAL SCHOOL TO EXAMINE THE DEFINITION OF BRAIN DEATH; DEAD DONOR RULE; DETERMINATION OF DEATH.

CARDIOPULMONARY DEATH. The **clinical judgment**, following accepted criteria, that **death** has occurred when there is irreversible cessation of heart and lung function. This determination is a component of **donation after cardiac death**. Legally, the determination on the basis of cardiopulmonary criteria that death has occurred does not require that the determination be made by a physician, except in cases of organ donation. There is concern that the use of the terms *cardiopulmonary death*, ***cardiac death***, and *circulatory death* can be confusing to the public by suggesting that each of these phrases names something different from the term ***brain death***. All these phrases refer to the death of a patient but determine that death has occurred using different clinically reliable criteria. *See also* AD HOC COMMITTEE OF THE HARVARD MEDICAL SCHOOL TO EXAMINE THE DEFINITION OF BRAIN DEATH; DEAD DONOR RULE; DETERMINATION OF DEATH.

CARDIOPULMONARY RESUSCITATION (CPR). Clinical intervention to reverse arrest of heart and lung function, with the intended outcome of restoration of spontaneous circulation. Cardiopulmonary resuscitation (CPR) is provided to patients by default, in other words, in the absence of a **Do-Not-**

Resuscitate Order, a **Do-Not-Attempt Resuscitation Order**, or an **Out of-Hospital Do-Not-Resuscitate Order.** Cardiopulmonary resuscitation is discontinued when in **deliberative clinical judgment** the concept of **physiologic futility** is invoked. In some **Advance Directives Acts**, CPR is defined as **life-sustaining treatment**. This makes possible refusal of CPR by a **surrogate** under conditions identified in the **statutory law**. *See also* END-OF-LIFE CARE; FUTILITY.

CARE ETHICS. Sometimes also care ethic. *See* ETHICS OF CARE.

CASE-BASED MEDICAL ETHICS. *See* CASUISTRY. *See also* ANALOGICAL REASONING; COMMON LAW; PLURALISTIC CASUISTRY.

CASTRATION. Surgical castration is removal of the testicles, bilateral orchiectomy, from a male **patient** to treat testicular diseases or to achieve **sterilization**. Chemical castration is the administration of medication that deactivates the testes, resulting in sterilization. When performed on the basis of the physician's **deliberative clinical judgment** and with the authorization of the patient in the **informed consent process**, sterilization is **ethically permissible** in **professional medical ethics**. There is a history of court-ordered chemical castration, including as an alternative to incarceration, for men who have been found guilty of rape. This calls into question whether the agreement of the convicted individual is **voluntary**. Depending upon one's **judgment** about the psychological strength of the inducement to avoid castration, agreement is in all cases **involuntary** and therefore not an agreement at all. This is a plausible position, given the inherently **coercive** nature of a judge's power in a criminal trial. In **Roman Catholic moral theology**, except when permitted under the concept of **double effect**, sterilization by castration is **ethically impermissible**.

CASTRO, RODRIGO DE (1550–1627). Portuguese Jewish physician and ethicist in the *medicus politicus* or politic physician tradition. This tradition is based on the concept that the virtue of **prudence** of the physician is subordinate to the power of the rich, royalty, and cities hiring municipal physicians. His *Medicus Politicus* (*The Politic Physician*) was published in 1614. He permits being untruthful with the sick when **truth-telling** would be so alarming to the sick individual that his or her condition would worsen. He thus anticipates the concept of **therapeutic privilege**.

CASUISTIC REASONING. *See* CASUISTRY.

CASUISTRY. Case-based **ethical reasoning**, a method of **ethical** reasoning about cases with deep roots in **Roman Catholic moral theology**. Casuistry deploys **analogical reasoning** to argue from paradigm cases of behavior that have already been reliably judged to be correct or incorrect behavior. One then compares a new case, which appears to be similar, to the paradigm case. If the new case is similar in all morally relevant respects, then the behavior described in the new case should be judged the same as in the paradigm case. If there are differences between the new case and the paradigm case in morally significant respects, the analogy from the new case to the paradigm case does not hold. While the word *casuistry* is not familiar to most physicians, case-based reasoning is common in the formation of **clinical judgment**. Casuistry is also deployed in **clinical ethics consultation**. *See also* PLURALISTIC CASUISTRY.

CAUTIONARY PRINCIPLE. *See* PRECAUTIONARY PRINCIPLE.

CCU. Critical care unit. *See* CRITICAL CARE.

CDCDD. Controlled donation after circulatory **determination of death**. *See also* DONATION AFTER CARDIAC DEATH.

CELSUS, AULUS CORNELIUS (14 BCE–50 CE). Roman encyclopedist. Like **Scribonius Largus** (ca. 1–ca. 50), he emphasizes the virtue of **compassion**, which, for the surgeon, must be managed carefully, so that the surgeon does not lose control and remains focused on benefiting the sick individual upon whom the surgeon is operating. *See also* EMPATHY; STEADINESS; SYMPATHY; TENDERNESS.

CESAREAN DELIVERY. Delivery of a **viable** fetus by means of abdominal surgery. This includes opening the pregnant woman's abdomen and then her uterus (by a cesarean section) followed by removal of the fetus and placenta from the uterus, transferring the care of the **neonatal patient** to a pediatrician in the delivery room for clinical evaluation and management, closing the surgical incisions, and recovery of the woman in the hospital. Ethical issues concerning cesarean delivery include the **right to refuse** cesarean delivery, **coerced cesarean delivery**, **cesarean delivery on patient request**, and **forced cesarean delivery**.

CESAREAN DELIVERY ON PATIENT REQUEST. A request by a pregnant woman for cesarean delivery when cesarean delivery is not a **medically reasonable alternative** in **deliberative clinical judgment**. This is the exercise of a **positive right**. The request may or may not be made as an outcome of the **informed consent process**. The **ethical justification** of a request made as an outcome of the informed consent process appeals to the **ethical principle of respect for autonomy** and ethically justified limits on it originating in the **ethical principle of beneficence** and the **professional virtue of integrity**. The weight to be given to an appeal to this ethical principle in an absence of the informed consent process is an **ethical controversy**.

CHARACTER. The set of **virtues** and **vices** that an individual exhibits in his or her patterns of **decision making, judgment,** and behavior. An individual of good character displays a preponderance of virtues over vices. An individual of bad character displays a preponderance of vices over virtues. A corrupt individual displays a preponderance of vices over virtues with little probability that the preponderance will change to a preponderance of virtues over vices. An evil individual appears to have no virtues and no probability of developing them.

CHARITY CARE. The provision without charge of **clinical management** to **patients** without a source of payment, including self-payment. This has been an **ethical obligation** for centuries in the **moral theologies** of diverse faith communities. For examples, monks in the monastic foundations of medieval Europe provided charity care to the sick poor of their communities. The creation of the **Royal Infirmaries** in the 18th century was motivated, in part, by an ethical obligation to care for the sick poor as a matter of Christian charity, with the cost of running an infirmary covered by its trustees. These hospitals became the model for the not-for-profit, private, and public hospitals in the United States, starting in the late 18th century. In the United States, hospitals sponsored by Christian and Jewish faith communities provided charity care to the sick poor. The scale of the lack of a source of payment for **patients** in the United States now far exceeds the capacity of hospitals and individual physicians to respond on the basis of charity. The recognition of this reality was among the motives for enacting the Affordable Care Act of 2010. *See also* ALTRUISM; HEALTH POLICY.

CHEMICAL CASTRATION. *See* CASTRATION.

CHILD. An individual who has not attained legal majority, either by reason of age or other provisions of the law. A child is under the protection of his or her parents, who have an **ethical obligation** to protect and promote their child's **interests**, including health-related interests. A child is also thought to have a **right to an open future**. The **professional medical ethics** of the care of children comes under **pediatric ethics**. There are also special provisions in the regulations of **human subjects research** on children. *See also* BEST INTERESTS OF THE CHILD STANDARD; INFORMED PERMISSION; PARENTAL PERMISSION; PARENTAL RESPONSIBILITY; PEDIATRIC ASSENT; PEDIATRIC ETHICS.

CHILDHOOD VACCINATION. The standard of care in pediatrics and in **public health** is that children should be immunized against communicable diseases for which there is a safe and effective vaccine. The only **ethically permissible** exception is biomedical: a **deliberative clinical judgment** that vaccination is medically contraindicated for the **patient**. This is a **beneficence**-based norm that protects individual children and also a **justice**-based norm that protects children who cannot be vaccinated for medical reasons.

Some states in the United States have adopted this norm and made vaccination mandatory except for medical reasons. The vaccination rates in these states approaches 100 percent. Some states allow for exceptions (e.g., on religious grounds), and their vaccination rates are much lower, increasing the risk of outbreaks of contagious diseases. Such outbreaks have occurred, resulting in preventable **morbidity** and **mortality**. There is **ethical controversy** about whether any such exceptions should be allowed and about whether parents who refused medically indicated childhood vaccination should be reported to child protection agencies of the government as child neglect or even abuse. *See also* BEST INTERESTS OF THE CHILD STANDARD; INFORMED PERMISSION; PARENTAL PERMISSION; PARENTAL RESPONSIBILITY; PEDIATRIC ETHICS.

CHORION VILLUS SAMPLING. *See* PRENATAL DIAGNOSIS.

CHRISTIAN BIOETHICS. Bioethics based on **Christian moral theology**. Like all medical ethics, it is based on **moral theology** (Amundsen 2009a, 2009b; Ferngren 2009), thus contributing to the pluralism of methods in bioethics. Christian moral theologians played a major role in the development of bioethics in the United States. Notables include **John Fletcher** (1931–2004), **Joseph Fletcher** (1905–1991), James Gustafson, **Richard A. McCormick** (1922–2000), and **Paul Ramsey** (1913–1988).

CHRISTIAN MEDICAL ETHICS. Medical ethics based on **Christian moral theology**. Like all medical ethics based on **moral theology**, the applicability of medical ethics based in moral theology beyond the original faith community is usually limited. Moral theology, because it is not secular, is not methodologically adequate to serve as the basis of **professional medical ethics** (Amundsen 2009a, 2009b; Ferngren 2009).

CHRISTIAN MORAL THEOLOGY. Moral theology based on sources of moral authority in Christian faith communities, including Sacred Scripture, tradition, and teaching. Given the variation in interpretation of these and other sources among Christian faith communities, Christian moral theology displays marked diversity. **Medical ethics** and **bioethics** based on Christian moral theology should be expected to display similar diversity (Amundsen 2009a, 2009b; Ferngren 2009). Christian moral theology is a major component of the **organizational culture** of hospitals, clinics, and other healthcare organizations supported by Christian faith communities. This culture is often expressed in the commitment of faith-sponsored healthcare organizations to provide **clinical management** to all **patients** independent of their source of payment or absence of such a source. *See also* CHARITY CARE.

CICERO, MARCUS TULLIUS (106–43 BCE). Roman politician, lawyer, and **Stoic** philosopher. His *De Officiis* appeals to **role-related ethical obligations** that originate in a social role or "office" that one has made the commitment to fulfill. Cicero's **Stoicism** emphasizes self-mastery, which is achieved, in part, by routinely fulfilling the **ethical obligations** of one's role. Cicero's **moral philosophy** was a source of influence on the **medical ethics** of **Thomas Gisborne** (1758–1846), **John Gregory** (1724–1773), and **Thomas Percival** (1740–1804) in the 18th century. For example, the influence of Cicero is evident in the title of the first version of Gregory's **professional medical ethics**; it was published in 1770 with the title *Observations on the Duties and Offices of a Physician*.

CIRCULATORY DEATH. *See* CARDIAC DEATH.

CIRCUMCISION. In males, cutting off the foreskin of the penis, often performed shortly after birth. This is a requirement in some faith communities. There is **ethical controversy** in **bioethics** about whether circumcision is **ethically permissible**. The American Academy of Pediatrics' position is the following: "After a comprehensive review of the scientific evidence, the American Academy of Pediatrics found the health benefits of newborn male circumcision outweigh the risks, but the benefits are not great enough to recommend universal newborn circumcision " (2012, https://www.aap.org/en-us/about-the-aap/aap-press-room/pages/newborn-male-circumcision.aspx, accessed 14 September 2017). This is an **evidence-based, beneficence**-based statement. In females, circumcision is a clitorectomy, a form of **genital mutilation**, which is **ethically impermissible**.

CIVIL DISOBEDIENCE. Public opposition to laws about which one has made an **ethical judgment** that the law is **unjust**. Civil disobedience requires that one publicly state or acknowledge that one has broken the law judged unjust, accept prosecution or civil court proceedings, and accept the outcomes of such proceedings. This process is a **conscience**-based effort to change **health policy** or **public policy**. Failure to meet these criteria means that an individual's law-breaking is not an act of conscience but, instead, undermines the rule of law, which violates one of the fundamental **ethical obligations** of citizenship in a republic of laws, respect for the rule of law. There is no **integrity** in such failure. *See also* CONSCIENTIOUS OBJECTION.

CLARITY. A requirement of **ethical reasoning** in **bioethics, medical ethics**, and **professional medical ethics** that a concept be as clearly stated as possible. If the concept is a **cluster concept**, clarity requires that the components invoked are clearly stated. Failure to meet this requirement disables ethical reasoning from its start, rendering all results of no value. *See also* CLINICAL ADEQUACY; CLINICAL APPLICABILITY; COHERENCE; CONSISTENCY.

CLINICAL ADEQUACY. A requirement of **ethical reasoning** in **bioethics, medical ethics**, and **professional medical ethics** that **judgments** made about clinical cases or ethical issues in the present have some applicability to future cases, if only to provide a point of departure. This requirement reflects a historically informed skepticism about claims that a clinical case or ethical issue is "new and unprecedented" and, therefore, threatens to outstrip ethical reasoning about it. *See also* CLARITY; CLINICAL APPLICABILITY; COHERENCE; CONSISTENCY.

CLINICAL APPLICABILITY. A requirement that the results of **ethical reasoning** in **bioethics, medical ethics**, and **professional medical ethics** provide concrete guidance for **clinical judgment** and **clinical management** of **patients** or the conduct of **clinical research**. *See also* CLARITY; CLINICAL ADEQUACY; COHERENCE; CONSISTENCY.

CLINICAL ETHICAL JUDGMENT. **Ethical reasoning** that classifies clinical care under ethical categories, which classification then focuses ethical reasoning on the components of the ethical category. Examples include an uninformed request by a patient for **clinical management** not supported in **deliberative clinical judgment** or **surrogate decision making** for a patient with a **terminal condition** who does not have an **advance directive**. Clinical ethical judgment is an essential component of **clinical ethics consultation**. *See also* JUDGMENT.

CLINICAL ETHICS. The application of **medical ethics** to **clinical practice**. Some make a sharp distinction between clinical ethics, on the one hand, and **bioethics** on the other, based on the claim that bioethics lacks a dedicated focus on clinical practice. *See also* CASUISTRY; CLINICAL ETHICS CONSULTATION; PLURALISTIC CASUISTRY.

CLINICAL ETHICS COMMITTEE. An **ethics committee** of a healthcare organization that limits its scope of responsibility to **clinical ethics**, omitting **organizational ethics** and **research ethics**. *See also* INSTITUTIONAL REVIEW BOARD (IRB).

CLINICAL ETHICS CONSULTANT. An individual or team who provides **ethics consultation** in the clinical setting about **clinical care** of **patients**. A process for certification of clinical ethics consultants is in development in the United States and other countries. *See also* RESEARCH ETHICS CONSULTANT; RESEARCH ETHICS CONSULTATION.

CLINICAL ETHICS CONSULTATION. Formal **consultation** with the **patient**'s physician and care team, the patient, or the patient's family about the responsible management of ethical issues in **clinical practice**. Clinical ethics consultation may be provided by an individual, team, or **ethics committee**. The **clinical ethics consultant** may be a physician, other healthcare professional, philosopher, theologian, lawyer, or someone from another discipline. In the United States, clinical ethics consultation is in the process of organizing itself into a profession. A crucial step in this process has been the approval in 2014 of a code of ethics, *Code of Ethics and Professional Responsibilities for Healthcare Ethics Consultations* (http://asbh.org/uploads/publications/ASBH%20Code%20of%20Ethics.pdf, accessed 14 September 2017), by the American Society for Bioethics and Humanities. A process for certification of clinical ethics consultants is in development in the United States and other countries. *See also* RESEARCH ETHICS CONSULTANT; RESEARCH ETHICS CONSULTATION.

CLINICAL JUDGMENT. Judgment that classifies the patient's **condition** as a **disability, disorder, disease**, or **injury**; assesses the seriousness of the patient's condition; and identifies **medically reasonable alternatives** for the clinical management of the patient's condition and his or her prognosis. Epistemologically, clinical judgment is evaluated prospectively for its reliability. Retrospective evaluation of whether a clinical judgment was true or false is meaningless. Clinical judgment should be evidence-based, rigorous, transparent, and accountable, resulting in **deliberative clinical judgment**.

CLINICAL MANAGEMENT. The provision by a physician to a **patient** of the components of **patient care**, including diagnosis, **risk assessment**, treatment planning, prognosis, the **informed consent process**, treatment provision and alteration as needed, and follow-up. Clinical management can also include planned **innovation** that has been prospectively reviewed and approved. *See also* RESEARCH.

CLINICAL PRACTICE. The prevention and management of an individual **patient**'s **condition**, **disease**, **disability**, **disorder**, or **injury** based on **deliberative clinical judgment**. Clinical practice should be based on reliable predictions of the outcomes of **clinical management**. When the outcomes of a clinical intervention cannot be reliably predicted, that clinical intervention becomes an **experiment**. Clinical experiments take two forms: **innovation** and **research**. *See also* PATIENT CARE.

CLINICAL RESEARCH. Research with **human subjects** to better understand and responsibly manage **conditions**, **disability**, **disease**, and **injury** in **clinical practice**. *See also* CLINICAL MANAGEMENT; ETHICS OF HUMAN SUBJECTS RESEARCH; EXPERIMENT; INNOVATION; PATIENT CARE.

CLINICAL TRIAL. Clinical **research** with **animal research subjects** or **human research subjects** to test a hypothesis about the improvement of the **clinical care** of a **condition**, **disability**, **disease**, **disorder**, or **injury**. Clinical trials come under **ethics of animal subjects research** and **ethics of human subjects research**. *See also* EXPERIMENT; INNOVATION; PHASE I CLINICAL TRIAL; PHASE II CLINICAL TRIAL; PHASE III CLINICAL TRIAL; PHASE IV CLINICAL TRIAL.

CLONING. The replication of a cell in the laboratory. Cloning can be therapeutic, in which a cell line is produced in the laboratory with the goal of replacing damaged tissue or a malfunction or missing organ in the **patient**'s body. Cloning can be reproductive cloning, in which an embryo is produced in the laboratory and transferred to a female's uterus with the goal of initiating pregnancy that results in live birth of a biological copy of the individual from whom the cell was taken to create the embryo. There is general agreement that therapeutic cloning should be undertaken in patients only after thorough study and evaluation in animal models of the clinical benefits and risks so that **Phase I trials** of efficacy and safety can be designed and conducted with prospective review and approval. Without this foundation, going directly to the use of therapeutic cloning in **clinical management** would be inconsistent with **professional integrity** and thus **ethically impermissible**. Reproductive cloning has been accomplished in animal models, which have shown the process to be inefficient (many embryos died and pregnancies failed) and resulting in unknown and potentially serious risks. There is **consensus** that reproductive cloning should not be undertaken with human beings, while **animal subjects research** continues. *See also* EMBRYONIC STEM CELL RESEARCH.

CLUSTER CONCEPT. A concept that has multiple components. Not all of the components have to be applicable for every successful application of the concept in different contexts. To meet the requirements of **clarity** and **consistency** in **ethical reasoning**, when a cluster concept is invoked, the components that are invoked must be clearly stated and used without addition or subtraction in ethical reasoning. The concept of **life** is an example. Its components include the capacities to maintain homeostasis, consume energy, secrete waste, reproduce, and locomote. A **patient** with the incapacity to produce sperm is still very much alive, as is a patient who has experienced quadriplegia. A patient may have lost the capacity to maintain homeostasis but can have this deficiency managed by **life-sustaining treatment**. It is philosophically challenging to determine when a cluster concept no longer applies. How many components must be absent becomes a vexed question known as the sorites problem or sorites paradox. This is especially the case for the concept of **death** and, therefore, for the **determination of death**.

CODE OF ETHICS. A document, usually containing general statements on **medical ethics**, created by a national or international association of physicians to guide and assess **judgments** about **clinical practice**, **innovation** and **research**, professional education, and **health policy**. Codes of ethics often form the basis for an association's **ethics statements**. Both are meant to be **clinically applicable** and therefore practical forms of medical ethics. Codes of ethics of specialty associations of physicians focus on the distinctive ethical concerns of physicians in that specialty. In French medical ethics of the 18th and 19th centuries, codes were known as *déontologie médicale*. *See also* OATH; PROFESSIONAL MEDICAL ETHICS.

COERCED CESAREAN DELIVERY. The use of **coercion** to perform cesarean delivery on a pregnant woman without her authorization in the **informed consent process**. Anyone who proposes to use coercion in any setting faces the **burden of justification** to provide an **ethical justification**

of coercion. While some state courts in the United States have approved cesarean delivery over the refusal of it by the pregnant woman, the majority of courts have not.

In most of the **bioethics** and **medical ethics** literature, especially work by legal scholars, court-ordered cesarean delivery is considered to be **ethically impermissible**. A counterview is that a pregnant woman has a **beneficence**-based **ethical obligation** to accept reasonable risk to herself to benefit the **fetal patient** and **neonatal patient**. This applies to conditions such as well-documented, intrapartum complete placenta previa, for which there are no reported cases of spontaneous reversion, and for which cesarean delivery eliminates the risk of **mortality** to the fetal patient and reduces the risk of morality to the pregnant woman to that of cesarean delivery. This risk is **judged** acceptable in **deliberative clinical judgment** (Chervenak and McCullough 2014). *See also* COURT-ORDERED CESAREAN DELIVERY; FORCED CESAREAN DELIVERY.

COERCED STERILIZATION. Sterilization without the **informed consent** of the **patient** accompanied with a threat. *See also* FORCED STERILIZATION; INVOLUNTARY STERILIZATION.

COERCION. Interference with **decision making** or the implementation of a decision by making threats to use force if the **patient** makes an undesired decision or implements such a decision. When the reason for making threats is to protect the patient from himself or herself, then coercion is a type of **paternalism**. *See also* INVOLUNTARY.

COERCIVE. *See* COERCION.

COGNITIVE UNDERSTANDING. *See* DECISION-MAKING CAPACITY.

COHERENCE. A requirement of **ethical reasoning** in **bioethics, medical ethics**, and **professional medical ethics** that the relationships between and among clearly stated concepts are identified, so that the appeal to **ethical principles** and **virtues** shows how *together* these components of ethical reasoning support implications that are the conclusions of ethical reasoning. Simply listing ethical considerations followed by a conclusion is not acceptable. *See also* CLARITY; CLINICAL ADEQUACY; CLINICAL APPLICABILITY; CONSISTENCY.

COMMODIFICATION. The reduction of the value of a living being or body part to its commercial value. This reductionism is considered **ethically impermissible** by those in **bioethics** who emphasize the importance of **dignity** and the **intrinsic worth** of each individual and by **moral theologies** that emphasize the **sanctity of life**. These lines of **ethical reasoning** are often deployed in arguments against the sale of human organs for **transplantation.** *See also* DEHUMANIZATION; PERSONALISM; RESPECT FOR PERSONS.

COMMON LAW. The law written by judges, especially in opinions issued by **appellate courts** in the states and by the federal government in the United States. The intellectual authority of court opinions is a function of the quality of their arguments, which should be based in the facts of the case being decided and the interpretation of relevant precedents, statutes, and state constitution (in state court cases) and the United States Constitution (in federal court cases). The common law has had strong influence on the development of **bioethics** and **medical ethics**, for example, **decision making** about **abortion** and **end-of-life care**. *See also* ADMINISTRATIVE LAW; REGULATORY LAW; STATUTORY LAW.

COMMON RULE. Regulatory law providing requirements for **Institutional Review Boards** and investigators to implement in **human subjects research**. The Common Rule is Part A of the federal regulations. *See also* 45 CFR 46; ETHICS OF HUMAN SUBJECTS RESEARCH; RESEARCH.

COMMUNITARIAN ETHICS. Ethical reasoning that replaces an emphasis on **rights** of individuals with an emphasis on the **ethical obligations** of individuals to their community. This is meant to provide an antidote to **individualism** in ethical reasoning. *See also* ALTRUISM; AUTONOMY; ETHICAL PRINCIPLE OF JUSTICE; ETHICS OF CARE; SOLIDARITY.

COMPASSION. The **virtue** that creates an **ethical obligation** to recognize when another human being is in **pain**, **distress**, or **suffering** and attempt to relieve it. This virtue also creates an ethical obligation to prevent pain, distress, and suffering in other human beings. *See also* PROFESSIONAL VIRTUE OF COMPASSION; VIRTUE ETHICS.

COMPELLING STATE'S INTEREST. A concept used in the common law that sets out a stringent test for justified limitations on constitutional **rights**. The scope of the concept is not clear in the **common law** but includes the state's obligation to protect the constitutional rights of persons (a living individual who is *ex utero* and under the jurisdiction of the U.S. Constitution) to life, liberty, and property.

This concept played a key role in the landmark decisions about **abortion** of the U.S. Supreme Court in abortion cases in 1973 (*Roe v. Wade* [410 U.S. 113] and *Doe v. Bolton* [410 U.S. 179]). The Court reached the **judgment** that the pregnant woman has a **privacy**-based right, rooted in the Bill of Rights and Due Process clauses, to make decisions with her physician about the disposition of her pregnancy. Because the fetus is not a legal person it does not have constitutional rights, including the **right to life**. The state, therefore, does not have a compelling interest in limiting the **decision making** of pregnant women and their physicians, and the implementation of those decisions, before **viability** based on an alleged **compelling state's interest** in protecting the life of the previable fetus. This does not mean that the state has no interest at all in the life of the fetus; the state does. However, this interest is not a compelling interest. *See also* PLANNED PARENTHOOD CASE.

COMPETENCE. The ability to complete a specific task at a specific time. There are two components of this ability: decisional autonomy and **executive autonomy**. *Competence* is therefore not a synonym for *decision-making capacity* but is sometimes used this way. For example, in the clinical setting the term *competence* is often used interchangeably with the term *decision-making capacity*. Some take the view that *competence* should be used only in the legal context, in other words, court proceedings to determine **legal incompetence**, meaning the loss of **decision-making capacity** or the loss of **executive capacity** to a degree that the individual should lose his or her right to control his or her own affairs.

Competence is task-specific, for example, the ability to manage one's own financial affairs without substantially damaging one's financial interests or the ability to make healthcare decisions without substantially putting one's health at risk serious, far-reaching, and irreversible loss or putting one's life at risk. The cognitive and affective demands of competence are a function of the complexity of the task. Simple decisions such as consenting to a needle stick are low demand while complex decisions such as consenting to heart catheterization to unblock coronary arteries are high demand. A **patient** may be competent to provide **simple consent** to a needle stick but not engage in the **informed consent process** for heart catheterization. Competence is also time-specific; it can wax or wane over time. In both **health law** and **medical ethics**, the assessment of competence should be guided by the **presumption of decision-making capacity**, which means that the **burden of justification** is on a court of law or physician to make a reliable **judgment** that a patient is **incompetent**. *See also* AUTONOMY.

COMPETENT. The state of having the ability to perform a specific task at a specific time. *See also* AUTONOMY; DECISION-MAKING CAPACITY; EXECUTIVE AUTONOMY.

COMPLEMENTARITY. A concept in **metaethics** that no one way of **ethical reasoning** is adequate to address the full range of topics in **ethics**, including **bioethics, medical ethics**, and **professional medical ethics**. Each way of ethical reasoning fails to address some issues that are adequately addressed by other ways of ethical reasoning. The diverse ways of reasoning complement or complete each other; hence the use of the term *complementarity*. When two or more ways of ethical reasoning are combined, comprehensiveness is achieved. For example, some take the view that **principlism** is inadequate and should be complemented with **virtues**.

CONCEPT OF HEALTH. *See* HEALTH, CONCEPT OF.

CONDESCENSION. Used today with a negative meaning, to refer to an attitude of feigned superiority to others that, on closer examination, is **biased**. This word was used very differently by **Thomas Percival** (1740–1804) in his *Medical Ethics* to identify one of the **virtues** of physicians. The physician, when caring for **patients** of lower social classes, should put aside class differences and not be biased by them. To achieve this, the physician should come down from his lofty social station and recognize the humanity of the patient. This was a crucial virtue for physicians to cultivate at the **Royal Infirmary** of Manchester, a hospital for the sick poor. Physicians then came from the middle class socioeconomically. The moral exemplar for this virtue is Jesus Christ: God condescended to become man in the form of his only begotten Son, Jesus. Percival was very familiar with this Christian theological concept. The other virtues that form the basis of Percival's **professional medical ethics** are **tenderness, steadiness**, and **authority**. *See also* VIRTUE ETHICS.

CONDITION. A general term used to describe the patient's state of health that meets two criteria: the patient does not have currently a **disease, disability, disorder**, or **injury** and that state of health intrinsically creates a risk of disease, disability, disorder, or injury. The term *condition* should therefore be understood to be **biopsychosocial** in its dimensions. These risks are significant in **beneficence**-based clinical judgment, supporting an **ethical obligation** to prevent and manage such risks. For example, pregnancy is a condition that is not a disease but that also intrinsically creates risks of mortality and morbidity for pregnant, fetal, and neonatal **patients**.

CONDRONCHUS, GIOVANNI (1547–1628). Italian physician and ethicist. He wrote *De Christiana ac Tuta Medendi Ratione* (*Christian and Careful Method of Medicine*, 1591), based on **virtues**; the most fundamental virtue is **justice**. He mainly focuses on what physicians should not do, for example, perform **abortions** (as one would expect of **medical ethics** based on **Christian moral theology**) or use poison. He also calls for physicians to care for the sick poor without charge, reflecting one of the "corporal works of mercy" in **Roman Catholic moral theology**.

CONFIDENTIALITY. The physician's **ethical obligation** to prevent unauthorized access to information about the **patient**'s condition, diagnosis, treatment plans and their outcomes, and prognosis with and without treatment. All healthcare professionals involved in the patient's care, as well as **clinical ethics consultants** who may not be healthcare professionals, are bound by confidentiality. Healthcare professionals not involved in a patient's care, who access information about such a patient, violate confidentiality and are subject to sanction by the healthcare organization. The ethical obligation of confidentiality originates in **professional medical ethics** and therefore independently of the **patient's rights**, in particular the patient's right to privacy. The terms *confidentiality*, on the one hand, and *privacy* and the *right to privacy*, on the other, are therefore not synonymous and therefore should not be used interchangeably.

CONFLICT OF COMMITMENT. Conflicts of commitment occur when an individual simultaneously occupies two social roles and **ethical obligations** generated by each role are mutually exclusive: to fulfill one of the two obligations requires one to violate the other. For physicians who are parents, there can be conflicts of commitment: fulfilling ethical obligations to a **patient** whose urgent care requires more time than anticipated may result in violating a promise to the physician's child to attend his or her athletic event. For physicians who are in the military, fulfilling the ethical obligation to use scarce resources according to **triage** may risk violating ethical obligations to patients. As a general rule, conflicts of commitment should be responsibly managed by giving priority to the physician's professional responsibilities to patients or **research subjects**. This means that the **burden of justification** is on giving priority to ethical obligations originating in the competing social role.

Conflicts of commitment are often conflated with **conflicts of interest**, which is a conceptual error. A conflict of interest exists when a **role-related ethical obligation** is not compatible with one or more **self-interests**.

CONFLICT OF INTEREST. A conflict of **interest** occurs when fulfilling a physician's **ethical obligations** to a **patient** are not compatible with **self-interest**. Some define conflict of interest as a conflict between the physician's interest in **patient care** or **research** and the interests of the physician in other matters. This is an error, because the moral relationship between a physician and patient is primarily professional, structured by ethical obligations, and not primarily contractual, structured by interests and **rights**.

For physicians, conflicts of interest are problematic because, if poorly managed, they cause bias to affect **clinical judgment**, which can result in clinical management that is not evidence-based. This problem was recognized as early as the 1770s by **John Gregory** (1724–1773), who was concerned that "men of interest" (i.e., men motivated primary by self-interest) engaged in biased clinical judgment that resulted in clinical management that was harmful to patients (Gregory 1772). He was also concerned that young physicians, ambitious to build their practices, would prematurely declare a patient's condition incurable to justify performing **experiments**, not to advance science but to advance their own reputations as leading physicians. Both are inconsistent with the **professional virtue of integrity**.

As a very strong general rule, therefore, conflicts of interest should be professionally managed by giving priority to fulfilling ethical obligations to patients or **research subjects**. This means that the **burden of justification** is on giving priority to fulfilling self-interest. This helps to explain why the **professional virtue of self-sacrifice** is an essential component of **professional medical ethics**. *See also* CONFLICT OF COMMITMENT; "STARK LAW".

CONFUCIUS (551–479 BCE). Chinese philosopher and sage. Confucius based his moral philosophy on the concept of *ren*, or humanity, and **filial piety**, the obedience to the decisions of one's parents. Confucian **medical ethics** is based on medicine as "the art of *ren*," emphasizing the physician's **virtues**. Confucian medical ethics was adopted by the Chinese government in 134 BCE (Fan 2009; Nie 2009).

CONSCIENCE. A fundamental set of beliefs and convictions about **values** that should define who an individual is and therefore support a life characterized by the **virtue** of **integrity**. Acting in ways inconsistent with the **ethical obligations** generated by these fundamental beliefs and convictions is not compatible with integrity and is therefore **ethically impermissible** for an individual. In **professional medical ethics**, a distinction is made between **individual conscience** and **professional conscience**. The **ethical justification** of **conscientious objection** appeals to conscience.

CONSCIENTIOUS OBJECTION. Refusal to fulfill an **ethical obligation,** usually a **role-related obligation,** based on **ethical reasoning** that doing so would violate **individual conscience** or **professional conscience.** *See also* CIVIL DISOBEDIENCE; INTEGRITY; PROFESSIONAL VIRTUE OF INTEGRITY.

CONSENSUS. An appeal to agreement on a **judgment** about whether an attitude, character trait, or behavior is **ethically justified** (Moreno 1995). The strength of such agreement varies, from 51 percent (the low end) to 100 percent (the high end). Strong consensus is usually set in the range of 67 percent (two-thirds) to 75 percent (three-quarters).

Studies in **empirical bioethics** and **empirical medical ethics** provide an important point of departure for subsequent **ethical reasoning.** Such studies can also challenge the results of ethical reasoning. For example, some have held that **physician-assisted suicide** (in the meaning of prescribing a life-taking medication to a patient who is capable of informed and **voluntary** decision making who then self-administers the medication) is incompatible with the **professional virtue of integrity** and is therefore **ethically imper-missible.** Empirical studies of physicians' attitudes have found consensus and even strong consensus support for this practice. These results can be interpreted in one of two ways: (1) these physicians are misguided; or (2) these physicians do not believe that physician-assisted suicide is incompat-ible with professional integrity. The second interpretation should prompt critical appraisal of the view that physician-assisted suicide is incompatible with professional integrity.

CONSENT. The authorization of the **patient** for a physician or other health-care professional to provide **clinical management** that has been offered or recommended to the patient. Consent can be either **simple consent** or **in-formed consent.** *See also* AUTONOMY; ETHICAL PRINCIPLE OF RE-SPECT FOR AUTONOMY; INFORMED CONSENT PROCESS; IN-FORMED REFUSAL.

CONSEQUENTIALIST ETHICS. Also known as consequentialism. **Ethi-cal reasoning** based the consequences of decisions and the behavior they support. The **ethical principle of beneficence,** the **ethical principle of jus-tice** (in some of its interpretations), and the **ethical principle of nonmalefi-cence** are consequentialist **ethical principles** in **bioethics, medical ethics,** and **professional medical ethics.** The principal form of consequentialist eth-ics is **utilitarianism.** *See also* DEONTOLOGICAL ETHICS.

CONSISTENCY. A requirement of **ethical reasoning** in **bioethics, medical ethics,** and **professional medical ethics** that a clearly stated concept be used with that meaning and no other. If the concept is a **cluster concept, clarity** requires that invoked components are the only ones used in ethical reasoning. Failure to meet this requirement by changing the meaning of terms in the course of ethical reasoning results in what is known as equivocation of terms, which disables ethical reasoning, rendering all results of no value. *See also* CLARITY; CLINICAL ADEQUACY; CLINICAL APPLICABILITY; CO-HERENCE.

CONSTITUTIONAL LAW. The provisions of the U.S. Constitution and state constitutions, as well as **common law** of courts that interpret the provisions of the applicable constitution. In the United States, state courts interpret state constitutions while federal courts interpret the federal constitution. In the United States, when there is conflict between state constitutional law and federal constitutional law, the latter always prevails. *See also* ADMINISTRATIVE LAW; REGULATORY LAW; STATUTORY LAW.

CONSULTATION. The process by which the patient's physician seeks the evaluation of the **patient** and proposals for **clinical management** from specialists. The ethics of consultation dates back to at least the **professional medical ethics** of **John Gregory** (1724–1773) and **Thomas Percival** (1740–1804). In the 18th century, the boundaries between physick (internal medicine) and surgery were disputed, to the detriment of the health and even life of patients. They called for an **ethics of cooperation** between physicians and surgeons, a radical idea in its time. In the ensuing centuries, the ethics of cooperation became the basis of the ethics of consultation.

The primary concern and focus of consultation should be on reaching a reliable diagnosis, an evidence-based treatment plan, and an evidence-based, unbiased division of labor in implementing the treatment plan based on an unbiased **judgment** about whose expertise is needed for each component of the treatment plan. The patient's attending physician, now usually a hospitalist for hospitalized patient, has the professional responsibility to coordinate the contributions of the consultants and to see to it that the patient authorizes the treatment plan on the basis of the **informed consent process**. *See also* BOUNDARY ISSUES.

CONTRACEPTION. The use of medication, both short-acting devices ("birth-control pill," spermicide, condom) and long-acting devices (implantable tubes that secrete medication over time, intrauterine device), or surgery (**sterilization**) to prevent pregnancy. Some agents work by creating a biologically hostile environment for sperm in the female reproductive tract, preventing ovulation, or preventing initiation of pregnancy (implantation of the embryo in the uterine wall). Surgery alters or removes female reproductive anatomy or alters male reproductive anatomy.

Contraception is understood in **professional medical ethics** to be a **medically reasonable alternative**, except when medically contraindicated. It therefore should be offered to both female and male patients as part of the **clinical management** of the **condition** of fertility when a **patient** expresses an interest in preventing pregnancy. Some, including the Roman Catholic Church, judge contraception to be **ethically impermissible** on the grounds of **moral theology** that it wrongfully separates sexual intercourse from procreation in violation of the natural purpose of sexual intercourse and therefore **natural law**. Because this **ethical reasoning** is not secular, it does not apply in professional medical ethics. *See also* PROCREATIVE LIBERTY.

CONTRACTUAL RELATIONSHIP. An exchange of goods and services between a buyer and seller, based on the pursuit of each party's **interests**, especially **self-interest**. Neither buyer nor seller has any **ethical obligation** to protect and promote the interests of the other party. Buyers, especially, need to be vigilant in protecting their self-interests in contractual exchanges, a point precisely expressed in the Latin phase *Caveat emptor*, or "Let the buyer beware." To protect themselves in what is a potentially predatory relationship with sellers, buyers assert their **rights**. Sellers then do the same. These rights are then expressed in the contract for goods or services. The resulting relationship is therefore one of distrustful, wary, strangers.

The contractual relationship differs sharply from a defining feature of a **professional relationship**: the professional has a **prima facie ethical obligation** to protect and promote the interests of the individual in a relationship with the professional for the provision of goods and services. As a result, the physician is trustworthy, and the **patient** need not be wary. The fundamental relationship between physician and patient in **professional medical ethics** is therefore not one of rights but of the physician's ethical obligation to protect the patient's life and health, creating a protected status for the patient independent of appeals to the patient's rights.

From the ancient world to the 18th century, in Western countries the relationship between a physician and a sick individual was contractual, which gave the sick individual power over the physician. The word used in the Latin literature is *aegrotus* or the "sick one." This was not a professional relationship governed by professional medical ethics. Instead, the ethical model of the relationship was based on the concept of *medicus politicus* or the "politic physician" who acted on the basis of the **virtue** of **prudence**. *See also* CASTRO, RODRIGO DE (1550–1627); ETHICAL CONCEPT OF MEDICINE AS A PROFESSION; HOFFMANN, FRIEDRICH (1660–1738).

CONTROLLED CLINICAL EXPERIMENT. An **experiment** is designed to test a hypothesis and should be conducted in a meticulous manner that fulfills the requirements for scientific excellence. This concept was introduced into the philosophy of science as early as the 16th century in the work of **Francis Bacon** (1561–1626). In contemporary biomedical science, achieving scientific excellence requires a **research** protocol that describes the significance and nature of the experiment, the hypothesis to be tested, the method by which the hypothesis will be tested, and the results evaluated. Controlled clinical experiments include at least two groups: a group of **animal research subjects** or **human research subjects** who receive either no intervention or an accepted intervention; and a group of animal or human research subjects who receive a new intervention. Alternatively, each group receives an accepted form of treatment, with the goal of identifying clinical superiority. The hypothesis states the expected difference or lack of difference between the two groups. When subjects are assigned randomly to the groups, the experiment is known as a **randomized controlled clinical trial**. When investigators do not know which treatment a subject has received, the clinical trial is known as a **blinded clinical trial**. *See also* CLINICAL TRIAL.

CONTROLLED CLINICAL TRIAL. A **clinical trial** with a control group and an intervention group of animal **research subjects** or **human research subjects**, to test hypotheses about improved **clinical management** of a **condition, disability, disorder**, or **disease**. *See also* CONTROLLED CLINICAL EXPERIMENT; HUMAN SUBJECTS RESEARCH; RESEARCH.

CONTROLLED DONATION AFTER CIRCULATORY DETERMINATION OF DEATH. *See* DONATION AFTER CARDIAC DEATH.

CONVENTION ON THE RIGHTS OF THE CHILD. Adopted by the General Assembly of the United Nations in 1989 and took force in 1990. Extends the **Universal Declaration of Human Rights** to children, especially in the context of the family and in response to the special needs of children for protection. *See also* CHILD; RIGHT.

COOPERATION, ETHICS OF. Disciplined study of the morality of cooperation, an essential component of modern team care of patients. *See* ETHICS OF COOPERATION.

COPPENS, FATHER CHARLES, SJ (1835–1920). American Jesuit priest of the Roman Catholic Church. He who wrote a **Roman Catholic moral theology** of medicine, titled *Moral Principles and Medical Practice: The Basis of Medical Jurisprudence* (1897). *See also* MEDICAL ETHICS; MEDICAL JURISPRUDENCE.

COSMESIS. The provision of clinical care, usually medication or surgery, in the absence of pathology that is therefore not a **medically reasonable alternative** but is acceptably safe, in response to a **patient**'s request. The **ethical justification** for cosmesis includes the following points: the patient's request should be informed, including information that the use of medication or surgery for the purpose desired by the patient is not medically reasonable; the medication or surgery should be expected to be physiologically or anatomically effective in fulfilling the goal of the patient's request, for example, remaining calm during a major presentation (which can be supported by the use of anti-hypertension medication) or improving the patient's facial appearance; and the risks of the medication or surgical procedure should be manageable to a minimum consistent with patient safety. *See also* ETHICAL PRINCIPLE OF RESPECT FOR AUTONOMY; PATIENTS' REQUESTS.

COSMETIC GENOMICS. The theoretical use of **gene editing** and other techniques in the attempt to produce desired traits. This is considered an **ethical controversy**. *See also* COSMESIS; ENHANCEMENT.

COSMETIC PHARMACOLOGY. The prescription of medication in **cosmesis**, usually to improve performance of specific tasks, for example, prescribing one dose of a beta blocker to help calm a **patient** who is not accustomed to public speaking and who must make a major presentation. *See also* COSMETIC GENOMICS; COSMETIC SURGERY.

COSMETIC SURGERY. The use of surgery in **cosmesis**. *See* COSMESIS.

COURAGE. A **virtue** that has an intellectual and physical component. Intellectual courage is the capacity to distinguish between what one ought not to fear and what one ought to fear. Intellectual courage requires one to ignore what one ought not to fear, so that it does not **bias** decision making, **judgment**, and behavior based on them. Physical courage is the capacity not to let what one ought to fear take mastery of one's **decision making**, judgment, and behavior based on them. Courage does not require that one develop or act upon reckless disregard for one's **legitimate self-interest**.

COURT-ORDERED CESAREAN DELIVERY. The order of a judge in a civil proceeding that a pregnant woman have her baby delivered by cesarean section, after she has refused the recommendation of her physician for cesarean delivery. This is a form of **coerced cesarean delivery**.

In most of the **bioethics** and **medical ethics** literature, especially work by legal scholars, court-ordered cesarean delivery is considered to be **ethically impermissible**. A counterview is that a pregnant woman has a **beneficence-**based **ethical obligation** to accept reasonable risk to herself to benefit the **fetal patient** and **neonatal patient**. This applies to conditions such as well-documented, intrapartum complete placenta previa, for which there are no reported cases of spontaneous reversion, and for which cesarean delivery eliminates the risk of **mortality** to the fetal patient and reduces the risk of morality to the pregnant woman to that of cesarean delivery. This risk is **judged** acceptable in **deliberative clinical judgment** (Chervenak and McCullough 2014). *See also* FORCED CESAREAN DELIVERY.

COVENANT RELATIONSHIP. Modeled on the relationship of God to the Israelites and His promise to protect them: a relationship of the physician to the **patient** based on a promise to protect and promote the health **interests** of the patient. The second commitment of the physician in the **ethical concept of medicine as a profession** can be interpreted as creating a covenant relationship.

COWART, DAX. *See* DAX COWART CASE.

CPR. *See* CARDIOPULMONARY RESUSCITATION (CPR). *See also* DO-NOT-ATTEMPT RESUSCITATION ORDER (DNAR ORDER); DO-NOT-RESUSCITATE ORDER (DNR ORDER); LIFE-SUSTAINING TREATMENT; OUT-OF-HOSPITAL DO-NOT-RESUSCITATE ORDER.

CREPE HANGING. A form of **deception** (creating a false impression) in which a physician is confidant that a procedure will go well for the **patient** but exaggerates the risks of the procedure with two goals in mind: (1) protecting the physician from the patient's disappointment when unexpected adverse outcomes occur; and (2) attempting to make the patient very grateful when things go well, as the physician expects them to do. Because it leads the patient to have a false belief and because it is motivated primarily by **self-interest**, crepe hanging is **ethically impermissible** in the **informed consent process**. In his **professional medical ethics**, physician-ethicist **Thomas Percival** (1740–1804) argued that engaging in "gloomy prognostications" (his phrase for crepe hanging) are ethically impermissible (Percival 1804, Chapter III, Section III). Crepe hanging has been characterized as "corrupt" in the **surgical ethics** literature (Jones, McCullough, and Richman 2007).

CRITICAL APPRAISAL. A tool for routinely achieving **deliberative clinical judgment** about **clinical management**. Critical appraisal starts with a focused question and then turns to a literature review to identify answers to the focused question and the level of evidence that supports the answers. The physician should then answer the focused question by appealing to the best available evidence. The physician should then ask how this answer will help him or her in **clinical practice**. The physician should periodically revisit the focused question, as it arises in other clinical cases. **Argument-based ethics** is modeled on critical appraisal. *See also* EVIDENCE-BASED MEDICINE.

CRITICAL CARE. The provision of medically, surgically, and technologically advanced intervention for patients at high risk of death. Critical care of adult **patients** is known as **adult critical care** and provided in critical care units or in intensive care units. Critical care of infants is known as **neonatal critical care** and provided in neonatal intensive care units. Critical care of other children under the age of 18 is known as pediatric critical care and provided in pediatric intensive care units. Critical care is sometimes further subdivided into cardiovascular intensive care, medical intensive care, neurologic intensive care, and surgical intensive care.

Critical care is provided with the short-term goal of preventing imminent death and the long-term goal of survival with an acceptable outcome. An acceptable outcome can be understood in two ways. The first is a clinical, **beneficence**-based perspective that values survival with at least some interactive capacity. Mere survival (i.e., survival without interactive capacity) is not **ethically justified** as a clinical goal in **professional medical ethics** because ethics are *not* based on **vitalism**. The second is a **patient**-oriented, **autonomy**-based perspective that values survival with a **quality of life** acceptable to the patient.

The **ethical obligation** to provide critical care is a **prima facie ethical obligation**. Justified limits on critical care exist when the short-term goal and therefore the long-term goal of critical care are not expected to be achieved. The **ethical justification** for such limits may appeal to a patient's **advance directive, anatomic futility, imminent demise futility, physiologic futility, qualitative futility, quantitative futility**, or **quality-of-life futility**. Ethically justified limits on critical care also exist when the first goal is expected to be achieved but the second is not, either from a clinical perspective or the patient's perspective. The ethical justification for limits from the patient's perspective may appeal to a patient's advance directive or quality-of-life futility. *See also* LIFE-SUSTAINING TREATMENT; OPPORTUNITY COST.

CRUZAN CASE. Ms. Nancy Beth Cruzan was diagnosed in 1983, after a severe head injury in an automobile accident, to be in a **permanent vegetative state**. In 1988, her parents asked that artificial nutrition and hydration, both forms of **life-sustaining treatment**, be discontinued based on the **substituted judgment standard** of **surrogate decision making**. The parents' argument was based on comments made by Ms. Cruzan to a friend that she would not want to be kept alive in such a condition. **Advance directive** law in the state of Missouri requires that the evidence for the wishes of an incompetent patient with an **irreversible condition** be based on "clear and convincing" evidence (a 75 percent probability of being correct), a higher standard than used in most states (more likely to be true than not). The physicians refused, and the case was litigated to the U.S. Supreme Court. In its 1990 decision (*Cruzan v. Director, Missouri Department of Health* 497 U.S. 261), the Court found that the **right to refuse treatment** is based in the Due Process clauses. The Court then ruled that (a) the clear and convincing evidence standard was constitutionally permissible and that (b) the U.S. Constitution does not require this standard. The result was to leave the matter of level of evidence for implementation of the substituted judgment standard to the states.

Associate Justice Antonin Scalia (1936–2016; term on Court 1986–2016) wrote a separate opinion in which he argued that withholding nutrition and hydration at the patient's request was a form of **suicide**. In doing so, he departed from **statutory law** on advance directives that state explicitly that discontinuing artificial hydration and nutrition and hydration, as well as other forms of life-sustaining treatment, from patients with a **terminal condition** or an irreversible condition, under the provisions of the statute, is not homicide or suicide. *See* END-OF-LIFE CARE.

CVICU. Cardiovascular critical care unit. *See* CRITICAL CARE.

D

DATA AND SAFETY MONITORING BOARD (DSMB). A committee of physicians, scientists, methodologists (experts in clinical trial design and execution), statistician(s), and ethicist(s) charged with independent prospective oversight of a **clinical trial**. For federally funded **clinical research**, the DSMB reports to the director of the National Institutes of Health that has funded the trial. The DSMB periodically evaluates the progress of the trial, trends in data, adverse events, and ethical issues and makes recommendations to the institute's director about continuation of the trial. For industry-funded trials and organizationally funded trials, the DSMB may report to organizational leadership. *See also* RESEARCH.

DATA AND SAFETY MONITORING COMMITTEE. *See* DATA AND SAFETY MONITORING BOARD (DSMB).

DAX COWART CASE. In 1973, Mr. Donald (a name he later changed to Dax) Cowart suffered severe, extensive, and life-threatening burns when a leaking propane gas transmission line exploded in Texas. He refused treatment from the beginning and consistently thereafter. At one point during his hospitalization, he undertook what his physicians **judged** to be a **suicide** attempt, which called into question the **presumption of decision-making capacity**. He was seen by a psychiatrist, possibly at the request of his mother, his next of kin, in whose **deliberative clinical judgment** Mr. Cowart had **decision-making capacity**. He subsequently authorized medical and surgical **clinical management** and was discharged from the hospital.

This case became public, with Mr. Cowart's permission, and was taken to be a **paradigm case** of **medical paternalism**. This judgment makes sense only if Mr. Cowart's physicians considered him to have decision-making capacity when they continued to treat him over his repeated objections. At that time, given the severity of his burns and his suicide attempt, it is doubtful that they did so. If that indeed was the case, then the Dax Cowart Case was not a paradigm case of medical paternalism, because his diminished **autonomy** meant that one of the two criteria for medical paternalism was not satisfied. It is important to keep in mind that this case occurred before **statutory laws** about medical decision-making were enacted, much less **Natural Death Acts** and **Advance Directives Acts**. In addition, the subspecialty of psychiatry known as consultation-liaison psychiatry, which was developed in hospitals to provide rapid evaluation of a patient's decision-making capacity, justifiably calls the presumption of decision-making capacity into question when evaluating patients expressing suicidal ideations or attempting suicide while hospitalized. There are not well understood clinical and ethical **norms** that would guide responses to a case like the Dax Cowart Case. *See also* END-OF-LIFE CARE; RIGHT; RIGHT TO REFUSE TREATMENT.

DEAD DONOR RULE. A rule based on the concept that **organ procurement** intended to occur after **death** has occurred not **kill** the human being from whose cadaver the organ is being taken; that human being must already be dead. This is known as the dead donor rule. This rule underscored the importance of following accepted clinical criteria for the **determination of death**, either by cardiopulmonary criteria or brain function criteria. **Donation after cardiac death** can challenge the dead donor rule because the time chosen before cardiopulmonary arrest is **judged** to be irreversible may be too short. Some have proposed abandoning the dead donor rule for procuring organs from a **patient** who is still alive by these two sets of criteria but for whom awareness has been irreversibly lost. There is **ethical controversy** about this proposal.

DEATH. The irreversible absence of **life**. Inasmuch as the concept of life is a **cluster concept**, the concept of death is also a cluster concept. There is philosophical controversy about which components of the concept of life must no longer be applicable for the concept of death to apply. *See also* DETERMINATION OF DEATH.

DEATH AND DYING. *See ARS MORIENDI*; DEATH; DYING; END-OF-LIFE CARE.

DECEPTION. Misleading the **patient** by creating a false impression with the goal of creating a false belief in the patient. A false impression can be created in one of two ways. Both are **ethically impermissible** in the **informed consent process**. First, the physician **lies** to the patient (i.e., represents as true what the physician knows to be false). Second, the physician provides information that is truthful but incomplete, framed in such a way that the patient draws a logical conclusion from the information that is inaccurate. Deception in this second meaning is not equivalent to lying. Nonetheless, this is colloquially called lying or lying by telling less than the whole truth. For example, in the Tuskegee Syphilis Experiment, potential subjects were told that they had "bad blood." This phrase had a wide range of meanings, which include benign conditions but also diagnoses such as syphilis, which was untreatable at that time. The goal was to have potential subjects think that their condition was benign, thus creating a false belief (Jones 2003 [1993]). *See also* CREPE HANGING; TRUTH-TELLING.

DECISION. A cognitive, evaluative, and affective process in which four steps can be distinguished from each other: setting a goal; compiling the options for producing that goal; ranking the options in the order of preference based on the individual's values and beliefs; and selecting the highest ranked alternative. In everyday life and in the clinical setting, **decision making** is more dynamic and recursive than simply done in discrete steps. For **patients**, the goal is effective management of the patient's condition, with the options for pursuing this goal being the medically reasonable alternatives for managing the patient's condition. The patient evaluates these alternatives based on his or her values and beliefs and selects the highest-ranked alternative (Braun et al. 2009). The affective dimensions of a decision have been overlooked, a shortcoming that **behavioral psychology** has begun to correct. *See also* DECISIONAL AUTONOMY; DECISION-MAKING CAPACITY.

DECISION AID. A structured approach to the **informed consent process** that provides the **patient** with information from **evidence-based medicine** with the goal of responsibly managing the variation in the informed consent process, thus improving its **quality** and enhancing the patient's exercise of his or her **autonomy**. Recent research has focused on incorporating the insights of **behavioral psychology** about the role of **bias**, including subtle bias that may be undetected by the patient in even a well-informed consent process. There is **ethical controversy** about how to reduce the influence of these biases without engaging in **manipulation** of the patient's thought processes and **judgment**. *See also* DECISION MAKING; ETHICAL PRINCIPLE OF RESPECT FOR AUTONOMY; NUDGE.

DECISION MAKING. The cognitive, evaluative, and affective process of identifying options for current and future behavior, evaluating these alternatives, selecting one for implementation, and implementing the selected option. The first three components are accomplished by exercising **decision-making capacity**, decisional capacity, or decisional autonomy, and the fourth component is accomplished by exercising **executive capacity** or decisional autonomy. The affective dimensions of decision making have been overlooked, a shortcoming that **behavioral psychology** has begun to correct. *See also* DECISION; ETHICAL PRINCIPLE OF RESPECT FOR AUTONOMY.

DECISION-MAKING CAPACITY. The ability of a patient to adequately meet the criteria for making **decisions** to authorize or refuse to authorize **clinical management** in the **informed consent process**, also known as decisional autonomy or decisional capacity. In shorthand, some patients are referred to as "decisional," meaning that they have decision-making capacity.

The criteria for decision-making capacity include paying attention to information that is provided to the patient about the patient's **condition, disability, disease, disorder,** or **injury** and the **medically reasonable alternatives** for clinical management; retaining and recalling pertinent clinical information (memory functions, which can be formally assessed using accepted clinical tools such as the mini mental state examination); reasoning from present events (treatment) to their likely outcomes (which is called cognitive understanding and has an affective component); believing that these outcomes could happen to oneself (which is called appreciation); evaluating those outcomes (i.e., determining whether one should want or reject them based on one's values and beliefs, which is called evaluative understanding and has an effective component); and expressing authorization or refusal of authorization of clinical management that has been offered or recommended. These components of decision-making capacity are iterative: any deficit in a component will be compounded by deficits in subsequent components. Decision-making capacity is task-specific, with simple decisions creating lower cognitive and affective demands than complex decision. Decision-making capacity is time dependent: it can wax or wane and therefore should be assessed when it is waxing.

The assessment of decision-making capacity is a matter of **deliberative clinical judgment** guided by the **presumption of decision-making capacity,** which puts the **burden of justification** on the physician to conclude that the patient lacks decision-making capacity. The goal of assessment is to determine whether the patient does not meet a threshold for each of the components. This threshold is set low to respect the patient's **autonomy** and to prevent arbitrary removal of the patient's authority over himself or herself. Concerns about a patient's decision-making capacity should be triggered by clinical signs and symptoms of impaired components. Refusal of offered or recommended clinical management is not evidence of loss of decision-making capacity. If the consequences of implementing such a refusal include serious, far-reaching, and irreversible clinical harm to the patient, assessing decision-making capacity is **ethically permissible**. Any physician can assess a patient's decision-making capacity, although psychiatrists who serve as consultation-liaison psychiatrists may have more experience in assessing decision-making capacity.

When a patient has been determined in deliberative clinical judgment to lack decision-making capacity, decisions for the patient should be made by a **surrogate**. When the patient retains some measure of the component of evaluative understanding, decisions should be made by the surrogate with the patient. In geriatric medicine, this is known as **geriatric assent**. *See also* ETHICAL PRINCIPLE OF RESPECT FOR AUTONOMY.

"DECISIONAL". A neologism that describes a patient who has intact **decision-making capacity**.

DECISIONAL AUTONOMY. *See* DECISION-MAKING CAPACITY.

DECISIONAL CAPACITY. *See* DECISION-MAKING CAPACITY.

DECISIONAL RIGHT. The **right** of an adult **patient** or (where permitted by law) mature minor to participate in the **informed consent process**. This is a **prima facie positive right** to information that should be provided in the informed consent process. This is also a **prima facie negative right** to non-interference with the patient's **decision-making process**, to ensure that this process is **voluntary**. *See also* ETHICAL PRINCIPLE OF RESPECT FOR AUTONOMY.

DECLARATION OF GENEVA. An **oath** for physicians created by the **World Medical Association** originally in 1948 with the most recent revision appearing in 2006 (https://www.wma.net/policies-post/wma-declaration-of-geneva/, accessed 14 September 2017). The oath comprises a set of commitments that a physician should make "at the time of being admitted as a member of the medical profession." These include protecting the life and health of **patients**; **clinical care** free of **bias** based on race, sex, and other human traits; and **confidentiality**. The oath is based upon the oath-taker's "honor."

DECLARATION OF HELSINKI. A statement on the **ethics of human subjects research** from the **World Medical Association**. The statement, first issued in 1975, has been revised seven times, with the most current version dating from 2013 (World Medical Association 2013). The statement enumerates "ethical principles for medical research involving human subjects." The statement appeals to the primary **professional responsibility** of physicians to "protect and safeguard the health, well-being, and rights of patients" and requires, among a comprehensive set of provisions, the informed and **voluntary** consent of research subjects, and oversight of research. This statement is widely used by **Institutional Review Boards** and **Research Ethics Committees** in many countries to guide and evaluate the prospective oversight of **human subjects research**. *See also* RESEARCH ETHICS.

DECORUM. The comportment of a physician with **patients** and other physicians and healthcare. This can be addressed based on **self-interest**, as appears to be the approach in *On Decorum* in the **Hippocratic Corpus**. This can also be addressed based on the principle of **respect for persons**, for example, not addressing a patient, especially patients of color, by his or her first name without permission. (In the era of legal segregation in the United States, the use of first names with people of color without their permission was a tool of oppression and disrespect.) This can also be addressed based on the **ethical principle of beneficence**, for example, in **John Gregory**'s (1724–1773) admonition to avoid forms of dress that can terrify children, still a rule for behavior in **pediatric ethics**. *See also* ETIQUETTE; MEDICAL ETIQUETTE.

DEHUMANIZATION. Treating a **patient** or **research subject** as an object or thing. Based on the **ethical principle of respect for persons**, **dignity**, and **the professional virtue of compassion**, dehumanization is **ethically impermissible**. *See also* CARE ETHICS; COMMODIFICATION.

DEISM. A metaphysics in which a creator God has caused all of physical reality to exist and has ordered it by laws, which are known as **natural laws**. Natural laws thus have the **moral status** of being oriented to human good. The ethical dimension of natural laws is expressed in the concept of **natural rights**. *See also* THEISM.

DELIBERATIVE CLINICAL JUDGMENT. Clinical judgment that is evidence based, rigorous, transparent, and accountable. Deliberative clinical judgment serves as a corrective to subjective clinical judgment and **enthusiasm** and an antidote to **bias**. *See also* EVIDENCE-BASED MEDICINE.

DEMENTIA. The progressive loss of cognitive and/or executive function, resulting in progressively diminished decisional autonomy and sometimes also (or separately) **executive autonomy**. **Decision making** *by* such patients begins while they retain the capacity to participate in the **informed consent process**. Decision making transitions to being *with* patients who have the capacity for **geriatric assent**, or **assisted decision making**. The final stage of decision making is *for* such patients by the legally designated **surrogate** in the **surrogate decision-making** process. Patients in the early stages of dementia who retain decisional autonomy should be urged to complete **advance directives** so that the geriatric assent and surrogate decision-making processes can be guided by the patient's **values** and beliefs. *See also* DECISION-MAKING CAPACITY; IMPAIRED DECISION-MAKING CAPACITY.

DEONTOLOGICAL ETHICS. **Ethical reasoning** based on considerations other than consequences, such as being a **person** protected by Kant's categorical imperative that all persons should be treated as ends in themselves and never as means merely to the interests of others. The **ethical principle of respect for autonomy** is often treated as a deontological **ethical principle** in **bioethics**. Deontological ethics should not be confused with *déontologie médicale*. *See also* CONSEQUENTIALIST ETHICS.

DÉONTOLOGIE MÉDICALE. A form of **medical ethics** developed in France in the 19th century that conceptualized medical ethics as a "science of duties," taken from the **moral philosophy** of British utilitarian **Jeremy Bentham** (1748–1832). In the French 19th-century literature on medical ethics, "medical deontology" comprised rules of conduct for physicians, similar to a **code** of medical ethics. These are not based on **utilitarianism**. A potential source of confusion is that these rules were not always based on utilitarianism. The term *déontologie médicale* should therefore not be taken to be synonymous with **deontological ethics**. *Déontologie médicale* by **Maximilien Isidore Amand Simon** (1807, fl. 1845–1865) is regarded as the most important text of *déontologie médicale*. It is based on "Christian social romanticism peculiar to the times" (Nye 2009, 422). Simon's medical ethics emphasized good character, and its opposition to euthanasia and abortion was based on Simon's "Catholic outlook" (Nye 2009, 422).

DEPENDENT MORAL STATUS. **Moral status** that is generated by a role that an entity occupies (e.g., the moral status of being a **patient)**, rather than originating in some constitutive property or properties of an entity. Dependent moral status contrasts with **independent moral status**, which is entirely self-generated and therefore not a function of a social role.

DEPRESSION. A mental **disorder** that negatively affects **decision making**, emotions, and well-being. The American Psychiatric Association distinguishes minor from major depression. A diagnosis of minor depression does not by itself defeat the **presumption of decision-making capacity**, whereas a diagnosis of major depression should at the very least cause this presumption to be questioned and the patient being formally evaluated by an experienced psychiatrist, psychologist, or other mental health professional. Decision making, therefore, should begin with decision making *by* the patient in the **informed consent process** and proceed to **assisted decision making** for patients who have diminished but not absent **decision-making capacity** and, finally, to **surrogate decision making** for patients who have lost decision-making capacity (which applies to major depression but not to minor depression). *See also* IMPAIRED DECISION-MAKING CAPACITY.

DESCRIPTIVE BIOETHICS. *See* EMPIRICAL BIOETHICS.

DESCRIPTIVE MEDICAL ETHICS. *See* EMPIRICAL MEDICAL ETHICS.

DETERMINATION OF DEATH. A clinical judgment that a **patient** is **dead** based on of brain-function criteria (**brain death**) or based on cardiopulmonary criteria (**cardiac death**, **cardiopulmonary death**, or circulatory death). *See also* AD HOC COMMITTEE OF THE HARVARD MEDICAL SCHOOL TO EXAMINE THE DEFINITION OF BRAIN DEATH.

DIALYSIS. A form of **life-sustaining treatment** that supplements or replaces kidney function. This typically takes the form of hemodialysis, in which blood is circulated through a machine to cleanse it of toxins. This can also take the form of peritoneal dialysis in which blood is circulated through the peritoneum to cleanse it of toxins. Dialysis is used to treat **end-stage renal disease**. *See also* END-OF-LIFE CARE.

DIGNITY. A **cluster concept**. Its components include the fundamental worth of each individual, the sacredness of each human being (drawn from **moral theology**), respect for each individual's uniqueness, enabling individuals with power, promoting the well-being of each individual, showing regard and even affection for each individual, and recognizing the potential and skill of each individual (Shestack 1998). Like all cluster concepts, when it is deployed in **ethical reasoning**, the components to which an appeal is being made should be clearly stated and then used with **consistency**. Dignity may originate in an individual, for example, in how he or she comports himself or herself in response to oppression. However, dignity also refers to the attitudes of respect of others toward an individual, resulting in dignity being attributed to that individual. In this respect, it is reasonable to say that a patient who is anesthetized or who is in a vegetative state nonetheless has dignity. *See also* ETHICAL PRINCIPLE OF RESPECT FOR PERSONS; PERSONALISM.

DIRECTIVE COUNSELING. In the **informed consent process**, the physician presents all the **medically reasonable alternatives** and recommends one, either because there is only one medically reasonable alternative or because among two or more medically reasonable alternatives one is clinically superior in **deliberative clinical judgment**. The goal is to influence the **decision making** of the **patient** without controlling it. The patient's decision making is therefore **voluntary**. This is a **beneficence**-based approach to the informed consent process. *See also* NON-DIRECTIVE COUNSELING; SHARED DECISION MAKING.

DIRECTIVE TO PHYSICIANS. An **advance directive** that instructs a patient's physician and care team about the patient's decisions regarding the provision of **life-sustaining treatment**. The directive may be implemented when the patient no longer has **decision-making capacity** as determined by the **clinical judgment** of the attending physician and the patient has either an **irreversible condition** or a **terminal condition**, as these are defined in applicable **statutory law** (i.e., **Advance Directives Acts**) and **common law**. A Directive to Physicians should be understood as an exercise by the patient of his or her **autonomy** in advance of the time at which the patient will have lost decision-making capacity and also has an irreversible or terminal condition. The **ethical obligation** to implement the patient's Directive to Physicians is based on the **ethical principle of respect for autonomy**. *See also* LIVING WILL.

DIRECT-TO-CONSUMER ADVERTISING. Advertising to consumers of drugs, devices, healthcare equipment, and healthcare services directly to individuals, bypassing physicians. In **ethical reasoning**, direct-to-consumer advertising, like all advertising of healthcare goods and services, should be understood as the beginning of the **informed consent process**. Physicians have the **professional responsibility** to prevent such advertising from unduly influencing the informed consent process and to recognize that **patients' requests** for advertised goods or services is the exercise of a **positive right**. All positive rights are **prima facie rights** that create a **prima facie ethical obligation** to implement the patient's request, but only when that request is supported in **deliberative clinical judgment**. Explaining this limitation on the patient request is part of the **professional responsibility** of a physician to protect the patient from herself or herself when the patient is making a clinically unwise decision (i.e., a decision that is incompatible with the patient's health-related **interests**).

DISABILITY. Abnormal anatomy or physiology that results in reduced affective, cognitive, motor, or sensory function that interferes with activities of daily living; self-care such as eating, dressing, or toileting; or with social activities such as attending school or work or is perceived to have one or more of these effects. Disability often results from **injury**. In **professional medical ethics**, disability, like **disease**, is in **deliberative clinical judgment** clinically abnormal. This means that there is a **beneficence**-based, **ethical obligation** to prevent disabilities, to provide effective **clinical management** of them, to conduct **research** to better understand and manage disabilities, and to teach trainees and practicing physicians how to fulfill their specialty-related **professional responsibility** to these **patients**. This management includes preventing the disability from worsening, ameliorating the disability, and, when possible, safely eliminating the disability.

This limited clinical perspective on disability is not the only perspective, as is clear from the disabilities studies literature. Some in this literature do not accept the classification of disability as abnormal. The consequences of this view for professional medical ethics are systemic: the ethical obligation to prevent and effectively manage disability, to conduct research, and to teach becomes very weak or even nonexistent. At best, only disabilities regarded as conditions implicating major risks to health and life would receive priority. In the United States, individuals with disabilities are protected by the **Americans with Disabilities Act**, enacted into law during the administration of President George H. W. Bush (term of office: 1989–1993), a Republican from Texas.

DISCRIMINATION. Often used to mean **invidious discrimination** (the most common use in **bioethics** and **medical ethics**). In this meaning, discrimination is making **ethically impermissible** distinctions among individuals or groups. In its benign sense, the term *discrimination* also means making **ethically permissible** distinctions between individuals based on defensible criteria. *See also* ETHICAL PRINCIPLE OF RESPECT FOR PERSONS; JUSTICE.

DISEASE. Abnormal anatomy (morbid anatomy) or physiology (pathophysiology) that should result in **clinical management** based on **deliberative clinical judgment**. Some take the view that the concept of disease is value neutral, inasmuch as the concept of abnormal is based on observed deviation from species-typical anatomy (e.g., polydactyly, bilateral renal agenesis in a fetus or newborn) or species-typical physiology (e.g., advanced dementia in a geriatric patient). Others take the view that the concept of disease is value laden, inasmuch as the concept of abnormal is based on value judgments about how much deviation from species-typical anatomy or species-typical physiology is enough to warrant clinical management. *See also* CONDITION; DISABILITY; DISORDER; HEALTH, CONCEPT OF.

DISORDER. A recognized pattern of abnormal anatomy or physiology that results in increased risk of outcomes that are **biopsychosocially** challenging to manage. Its pathology is not well understood. The application of the label *disorder* provides an **ethical justification** to develop, offer, and be paid for **clinical management** and **research**. *See also* CONDITION; DISABILITY; DISEASE; HEALTH, CONCEPT OF; INJURY.

DISORDERS OF SEXUAL DEVELOPMENT. Disorders that result from atypical development of anatomic **sex** as a result of nonalignment of the components of sex on a single sex and therefore atypical sexual development and function, as well as in some cases **gender** identity. These components include genomic sex, chromosomal sex, hormonal sex, brain sex, and parents' gender assignment. This nomenclature has replaced **intersex condition** in clinical discourse. There is **ethical controversy** about the **professionally responsible** clinical management of **patients** with disorders of sexual development, especially disorders in which the nonalignment of the components of sex reduces the reliability of a prediction of long-term **gender**. Some take the view that irreversible surgical management is **ethically permissible**. Some take the view that irreversible surgical management is **ethically impermissible** and, therefore, should be postponed until the patient is old enough to **consent** to such surgical management. *See also* GENDER IDENTITY DISORDER.

DISTRESS. Unwelcome experience of the disruption in one's normal behavioral repertoire accompanied by awareness. **Pain** can cause distress, but distress can occur in the absence of pain (e.g., the distress resulting from fear). Distress can cause **suffering**, especially prolonged distress, but distress can occur in the absence of suffering. The term *distress* is therefore not synonymous with the terms *pain* or *suffering*. The phrase *mental pain* is imprecise and sometimes has the same meaning as the term *distress*. When this is the case, the term *distress* should be used. In **professional medical ethics**, there is an **ethical obligation** to prevent distress and to manage distress effectively. This obligation, which has been recognized in the history of professional medical ethics, especially since the beginnings of neurology as a specialty in the 18th century and the beginnings of psychiatry as a specialty in the 19th century, is based on the **ethical principle of beneficence** and the **professional virtue of compassion**.

DISTRIBUTIVE JUSTICE. A **specification** of the **ethical principle of justice** that focuses on the fair outcome of allocation of a scarce resource or, in more colloquial terms, who gets what. The allocation of scarce clinical resources such as organs for **organ transplantation** or of **critical care** beds is a matter of distributive justice. What is termed *fair* may be understood variously, depending on which additional specification of the ethical principle of justice is invoked, including equality of outcomes (so far as practically possible), or **egalitarian justice**; outcomes that meet the basic needs of the least well off, or **Rawlsian justice**; outcomes based on ability to pay, or **libertarian justice**; outcomes that maximize the overall social good, or **utilitarian justice**; or outcomes that meet clinical needs as defined in **deliberative clinical judgement** or **healthcare justice**.

DNAR ORDER. Do-Not-Attempt Resuscitation Order. *See also* DO-NOT-RESUSCITATE ORDER (DNR ORDER).

DNR ORDER. *See* DO-NOT-RESUSCITATE ORDER (DNR ORDER).

"DO NOT GO GENTLE INTO THAT GOOD NIGHT". A poem by **Dylan Thomas** (1914–1953) famous in the literature on **death and dying**, **end-of-life care**, and **geriatric ethics** for lines from its first verse:

> Do not go gentle into that good night,
> Old age should burn and rave at close of day;
> Rage, rage against the dying of the light. (Thomas 2003, 239)

DOE V. BOLTON. The companion case to *Roe v. Wade* (410 U.S. 113) decided by the United States Supreme Court in 1973 about the legal permissibility of an **induced abortion**. *See also* ABORTION.

DONATION AFTER CARDIAC DEATH. A clinically specialized application of the concept of **cardiopulmonary death** in **organ procurement** and **organ transplantation**. Permission is obtained for the procurement of a **patient**'s organs after a **determination of death** has been made, when it is **ethically permissible** and legally permissible to discontinue **life-sustaining treatment** under an applicable **Advance Directives Act**. The patient is taken to an operating room where the life-sustaining treatment is discontinued, and a determination of death is made by the attending physician using cardiopulmonary criteria. The patient is declared dead. This approach is taken to satisfy the **dead donor rule**. The surgical transplant team then enters the operating room and removes organs to be donated to patients who need them. There is scientific, clinical, philosophical, and therefore **ethical controversy** about how long the attending physician should wait after cardiopulmonary arrest for it to be considered irreversible in **deliberative clinical judgment**. There is, therefore, ethical controversy about whether donation after cardiac death is ethically permissible.

DONNE, JOHN (1572–1631). English poet and cleric of the Church of England. His work on ethics included an argument against regarding **suicide** as an "irremissible" sin.

DONOR EGG. An ovum obtained from one woman to be fertilized. The resulting embryo becomes a candidate for **embryo transfer** to another woman, who is initiating the pregnancy as a component of **in vitro fertilization**. The **patient** who provides the ovum typically takes a superovulatory medication to stimulate multiple ovarian follicles from which ova are retrieved in an invasive procedure. These create increased **biopsychosocial** risks that include **morbidity**, blurred parenthood, and the possibility of a future child wanting to contact his or her genetic parent. These risks must be described in the **informed consent process** and, as a matter of **prudence**, carefully evaluated by the patient. The patient using resulting embryos must be informed about the biopsychosocial risks as well, including genetically based risk of **disease, disorder,** or **disability** in the future child and managing the wish of the future child to identify and contact his or her genetic mother. Egg donors are sometimes compensated monetarily. There is **ethical controversy** about setting limits on such compensation. Nonidentifying information about the donor is typically provided, which may result in the patient and her partner or spouse applying this information to make predictions about the characteristics of a possible future child, which is not evidence-based reasoning. *See also* ASSISTED REPRODUCTION.

DONOR EMBRYO. An embryo created by **in vitro fertilization** with the ovum of another woman and the sperm of the **patient**'s partner or spouse or of a known or unknown donor. The patient must be informed about the **biopsychosocial** risks, including blurred parenthood, genetically based risk of **disease** or **disability** in the future child (especially when such risk is identified by **preimplantation genetic diagnosis**), and managing the wish of the future child to identify and contact his or her genetic mother, and the possibility of a future child wanting to contact his or her genetic parent. These risks must be described in the **informed consent process** and, as a matter of **prudence**, carefully evaluated by the patient. *See also* ASSISTED REPRODUCTION.

DONOR SPERM. Sperm obtained from a known or unknown donor used to initiate a pregnancy, either by **artificial insemination** or by **in vitro fertilization**. Anonymous sperm donors are typically compensated. They must be informed about the **biopsychosocial** risks, including breach of confidentiality by the sperm bank when a future child is successful in obtaining a court order or is allowed by law to learn the identity of his or her biological father. *See also* ASSISTED REPRODUCTION.

DO-NOT-ATTEMPT RESUSCITATION ORDER (DNAR ORDER). The equivalent of a **Do-Not-Resuscitate Order**. A Do-Not-Attempt Resuscitation Order is thought to ease the emotional burden on families and care teams of not performing cardiopulmonary resuscitation and **letting the patient die**. *See also* END-OF-LIFE CARE; OUT-OF-HOSPITAL DO-NOT-RESUSCITATE ORDER.

DO-NOT-RESUSCITATE ORDER (DNR ORDER). A written order by a physician that states that **cardiopulmonary resuscitation** (CPR) will not be provided to a **patient** who experiences cardiopulmonary arrest. Inasmuch as CPR is the default treatment when a patient experiences cardiopulmonary arrest, CPR must be provided unless there is a Do-Not-Resuscitate Order in the patient's record. A DNR Order is typically suspended during surgery and is reinstated postoperatively when it is expected that cardiopulmonary arrest will be due to the patient's **condition** and not to surgery or anesthesia. There is **ethical controversy** about whether organizational policy should allow a physician to write a DNR Order unilaterally (i.e., without the consent of the patient or the patient's **surrogate**). *See also* ADVANCE DIRECTIVE; END-OF-LIFE CARE; LIFE-SUSTAINING TREATMENT.

DOUBLE-BLINDED CLINICAL TRIAL. A **clinical trial** using **blinding** in which neither the **research subjects** nor the investigators know what treatment the subject is receiving. This method is used to prevent **bias** in self-reporting by subjects of symptoms and other outcomes that are end-points of the trial. The **informed consent process** must disclose and explain the nature and purpose of such blinding. See also CLINICAL RESEARCH; HUMAN SUBJECTS RESEARCH.

DOUBLE EFFECT, PRINCIPLE OF. A rule for **ethical reasoning** that originated in **Roman Catholic moral theology** (McCormick 1977) to guide ethical reasoning about forms of **clinical management** that have two outcomes, one **ethically permissible** and the other **ethically impermissible**, hence "double effect," and with the benefit of the first outcome outweighing the harm of the second (the test of "proportionality"). A classic example is surgical management of uterine cancer for a pregnant woman that results in removal of the cancerous uterus (the ethically permissible outcome) and that also results in **feticide** (the ethically impermissible effect). (If one does not **judge** feticide to be ethically impermissible in such clinical circumstances, then there is no need to appeal to double effect in one's ethical reasoning.) The principle of double effect allows for such clinical management when the physician does not intend the ethically impermissible outcome.

Intend can be interpreted in two ways. The first, and most stringent, interpretation applies when there is no causal connection between the ethically impermissible outcome (as cause) and the ethically permissible outcome (as result). When there is such a connection, one necessarily intends the ethically impermissible outcome as the means to bring about the ethically permissible outcome. When this causal connection exists, then the principle of double effect does not apply and, therefore, cannot be appealed to in ethical reasoning. Crushing the fetal skull in a way that is in **deliberative clinical judgment** expected to cause feticide to manage severe cephalopelvic disproportion in the era before safe cesarean delivery is not acceptable under the principle of double effect. The second, and less stringent, application is a purely epistemological appeal, independent of causal analysis, of the physician's state of mind.

The principle of double effect is also invoked in the use of analgesia (pain relief) in **palliative care**. The dying human body can tolerate very high levels of analgesic medication without that level of medication causing **death** by **killing** the **patient**. It is considered ethically permissible to titrate analgesic medications upward, to gain effective pain relief, at the increased risk of complications such as compromised respiratory function. The death of a patient from such complications is causally independent of pain relief and is therefore ethically permissible under the principle of double effect. *See also* END-OF-LIFE CARE.

DSD. *See* DISORDERS OF SEXUAL DEVELOPMENT.

DSMB. *See* DATA AND SAFETY MONITORING BOARD (DSMB).

DUELING IN THE CHART. The practice of one member of the **patient**'s care team criticizing other members of the care team in the patient's record. This is done from **mere self-interest** in avoiding the discussions required by the commitment to **quality** and its improvement of **patient care**. Dueling in the chart is therefore **ethically impermissible**. *See also* FLYTING.

DURABLE POWER OF ATTORNEY. The assignment of an individual to act as one's **surrogate** when one has been declared **legally incompetent** by a court or to lack **decision-making capacity** by a physician. The assignment of one's powers of **decision making** to this individual is durable in the sense that it persists after **incompetence** or loss of decision-making capacity. *See also* ADVANCE DIRECTIVE.

DURABLE POWER OF ATTORNEY FOR HEALTHCARE. An **advance directive** in which a **patient** assigns an individual to act as one's **surrogate** when one has been declared **legally incompetent** by a court or to lack **decision-making capacity** by a physician. The assignment of one's powers of **decision making** to this individual is durable in the sense that it persists after **incompetence** or loss of decision-making capacity. *See also* MEDICAL POWER OF ATTORNEY.

DUTY. A cause of action that must be completed. The words *duty* and *obligation* are often used interchangeably. When they are not, the reason(s) for doing so should be made clear, to distinguish clearly that *duty* and *obligation* have a different meaning.

DUTY TO TREAT. This is a subcategory of the physician's **ethical obligation** to provide **clinical management** that is **medically reasonable** and that the **patient** has authorized in the **informed consent process**. The logic of **professional responsibility** is that this ethical obligation overrides the physician's **self-interests**, including the physician's **legitimate self-interests** in such matters as life and health when risks to life, health, and other forms of legitimate self-interest can be protected by following accepted protocols for self-protection. Specifically, if the patient has a communicable disease and there exist accepted protocols for self-protection, then there is a duty to treat.

This arose as an ethical challenge in the 1980s when **AIDS** was first characterized and there was no treatment for it. Some physicians and other healthcare professionals refused to treat **HIV**-infected patients on the grounds that doing so exceeded the limits of the **professional virtue of self-sacrifice**. Once the vectors of infection and effective precautions were identified, this line of reasoning became unacceptable in **professional medical ethics**, creating the duty of treating HIV-infected patients provided that the materials required for universal infection control are available.

DUTY TO WARN. There is **ethical controversy** about whether a physician who learns that a **patient** who poses a danger to an identified individual or individuals has an **ethical obligation** to warn those endangered parties and thus violate the **professional obligation** of **confidentiality**. Ethical reasoning about this matter must consider that violating the professional obligation of confidentiality and the patient's **right to privacy** bears the **burden of justification**. Whether this burden can be met is a function of the reliability of the physician's prediction of dangerousness, the potential for greater harm if the other parties are warned, and the damage to the patient's trust in the physician and healthcare professionals generally. In addition, in **deliberative clinical judgment** in psychiatry, relying on talk therapy to help defuse the patient's violent ideations may be a more reliable way to protect innocent others.

There is general agreement that, if the risk to identified others is death and that the patient has detailed plans to kill them, it is **ethically permissible** to prevent this serious, far-reaching, and irreversible harm by warning them. Inasmuch as doing so violates the patient's right to privacy, some have also argued that the patient must be informed. In 1976, the California Supreme Court went further and, in *Tarasoff v. Regents of the University of California* (17 Cal.3d 425) held that, when a clinician believes that a patient poses a danger to identified others, the clinician has a **legal obligation** to warn them. This ruling holds only in the state of California.

DYING. An imprecise term to characterize an individual's final hours or days as the organs in his or her body irreversibly cease to function, culminating in **death**. **Ethical reasoning** about dying focuses on setting **ethically justified** limits on **life-sustaining treatment** and **palliative care**. This topic is sometimes referred to by the phrase "death and dying." *See also ARS MORIENDI*; END-OF-LIFE CARE; EUTHANASIA.

E

ECMO. *See* EXTRACORPOREAL MEMBRANE OXYGENATION (ECMO).

ECT. *See* ELECTROCONVULSIVE THERAPY (ECT).

EGALITARIAN JUSTICE. A **specification** of the **ethical principle of justice** with implications for both **procedural justice** and **distributive justice**. Procedurally, egalitarian justice requires that everyone counts for one and no one for more than one, which means that the needs of all should be given equal consideration. This approach applied to healthcare encounters the difficulty that there is wide variation in the health status of individuals in a population. Distributively, egalitarian justice requires that each individual's needs be met equally, insofar as possible. This approach applied to healthcare encounters the difficulty that there is wide variation in the health needs of individuals in a population. One way to respond to this difficulty is to treat each individual equally with respect to his or her health status. The goal of doing so is to preserve, insofar as possible, equal opportunity of access to opportunity to pursue one's life goal insofar as possible. This approach provides an **ethical justification** for disproportionately more resources for individuals with **disabilities**, to equalize opportunity vis-à-vis individuals without disability. *See also* HEALTHCARE JUSTICE; LIBERTARIAN JUSTICE; RAWLSIAN JUSTICE; UTILITARIAN JUSTICE.

ELECTROCONVULSIVE THERAPY (ECT). A procedure performed under general anesthesia in which a current of electricity is passed through the brain, which can cause a small seizure. ECT is now considered to be safe and effective for treatment of morbid major depression, a condition that can lead to extreme self-neglect and therefore become life-threatening in geriatric patients and other serious mental illnesses. ECT was (negatively) popularized in the 1975 movie *One Flew over the Cuckoo's Nest*, directed by Miloš Forman and based on the book *One Flew over the Cuckoo's Nest* from 1962 by Ken Kesey. The movie includes the use of ECT in the 1950s in a way that is now considered primitive and clinically unacceptable. This depiction is clinically inaccurate and therefore of questionable relevance (at best) for **ethical reasoning** about ECT.

ELSI. Ethical, Legal, and Social Implications Research Program of the National Human Genome Research Institute (https://www.genome.gov/elsi/, accessed 14 September 2017). The acronym is also used generally to refer to scholarship and teaching on ethical, legal, and social implications of a field of biomedical science. *See also* GENETHICS.

EMBRYO DONATION. The provision of an embryo by a couple to permit a woman to initiate a pregnancy as part of **assisted reproduction**. Embryos may be already created through **in vitro fertilization** and be cryopreserved. Embryos may be created for the purpose of donation, with the gamete donors already known to the recipient couple, known as directed donation. There is agreement that the couple providing the embryo(s) must provide **informed consent**. This should include the **biopsychosocial** risks, such as the child who may result attempting to contact his or her genetic/biological parent(s) and legal risks such as unexpected claims on the estate of the donors. There is also a **prudence**-based concern that, given these psychosocial risks, embryo donation is unwise and therefore should be discouraged.

EMBRYO RESEARCH. Research on embryos created by **in vitro fertilization**. There is **ethical controversy** about embryo research, starting with whether it is **ethically permissible** to create embryos for this purpose. Such research is essential for an improved understanding of the early stages of human gestation and to improve techniques of genetic and genomic analyses of embryos to improve **preimplantation genetic diagnosis**. The **ethical justification** for such research is **beneficence** based. Some have objected to embryo research on the grounds that during or at the end of the research the embryo will be destroyed, which is not ethically permissible given the **moral status** of the embryo. Such objections originate for the most part in some variants of **Christian moral theology**, especially **Roman Catholic moral theology**. These objections are limited by the fact that other faith communities do not regard embryo research as ethically impermissible. In **moral philosophy**, there is agreement that an embryo does not have **independent moral status** and, therefore, does not have **rights**. In **professional medical ethics** of obstetrics and gynecology, an embryo that is not going to be transferred to a woman's uterus is not a **patient**, which means that **embryocide** is not the **killing** of a patient. There is also ethical controversy about the cut-off date (in days of gestation) beyond which embryo research should be judged **ethically impermissible**.

EMBRYO TRANSFER. In vitro embryos created in the laboratory are transferred into a woman's uterus as a component of **in vitro fertilization**. If two embryos are transferred, a twin pregnancy can result, with increased perinatal risks from prematurity and additional care burdens if a twin pregnancy results. If three or more embryos are transferred, a higher-order multiple or multi-fetal pregnancy can result, with greatly increased perinatal risks from prematurity, including extreme prematurity, and greatly increased care burdens if a higher-order multiple pregnancy results.

There are two approaches to managing the risks of twin and higher-order pregnancy. The first is to restrict the number of embryos transferred to one or, at most two, despite evidence that at more advanced maternal ages transferring more embryos may increase the probability of pregnancy and live birth. Some countries restrict the number as a matter of health policy. For example, the Human Fertilisation and Embryology Authority in the United Kingdom recommends that for most women only one embryo be transferred. In the United States, there is no direct regulation by the government. However, the American Society for Reproductive Medicine has published guidelines that discourage transfer of more than one embryo.

The second approach is to offer **selective termination** down to twins or a singleton. This approach is **autonomy** based because the decision about how many children to have is a personal decision. To be sure, there is a medical component to that decision, but the medical component is, as a rule, not decisive. *See also* ASSISTED REPRODUCTION.

EMBRYOCIDE. The **killing** of a human embryo. Some object to embryocide on the grounds that the embryo has **moral status**, but often fail to distinguish between **dependent moral status** and **independent moral status**. There is a metaphysical problem with this position. The embryo is capable of twinning (i.e., dividing into two embryos). This means that the embryo is not an individual. In metaphysics, to be an individual requires that an entity meet two criteria: the entity is distinct from other entities; and the entity is not divisible into two entities of the same species (Gracia 1988). These are known as *distinction* and *indivisibility*. An entity can be distinct but divisible, in which case it is classified as a particular not an individual. The embryo meets only the criterion of distinction, which means that it is a particular. Only individuals can generate their own moral status (i.e., have independent moral status). Moreover, only individuals can be **ensouled** by a creator God (i.e., have dependent moral status). At best, the embryo, as a particular, can have dependent moral status as a non-ensouled creature of God. This **moral theological** position is distinctive only to some faith communities and not all. This moral theological position is not secular and, therefore, is not the basis for an account of the moral status of the embryo in **professional medical ethics**. Because this moral theological position is not widely shared (e.g., Islam and Judaism do not endorse it), it has very limited applicability as the basis for **public policy**. *See also* ABORTION; FETICIDE.

EMBRYONIC STEM CELL RESEARCH. The use of stem cells for research, taken from embryos, a process that destroys the embryo. The stem cells of an embryo are totipotent, which means that they can become a wide variety of cell types and therefore organs. Stems cells thus hold the potential to improve **clinical care** in the emerging field of **regenerative medicine**. There is **ethical controversy** about embryonic stem cell research. Some have objected to embryonic stem cell research on the grounds that at the end of the research the embryo will be destroyed, which is not **ethically permissible** given the **moral status** of the embryo. Such objections originate for the most part in some variants of **Christian moral theology**, especially **Roman Catholic moral theology**. These objections are limited by the fact that other faith communities do not regard embryo research as ethically impermissible. In **moral philosophy**, there is agreement that an embryo does not have **independent moral status** and therefore does not have **rights**. In **professional medical ethics** of obstetrics and gynecology, an embryo that is not going to be transferred to a woman's uterus is not a **patient**, which means that **embryocide** is not the **killing** of a patient. Others object on the grounds that adult stem cells can be engineered to be used in regenerative medicine and that research should start with them until the safety and efficacy of proposed techniques of stem cell therapy are better understood. *See also* EMBRYO RESEARCH.

EMERGENCY. A clinical **condition** that must be treated immediately in order to prevent the **death** of a **patient**, or serious, far-reaching, and irreversible harm to the patient's **health**, leaving no time for the **informed consent process** or for **informed refusal**. *See also* EMERGENCY EXCEPTION TO INFORMED CONSENT.

EMERGENCY EXCEPTION TO INFORMED CONSENT. The ethical and legal requirement to obtain the **informed consent** of the **patient** for clinical management is suspended in the case of medical **emergencies**. These occur when the patient's life is in imminent danger and **clinical management** must be initiated to prevent imminent death, meaning that there is no time for the **informed consent process** or **informed refusal** should the patient refuse. These also occur when the patient's health is at immediate risk of serious, far-reaching, and irreversible harm and clinical management must be initiated to prevent imminent death, meaning that there is no time for the informed consent process or informed refusal should the patient refuse. The

ethical justification for this exception appeals to the **beneficence**-based **ethical obligation** in **professional medical ethics** of the physician to protect and promote the health-related interests of the patient. In medical emergencies as defined here, there is also no time for the informed consent process or informed refusal with the patient's **surrogate**, should he or she be available.

EMERGENCY MEDICAL TREATMENT AND ACTIVE LABOR ACT (EMTALA). A federal **statutory law** enacted in 1968 that requires all emergency centers to work up and stabilize **patients**, regardless of the source of payment. The federal government has provided no funding for this mandate, thus exploiting the concept of being a patient, which includes no reference to source of payment. Hospitals and physicians have the **professional responsibility** to admit patients who cannot be stabilized in the emergency and continue **clinical management** of their **condition(s)** until they are stable enough for safe discharge. *See also* HEALTH POLICY; PUBLIC POLICY.

EMPATHY. Names a psychosocial, cognitive, but not affective process by which the physician identifies the affective state of the **patient** and, out of **beneficence**-based concern for the patient's well-being, becomes concerned and offers **clinical management** motivated by this concern. This has been called "detached concern." The concept of empathy makes the implicit assumption that entering directly into the experience of the patient is intrinsically unmanageable and will therefore **bias** and even disable **deliberative clinical judgment**. This assumption differs from the account of **sympathy** in the **professional medical ethics** of **John Gregory** (1724–1773), where the physician enters directly into the experience of the patient, a process that is regulated by the twin virtues of **tenderness** and **steadiness**. Steadiness prevents the physician's affective response from biasing deliberative clinical judgment. Empathy also differs from **Sir William Osler**'s (1849–1919) concept of *aequanimitas*, which is a condition of imperturbability, insulating the physician from the affective dimensions of clinical management.

EMPIRICAL BIOETHICS. The use of methods of qualitative and quantitative social sciences to describe attitudes and behaviors of healthcare professionals; **patients**; organizational leaders; clinicians engaged in **innovation**; investigators in **animal subjects research** and in **human subjects research**; those with oversight responsibility for such research, such as members of **Institutional Review Boards** or **Research Ethics Committees**; and policy makers and administrators as these attitudes and behaviors bear on the **morality** of the healthcare professions, patients, organizational policy and practice, innovation and research, and health policy. Well-designed, well-conducted, and well-reported empirical studies of these attitudes and behaviors become an indispensable starting point for **normative bioethics**. *See also* EXPERIMENTAL PHILOSOPHY.

EMPIRICAL MEDICAL ETHICS. The use of methods of qualitative and quantitative social sciences to describe attitudes and behaviors of physicians; patients; physician leaders; physicians engaged in **innovation**; physician-investigators in **animal subjects research** and in **human subjects research**; those with oversight responsibility for such research, such as members of **Institutional Review Boards** or **Research Ethics Committees**; and physician policy makers and administrators as these attitudes and behaviors bear on the **morality** of the physicians, patients, organizational policy and practice, innovation and research, and health policy. Well-designed, well-conducted, and well-reported empirical studies of these attitudes and behaviors become an indispensable starting point for **normative medical ethics**. *See also* EXPERIMENTAL PHILOSOPHY.

EMTALA. *See* EMERGENCY MEDICAL TREATMENT AND ACTIVE LABOR ACT (EMTALA).

ENCYCLICAL. A formal letter issued by the Roman Catholic pope to guide the faithful in matters of faith and morals (i.e. **Roman Catholic moral theology**). Encyclicals on moral theology have direct relevance to **Roman Catholic medical ethics** and to **bioethics**.

END-OF-LIFE CARE. Clinical management of end-stage, life-taking **disabilities, diseases**, and **injuries** with the goal of reducing disease-related and iatrogenic burdens, especially **pain, distress**, and **suffering**. Major ethical concerns include initiating and discontinuing **life-sustaining treatment** and the preparation and implementation of **advance directives. Palliative care** is a major component of end-of-life care. Ethical issues focus on setting **ethically justified** limits on life-sustaining treatment. *See also* EUTHANASIA; PHYSICIAN-ASSISTED SUICIDE.

END-STAGE RENAL DISEASE (ESRD). End-stage disease of the kidneys, a life-threatening **condition** that is treated with **dialysis** or with **transplantation** of a kidney from a cadaveric or living donor. The treatment of ESRD is covered in the United States by **Medicare**, the only disease with such coverage.

ENGINEERING MODEL OF MEDICAL ETHICS. A simple approach to **ethical reasoning** in **medical ethics**, typically about clinical cases. **Ethical principles** are deployed, and their implications are identified. **Virtues** are usually omitted. Critics have pointed out that ethical principles should be interpreted in context and not abstractly applied. Failure to do so puts the engineering model at risk of becoming simplistic or, worse, applied in a rote fashion, which is a caricature of ethical reasoning. *See also* CLINICAL APPLICABILITY; "GEORGETOWN MANTRA"; PRINCIPLISM.

ENGLISH ENLIGHTENMENT. An intellectual, scientific, social, and political movement during the 18th century to improve many branches of human endeavor on the basis of experience as explicated by **Francis Bacon** (1561–1626) and **intuition** as explicated by **Richard Price** (1723–1791). This methodological approach differs from the Enlightenments that occurred in the countries of continental Europe, which emphasized **reason**. **Thomas Percival** (1740–1804) was the major figure in **medical ethics** of the English Enlightenment. *See also* SCOTTISH ENLIGHTENMENT.

ENHANCEMENT. The use of medical, surgical, and genomic interventions to create or strengthen traits in **patients** that are thought to be desirable. These interventions are not unique in that they should be categorized as **cosmesis, cosmetic genomics,** or **cosmetic surgery**. Genomic enhancement differs from other forms of cosmesis because it can alter not just an individual's traits (**somatic cell genetic engineering**) but also the traits of that individual's genetic descendants (**germ line genetic engineering**). The latter is an **ethical controversy** because the future individuals affected cannot **consent** to this change or to its risks. Enhancement of embryos is ethically controversial for the same reasons. Finally, there are perils of biomedical reductionism of an individual to his or her genome, which is a scientific error because desired traits are complex and thus subject to variation of their expression as the genome interacts with the epigenome, and larger environment. Prediction of traits and hopes for them should therefore be tempered by the unavoidable limits that are emphasized in a **biopsychosocial** approach to enhancement.

ENSOULMENT. The placing of a soul (an individual, nonmaterial entity created by God) into a human body, resulting in **dependent moral status** as one of God's creatures. The world's religions that deploy this concept do not agree on when during human gestation the developing human life form is ensouled. **Roman Catholic moral theology** places this event at the "moment of conception" whereas **Islamic moral theology** places the event later (with some differences among the schools of Islamic moral theology). The problem for Roman Catholic moral theology is that the embryo can twin, which means that, in Aristotelian metaphysics (which Roman Catholic moral theology accepts), the embryo is divisible and therefore not an **individual**. In general, moral theological views on the dependent moral status of human gestational life forms are limited in their applicability beyond the faith community in which each such view originates and the fact of wide disagreement among faith communities about when ensoulment occurs. *See also* MORAL STATUS.

ENTHUSIASM. A belief that lacks a basis of evidence and is therefore incompatible with **deliberative clinical judgment** and **ethical reasoning**. The problem of enthusiasm was recognized as early as the late 18th century when **John Gregory** (1724–1773) rejected enthusiasm as incompatible with experience as explicated by **Francis Bacon** (1561–1626). Gregory pointed out that, because many patients have lost their health and lives to enthusiasm, it is not clinically benign. Enthusiasm is a source of powerful **bias** in clinical judgment. *See also* EVIDENCE-BASED MEDICINE.

ENTRALGO, PEDRO LAÍN (1908–2001). Spanish medical scientist and historian of medicine; a major source of influence on **bioethics** and **medical ethics** in Latin America. In that region of the world, the approach to **philosophy of medicine** based on medical anthropology has been very influential. He is therefore regarded as the "patriarch of Ibero-American medical humanism" (Mainetti 2009, 502). *See also* MEDICAL HUMANITIES.

ENVIRONMENTAL ETHICS. The disciplined study of the **morality**—what is **ethically permissible, ethically impermissible**, and **ethically obligatory**—of the relationship between human beings and the environment, including especially other living things (plants and animals) and natural resources vital to the well-being of living things, such as the quality of air and water. An important connection between environmental ethics and **bioethics** is **ethical reasoning** about the impact of changes in the environment—both natural changes and changes resulting from human behavior—on health. Environmental ethics was a component of **bioethics** early in its history but was displaced by an emphasis on **biomedical ethics**. This is now changing as the original understanding gains increasing traction. *See also* POTTER, VAN RENSSELAER (1911–2001).

EPIDEMICS. A text in the **Hippocratic Corpus**. Mistakenly cited as the origin of the dictum "**First do no harm**" (later Latinized as *Primum non nocere*). The text reads: "Declare the past, diagnose the present, foretell the future; practice these acts. As to diseases, make a habit of two things—to help or at least to do no harm." *See also* ETHICAL PRINCIPLE OF NON-MALEFICENCE.

EQUIPOISE. A necessary condition for the initiation of a **Phase III clinical trial** (i.e., the use of **randomization** to assign **research subjects** to arms of the trial). Equipoise means that there is uncertainty about which arm of a controlled trial is clinically superior to the other. When this is the case, it is **ethically permissible** for physicians to refer their **patients** to the clinical trial without violating their **ethical obligation** to provide **clinical management** on the basis of **deliberative clinical judgment**.

There are two concepts of equipoise. The first is empirical: the majority of the relevantly informed and experienced clinical community is uncertain about clinical superiority of the competing arms of a trial. This is known as "opinion-based equipoise." The second is evidence-based reasoning: a **critical appraisal** of reported experience in the peer-reviewed scientific and clinical literature requires physicians to become uncertain about clinical superiority. This is known as "evidence-based equipoise." While opinion-based equipoise is the older of the two concepts, it is now regarded to be at unmanageable risk of bias, resulting in evidence-based equipoise being considered the superior understanding of the concept.

ESRD. *See* END-STAGE RENAL DISEASE (ESRD).

ETHICAL. Ambiguous between **ethically obligatory** and **ethically permissible**. *See also* IMMORAL; MORAL; UNETHICAL.

ETHICAL ANALYSIS. The discipline of becoming as clear as possible about the meaning of concepts that should guide **judgment** about what is **ethically permissible, ethically obligatory**, and **ethically prohibited**. Ethical analysis is one of the two required components of **ethical reasoning**, the other being **ethical argument**. Once a concept has been clarified, it should always be used explicitly with this meaning, to achieve consistency and coherence in one's subsequent ethical reasoning in ethical argument. Ethical analysis in **professional medical ethics** seeks to be clear about the meaning of **ethical principles, professional virtues**, and clinical ethical concepts such as **futility**.

ETHICAL AND RELIGIOUS DIRECTIVES FOR CATHOLIC HEALTH CARE SERVICES. A comprehensive guide, from the United States Conference of Catholic Bishops, to **Roman Catholic moral theology** pertaining to many topics in **bioethics** and **medical ethics**. "The purpose of these Ethical and Religious Directives then is twofold: first, to reaffirm the ethical standards of behavior in health care that flow from the Church's teaching about the dignity of the human person; second, to provide authoritative guidance on certain moral issues that face Catholic health care today" (http://www.usccb.org/issues-and-action/human-life-and-dignity/health-care/upload/Ethical-Religious-Directives-Catholic-Health-Care-Services-fifth-edition-2009.pdf, accessed 14 September 2017). *See also* EXTRAORDINARY MEDICAL TREATMENT; ORDINARY MEDICAL TREATMENT.

ETHICAL ARGUMENT. The discipline of identifying the implications of concepts that have been clarified by **ethical analysis** for **judgment** about what is **ethically permissible, ethically obligatory**, and **ethically prohibited**. Ethical argument is one of two required components of **ethical reasoning**. The discipline of ethical reasoning results from always going where these implications take one and nowhere else. It is a violation of the disciplined reasoning of ethics to start with conclusions and then go in search of supporting premises. Failure to adhere to the discipline of ethical analysis and argument results in what Plato (427–347 BCE) has Socrates in the *Dialogues* characterize—and rightly dismiss—as worthless—"**mere opinion**."

ETHICAL CONCEPT OF MEDICINE AS A PROFESSION. Requires three commitments of physicians: (1) become and remain scientifically and clinically competent; (2) make the protection and promotion of the **patient**'s health-related interests the physician's primary concern and motivation, keeping self-interest systematically secondary; and (3) sustain medicine as a **public trust** (the phrase is Thomas Percival's) that exists for the benefit of current and future patients, physicians, and society, rather than a guild, which medicine had been for centuries, that protects the economic, social, and political status and power of physicians as its primary concern and motivation.

The ethical concept of medicine as a profession was introduced into the history of medical ethics in the 18th century by the Scottish physician-ethicist **John Gregory** (1724–1773) and the English physician-ethicist **Thomas Percival** (1740–1804). Both drew on the **philosophy of science** and **philosophy of medicine** of **Francis Bacon** (1561–1626). Bacon called for a method of science and scientific medicine that minimized sources of **bias** (he called them "idols") and the minimally biased, careful observation of the results of **natural experiments** and **controlled experiments**. His word for these experiments was *experience*, by which he emphatically did not mean one's personal experience. Bacon's concept of experience-based medicine was a nascent form of **evidence-based medicine**. Gregory and Percival also drew on Baconian **moral science** to address the ethical dimensions of medical practice and research and health policy. Gregory drew on the moral science of **David Hume** (1711–1776), based on the **principle** of **sympathy** and the **virtues** that regulate it. Percival drew on the moral science of **Richard Price** (1723–1791), based on the **intuition** of moral truths.

The ethical concept of medicine is put into **clinical practice** and guides **innovation** and **research**, professional education, and **health policy** based on **professional virtues** and the **ethical principle of beneficence**. By physicians making and sustaining these three commitments, physicians make it true that medicine is a profession, which invokes the concept of truth in **pragmatism**.

The ethical concept of medicine, while it originates in Western philosophy, was invented by Gregory and Percival to bridge the religious and political differences of the increasingly pluralistic societies in which they lived. The concept achieves this status by being secular in nature: no appeal to divinity or sacred texts and traditions is required to understand and make the three commitments, and there is no necessary conflict between these three commitments and faith communities. Gregory taught a multinational group of medical students and thus created a concept that had no requirement of and therefore restriction to a specific national identity. The ethical concept of medicine as a profession is therefore transcultural, transreligious, and transnational. This crucial feature of the concept allows both national and international associations of physicians to write **codes of ethics** and **ethics statements** that are transcultural, transreligious, and transnational and thus have intellectual and moral authority for physicians in every country, faith community, and cultural setting. Refer to the introduction and *see also* PROFESSIONAL MEDICAL ETHICS.

ETHICAL CONCEPT OF THE FETUS AS A PATIENT. The fetus becomes a **patient** when the pregnant woman is presented for **clinical care**, and there exist forms of **clinical management** that in **deliberative clinical judgment** are reliably expected to benefit the fetus and future child clinically. Before **viability** (about 24 completed weeks with availability of advanced **neonatal critical care**), the fetus becomes a patient as a function of the pregnant woman's **autonomous decision** to confer the status of being a patient on her fetus(es), because her decision is the only link between the fetus and its becoming a future child (Chervenak and McCullough 2014).

After viability, the fetus becomes a patient when the pregnant woman is presented for clinical care, because viability establishes a link to the future child (Chervenak and McCullough 2014). Before viability, a pregnant woman's decision with her physician to have an **induced abortion** removes the moral status of being a patient from the fetus. This means that, while induced abortion results in the **killing** of the fetus, induced abortion does not result in the killing of a patient and is therefore not inconsistent with the **general prohibition against killing a patient** in **professional medical ethics**.

ETHICAL CONFLICT. *See* ETHICAL CONTROVERSY.

ETHICAL CONTROVERSY. Judgments about what is **ethically impermissible, ethically permissible**, or **ethically obligatory** that are incompatible with each other. Sometimes controversy is based on **argument** and sometimes not. When all positions in a controversy are based on argument, there is reasoned difference in judgment. When one or more positions in a controversy is not based on argument, reasoned difference is replaced with **mere opinion**. When an ethical controversy has existed for a long time (e.g., about the criteria required for a human being to have **independent moral status** or about the **moral status** of the fetus), resolution is unlikely because there is no method accepted by all parties to the controversy that could resolve the controversy. *See also* ETHICAL REASONING.

ETHICAL JUSTIFICATION. The use of the tools of **ethical reasoning, ethical analysis**, and **ethical argument** to reach a **judgment**. Ethical justification requires giving reasons (stating premises) that together support a conclusion that is then expressed as a judgment. Ethical justification is assessed for its reliability, which means that there can be degrees of strength of a specific justification.

ETHICAL, LEGAL, AND SOCIAL IMPLICATIONS (ELSI) RESEARCH PROGRAM. A research program of the National Human Genome Research Institute of the National Institutes of Health of the United States on the ethical, legal, and social implications of the human genome project, which is broadly understood to include genetics and genomics (https://www.genome.gov/elsi/, accessed 14 September 2017). *See also* GENETHICS.

ETHICAL OBLIGATION. An action or policy that **ethical reasoning** supports as the only **ethically justified** action or policy and, therefore, an **obligation** in a specific set of circumstances. For example, with the exception of life-threatening conditions in which treatment must be initiated immediately for such treatment to be effective in preventing imminent death of the **patient**, the **informed consent** of the patient is required for clinically risky procedures. *See also* LEGAL OBLIGATION.

ETHICAL PRINCIPLE. A general guide to **judgment** about what is **ethically permissible, ethically impermissible,** or **ethically obligatory** and to behavior based on such judgment. Four ethical principles are prominent in the **bioethics** literature: **ethical principle of beneficence, ethical principle of justice, ethical principle of nonmaleficence,** and **ethical principle of respect for autonomy.** The **ethical principle of respect for persons** is also invoked. Ethical principles sometimes require **specification** to make them applicable. *See also* ETHICAL REASONING; ETHICS.

ETHICAL PRINCIPLE OF BENEFICENCE. An **ethical principle** that creates an **ethical obligation** to act in a way that results in net benefit for another. Invoking the ethical principle of beneficence successfully in **ethical reasoning** requires one to have intellectual **authority** to identify reliably for another individual or group what is beneficial and harmful to that individual or group and to make reliable **judgments** about how to balance what is beneficial and harmful. The reliability of intellectual authority becomes the basis for the reliability of moral authority: acting on intellectually authoritative judgments. The identification of what is beneficial and harmful requires specifying the scope of benefits and harms about which intellectual and moral authority are claimed. The evidence-based reasoning for beneficence-based judgment should always be critically appraised.

In **bioethics,** there is a wide range of views, both implicit and explicit, on whether such intellectual authority exists and, when it exists, how its limits should be understood. Some deny that anyone other than the individual in question has the intellectual and moral authority to make beneficence-based judgments about himself or herself. This view is reflected in claims that each individual is an expert about his or her own values and that no one else possesses such expertise. Some accept limited intellectual and moral authority of healthcare professionals but are concerned about the potential of claims to such authority to result in **medical paternalism**. These reservations can be managed by appealing to a preference-based understanding of beneficence: patients, as a rule, are in the best position to make judgments about what forms of clinical management will result in net clinical benefit acceptable to the patient.

In **professional medical ethics,** physicians have the intellectual authority to identify clinical goods and harms for patients. The scope of the intellectual authority is restricted to the health-related interests of patients: prevention of premature death; prevention of death without morbidity that results in severe and irreversible loss of interactive capacity; and the prevention and effective management of **disease, disability, disorders, distress, injury, pain,** and **suffering**. These become the clinical goods identified in beneficence-based clinical judgment. The clinical harms for patients include disease, disability, disorders, distress, injury, pain, and suffering. Beneficence-based clinical judgment about net clinical benefit or net clinical harm should be **deliberative clinical judgment**. The moral authority to act on the intellectual authority of deliberative beneficence-based clinical judgment supports offering all **medically reasonable alternatives** to the patient (or the **surrogate** of a patient not able to make decisions for himself or herself) and making an evidence-based recommendation about a medically reasonable alternative when there is only one such alternative or when in deliberative clinical judgment one medically reasonable from among two or more medically reasonable alternatives.

In professional medical ethics, beneficence-based clinical judgment is **paternalistic** in the sense that the physician makes a justified claim to authority or superior knowledge about what forms of clinical management are medically reasonable and, therefore, are reliably expected to protect and promote the health-related interests of the patient. In professional medical ethics, beneficence-based clinical judgment is not **paternalism** because no interference with the patient's **autonomy** occurs. *See also* ETHICAL PRINCIPLE OF JUSTICE; ETHICAL PRINCIPLE OF NONMALEFICENCE; ETHICAL PRINCIPLE OF RESPECT FOR AUTONOMY; ETHICAL PRINCIPLE OF RESPECT FOR PERSONS; ETHICS.

ETHICAL PRINCIPLE OF JUSTICE. An **ethical principle** that creates an **ethical obligation** to achieve fairness in the distribution of benefits and burdens among a group of individuals. There are competing accounts of this ethical principle in history of philosophical ethics, resulting in **ethical controversy** about what should count as fair. There is agreement that there should be fairness in the process of deciding about how to distribute benefits and burdens, which is known as **procedural justice**. Procedural justice requires that the interests of all those affected by a distribution of benefits and burdens have their **interests** considered. There is also agreement that there should be fairness in the outcome of that **decision-making process**, which is known as **distributive justice**. In distributive justice, there is agreement that the distribution of benefits and burdens should prevent **exploitation**.

Invoking the ethical principle of justice in **ethical reasoning** requires one to be clear about which theory of justice one is adopting and why and to distinguish between procedural and distributive justice. In **bioethics, medical ethics**, and **professional medical ethics**, there are competing **specifications** of the ethical principle of justice, including **egalitarian justice, health-care justice, libertarian justice, Rawlsian justice**, and **utilitarian justice**. *See also* ETHICAL PRINCIPLE OF BENEFICENCE; ETHICAL PRINCIPLE OF NONMALEFICENCE; ETHICAL PRINCIPLE OF RESPECT FOR AUTONOMY; ETHICAL PRINCIPLE OF RESPECT FOR PERSONS; ETHICS.

ETHICAL PRINCIPLE OF NONMALEFICENCE. An ethical principle that creates an **ethical obligation** not to act in ways that result in *net* harm to others. In **professional medical ethics**, this ethical principle functions as a limiting condition on the **ethical principle of beneficence** by ruling out **clinical management** that is *only* harmful to a **patient** clinically and therefore **ethically impermissible**.

Invoking nonmaleficence successfully requires one to have intellectual **authority** to identify reliably for another individual or group what is harmful to that individual or group and to make reliable **judgments** about how to balance what is harmful against other outcomes. The reliability of intellectual authority becomes the basis for the reliability of moral authority: acting on intellectually authoritative judgments. The identification of what is harmful requires specifying the scope of harms about which intellectual and moral authority are claimed. The evidence-based reasoning for nonmaleficence-based judgment should always be critically appraised.

In **bioethics**, there is a wide range of views, both implicit and explicit, on whether such intellectual authority exists and, when it exists, how its limits should be understood. Some deny that anyone other than the individual in question has the intellectual and moral authority to make nonmaleficence-based judgments. This view is reflected in claims that each individual is an expert about his or her own values and that no one else possesses such expertise. Some accept limited intellectual and moral authority of healthcare professionals but are concerned about the potential of claims to such authority to result in **medical paternalism**. These reservations can be managed by appealing to a preference-based understanding of nonmaleficence: patients, as a rule, are in the best position to make judgments about what forms of clinical management will result in net clinical benefit acceptable to the patient.

In **professional medical ethics**, physicians have the intellectual authority to identify clinical harms for patients. The scope of the intellectual authority is restricted to the health-related interests of patients: prevention of premature death; prevention of death without morbidity that results in severe and irreversible loss of interactive capacity; and the prevention and effective management of **disease, disability, distress, disorders, injury, pain,** and **suffering**. These become the clinical goods identified in nonmaleficence-based clinical judgment. The clinical harms for patients include disease, disability, distress, injury, pain, and suffering. Nonmaleficence-based clinical judgment about net clinical harm should be **deliberative clinical judgment**. The moral authority to act on the intellectual authority of deliberative nonmaleficence-based clinical judgment supports recommending against clinical management that is net clinically harmful.

In professional medical ethics, nonmaleficence-based clinical judgment is **paternalistic** in the sense that the physician makes a justified claim to authority or superior knowledge about what forms of clinical management are net clinically harmful and, therefore, are reliably expected not to protect and promote the health-related interests of the patient. In professional medical ethics, nonmaleficence-based clinical judgment is not paternalism because no interference with the patient's **autonomy** occurs.

The ethical principle of nonmaleficence is sometimes stated as the ethical principle of "nonmalfeasance." This is an error because *malfeasance* means wrongdoing in a legal sense. *See also* ETHICAL PRINCIPLE OF JUSTICE; ETHICAL PRINCIPLE OF RESPECT FOR AUTONOMY; ETHICAL PRINCIPLE OF RESPECT FOR PERSONS; ETHICAL REASONING; ETHICS.

ETHICAL PRINCIPLE OF RESPECT FOR AUTONOMY. In **bioethics**, an **ethical principle** that creates an **ethical obligation** not to interfere with a **patient's decision making** and to implement the patient's decision about authorizing or refusing to authorize **clinical management** that has been offered or recommended. In much of the bioethics literature, the ethical principle of respect for autonomy is an **absolute ethical principle**.

In **professional medical ethics**, it is an ethical principle that creates an ethical obligation of the physician to empower the patient to engage in the **informed consent process** with the goal of the patient exercising his or her **autonomy** in the form of an informed and **voluntary** decision. There is **ethical controversy** in professional medical ethics about whether the ethical principle of respect for autonomy is an absolute ethical principle.

In bioethics, the ethical principle of respect for autonomy functions as an antidote to what is taken to be the long history of **paternalism** in medical ethics and **clinical practice**. Recent scholarship has called into question whether in the history of medical ethics paternalism was endorsed as an ethical **norm** (McCullough 2011). *See also* ETHICAL PRINCIPLE OF BENEFICENCE; ETHICAL PRINCIPLE OF JUSTICE; ETHICAL PRINCIPLE OF NONMALEFICENCE; ETHICAL PRINCIPLE OF RESPECT FOR PERSONS; ETHICAL REASONING; ETHICS.

ETHICAL PRINCIPLE OF RESPECT FOR PERSONS. An **ethical principle** related to but of broader scope than the **ethical principle of respect for autonomy**. The *Belmont Report* provides an account that continues to be in use: "Respect for persons incorporates at least two ethical convictions: first, that individuals should be treated as autonomous agents, and second, that persons with diminished autonomy are entitled to protection. The principle of respect for persons thus divides into two separate moral requirements: the requirement to acknowledge autonomy and the requirement to protect those with diminished autonomy" (U.S. National Commission 1979). The first conviction expresses the ethical principle of respect for autonomy. The second goes beyond this ethical principle. The basis for the second conviction might appeal to **dignity**. *See also* ETHICAL PRINCIPLE OF BENEFICENCE; ETHICAL PRINCIPLE OF JUSTICE; ETHICAL PRINCIPLE OF NONMALEFICENCE; ETHICAL PRINCIPLE OF RESPECT FOR AUTONOMY; ETHICAL REASONING; ETHICS.

ETHICAL REASONING. The use of **ethical analysis** and **ethical argument** to reach well-supported ethical **judgments** about what is **ethically permissible, ethically obligatory**, and **ethically impermissible**. To be valid and reliable, ethical reasoning must meet the following requirements: **clarity, consistency, coherence, clinical applicability**, and **clinical adequacy**. Meeting these requirements results in the disciplined study of **morality**, which is manifested by the commitment to go where argument takes one—to the conclusions supported by the implications of clear concepts consistently used—and nowhere else. Failure to submit to this intellectual and practical discipline results in **mere opinion**, which is never acceptable in ethical reasoning.

ETHICAL THEORY. *See* METAETHICS.

ETHICALLY IMPERMISSIBLE. An action or policy that is ruled out as unacceptable by **ethical reasoning** and therefore ought not to be undertaken. *See also* ETHICALLY OBLIGATORY; ETHICALLY PERMISSIBLE.

ETHICALLY OBLIGATORY. An action or policy that in **ethical reasoning** ought to be undertaken as a matter of **obligation**. *See also* ETHICALLY IMPERMISSIBLE; ETHICALLY PERMISSIBLE.

ETHICALLY PERMISSIBLE. An action or policy that is supported by **ethical reasoning** in the context in which competing actions or policies are also supported, including but not limited to **ethical controversy**. Competing supported actions or policies result in the freedom to engage on any one of such actions or implement any one of such policies. For example, there is ethical controversy about the justified scope of a **positive right** to healthcare, resulting in a wide range of justified policy options. *See also* ETHICALLY IMPERMISSIBLE; ETHICALLY OBLIGATORY.

ETHICALLY PROHIBITED. *See* ETHICALLY IMPERMISSIBLE.

ETHICS. The disciplined study of **morality** with the goal of continuous improvement. Ethics aims to improve mortality by asking and answering a single question: What should morality be? Two disciplines of the humanities, philosophy and theology, provide the methods of **ethical analysis** and **ethical argument** that are used to address this question in **ethical reasoning**. Theological ethics, known as **moral theology**, draws on the sacred texts and traditions of a specific faith community and thus has limited applicability outside of that faith community. Philosophical ethics, known as "moral philosophy," draws on intellectual resources available to anyone willing to engage in reasoned discourse, using ethical analysis and argument, to improve morality. Philosophical ethics aims to be transreligious, transcultural, and transnational. Notwithstanding, there are competing methods of ethics, in both theology and philosophy.

ETHICS COMMITTEE. An organizational committee with oversight responsibility for **ethics of patient care** and, sometimes, **organizational ethics**. Typically, the committee is multidisciplinary and sometimes also includes lay members from the community that the organization serves. A common approach is for the ethics committee to develop organizational policies pertaining to **clinical ethics** (e.g., regarding **advance directives** in **end-of-life care**) that physicians, nurses, and other clinicians are expected to follow and are supported by the organization's leadership when they do so. These policies are also used by the organization's **clinical ethics consultants**, whose work should be overseen by the committee. An ethics committee reports to the organization's leadership, for example, through the medical executive committee in a hospital or to a senior leader in patient safety and quality. An ethics committee does not have oversight responsibility for the **ethics of human subjects research**, which is the purview of an **Institutional Review Board** or **Research Ethics Committee**. In the **common law**, the New Jersey Supreme Court in *In re Quinlan* in 1976 called for the creation of ethics committees to provide guidance for **surrogate decision making** about end-of-life care for patients. Critics pointed out that the Court, in effect, called for a prognosis committee.

ETHICS CONSULTATION. An individual or team who provides **consultation** about **clinical ethics** or **research ethics**.

ETHICS MANUAL. The American College of Physicians first published its comprehensive *Ethics Manual* in 1989. The current sixth edition was published in 2012 (Snyder 2012). The *Manual* is based on an account of professionalism in medicine and comprises the following sections: "The Physician and Patient"; "Care of Patients Near the End of Life"; "The Ethics of Prac-tice"; "The Physician and Society"; and "Research." *See also* CODE OF ETHICS.

ETHICS OF ANIMAL SUBJECTS RESEARCH. Ethical reasoning about **research** with animals for the purposes of advancing biomedical sci-ence or improving the quality of veterinary or human medicine. The ethics of animal subjects research starts with inquiry about whether such research is ever **ethically permissible**. For those who hold that such research is ethically permissible, inquiry continues into such topics as the ethically permissible scope and purposes of research with animals; study design, including the sample size and nature, duration, and intensity of **pain** and **distress** that are necessary to test a hypothesis; the management of animals during research and after research has been completed; and the prospective review and ap-proval by an **Institutional Animal Care and Use Committee**. The ethics of animal subjects research has a history dating from at least the 19th century, spurred in part by concern to prevent cruelty to animals from such practices as **vivisection**. In the United States, research with animal subjects is gov-erned by **statutory law**, the **Animal Welfare Act**, and by **regulatory law**, including federal and state regulations. In the United States, there is also a certification process provided by the American Association for Laboratory Science (https://www.aalas.org/, accessed 14 September 2017) and the Asso-ciation for the Assessment and Accreditation of Laboratory Animal Care International (http://www.aaalac.org/, accessed 14 September 2017). *See also* ANIMAL CRUELTY; EXPERIMENT.

ETHICS OF CARE. Ethical reasoning based on the commitment of a human being to attend to another human being, to protect and promote the **interests** of that individual, and to protect that individual from harm. The ethics of care was developed as a response to the abstract nature of principle-based ethical reasoning that was taken to draw implicitly on the rule-orienta-tion of men. The ethics of care does not reject **ethical principles** but does not make them central. The **virtues** of the caregiver are central. The **professional medical ethics** of **John Gregory** (1724–1773) can be read as an early exam-ple of professional medical ethics based on an ethics of care. There is close affinity of an ethics of care to **feminine bioethics, feminine ethics,** and **feminine medical ethics**. *See also* PROFESSIONAL VIRTUE OF COM-PASSION.

ETHICS OF COOPERATION. Cooperation is an essential component of effective team care of **patients**. The ethics of cooperation is based on the **ethical concept of medicine as a profession** generalized to all of the healthcare professions, which are united in their three commitments: (1) to scientifically and clinically competent **patient care**; (2) putting the health-related **interests** of **patients** systematically first; and (3) sustaining their healthcare profession as a **public trust**. The second of these commitments blunts individual **self-interest**, and the third blunts group self-interest. Failure to blunt these two forms of self-interest results in competition for supremacy of self-interest, which undermines the safety and **quality** of patient care. In his *Medical Ethics* (1803), **Thomas Percival** (1740–1804) writes perhaps the first ethics of cooperation for three groups—physicians, surgeons, and apothecaries (pharmacists)—who were fierce competitors in the small market place for private practice, a rivalry that affected the **organizational culture** of the **Royal Infirmary** of Manchester. Percival defines a common **professional ethics** for the three groups and proposes the organizational structure of a committee to review hospital practice for its quality and also to prospectively review and approve **research with human subjects**.

ETHICS OF END-OF-LIFE CARE. Ethical reasoning about the **ethical obligations** of clinicians, healthcare organizations, family members, society, and government to patients with end-stage **disability**, **disease**, or **injury** that is expected to result in the patient's **death** in the near-term future. *See also* ADVANCE DIRECTIVE; ADVANCE DIRECTIVES ACT; END-OF-LIFE CARE; FUTILITY; INFORMED CONSENT; INFORMED REFUSAL; SURROGATE DECISION MAKING.

ETHICS OF HUMAN SUBJECTS RESEARCH. Ethical reasoning about **research** with humans for the purposes of advancing biomedical science or improving the quality of **patient** care. The ethics of human subjects research starts with inquiry about whether such research is ever **ethically permissible**. There is general agreement that such research is ethically permissible, provided that human subjects research is undertaken for valid scientific reasons and is undertaken only with prospective review and approval by an **Institutional Review Board** (IRB) (in the United States) or a **Research Ethics Committee** (REC) (in other countries). Inquiry is undertaken into such topics as the ethically permissible scope and purposes of research with humans; study design; ethically permissible iatrogenic burdens of participation (the risk-benefit ratio); the **clinical management** of subjects during research and after research has been completed; protection of **privacy**; and the **scientific integrity** of recording, analyzing, and reporting results. There is ethical inquiry into the four phases of human subjects research, **Phase I Research, Phase II Research, Phase III Research**, and **Phase IV**

Research. There is ethical inquiry about research with specific populations, including fetuses and pregnant women, prisoners, and individuals with **impaired decision-making capacity.**

Guidance for the ethics work of IRBs and RECs is provided by **statutory law** and **regulatory law.** In the United States, human subjects research is regulated by the U.S. Department of Health and Human Services' **Office for Human Research Protections** (http://www.hhs.gov/ohrp/, accessed 14 September 2017) on the basis of federal statutory law. *See also* 45 CFR 46. *See also* ETHICS OF INNOVATION; INNOVATION.

ETHICS OF INNOVATION. Ethical reasoning about **innovation** in **patient care.** There is now strong consensus that planned innovation, surgical (Biffl et al. 2008) as well as medical, should be undertaken only with the approval of a committee that has prospectively approved the innovation for its scientific justification, probability of success, and **informed consent process.** The informed consent process for innovation should make clear to the **patient** or **surrogate decision maker** that there is no **ethical obligation** to consent to innovation because its outcome cannot be reliably predicted. *See also* CLINICAL TRIAL; EXPERIMENT; HUMAN SUBJECTS RESEARCH; RESEARCH.

ETHICS OF PATIENT CARE. Ethical reasoning about all aspects of **patient care,** usually not including **ethics of human subjects research.** *See also* MEDICAL ETHICS; PROFESSIONAL MEDICAL ETHICS.

ETHICS OF SCIENTIFIC RESEARCH. Ethical reasoning about the design, conduct, funding, supervision, and reporting of scientific **research.** Topics include the **integrity** of investigators; responsible management of both **conflicts of interest** and **conflicts of commitment;** management of **bias;** maintaining **autonomy** over research, especially industry-funded research; the evaluation of findings; the reporting of findings at scientific conferences; the peer-reviewed literature and public media; and the prospective review, approval, and oversight of research by **Institutional Review Boards** (in the United States) or **Research Ethics Committees** (in other countries). *See also* INTEGRITY.

ETHICS STATEMENT. A document produced by a national or international professional association of physicians to guide and assess **clinical practice, innovation** and **research,** professional education, and **health policy.** These statements are often based on the association's **code of ethics.** *See also* PROFESSIONAL MEDICAL ETHICS.

ETIQUETTE. Proper manners and behavior among individuals. Perhaps as late as the early 18th century in the United Kingdom and its colonies and in countries in Europe, it was thought that one could reliably infer good character from consistently good behavior, including etiquette. Etiquette, therefore, had a moral content and was not mere manners, a common view in the literature of **bioethics** and **medical ethics**. In the United Kingdom, a crisis of manners emerged by the middle of the 18th century, characterized by a loss of confidence in this inference. This crisis was epitomized by the man of "false manners," who hid predation behind a veneer of good manners. Etiquette took on a different moral content, of caution and mistrust, not trust. This history informs skepticism about the ethical significance of **medical etiquette** in the literature of bioethics and medical ethics. *See also* BOUNDARY ISSUES.

EUGENICIST. An individual who is an advocate for **eugenics**.

EUGENICS. The use of breeding and laboratory techniques to improve the genetics of a species, especially humans. This concept was developed in the early 20th century and applied by Nazi Germany. **Negative eugenics** uses these techniques to blunt the expression of or remove what are considered as deleterious traits (such as developmental **disability**) or deleterious genes. **Positive eugenics** uses these techniques to enhance or add what are considered as traits or genes that improve genetics (such as increased intelligence), or genetic **enhancement**. The evidence base for the claims of **eugenicists** varies, from nonexistent (the use of phrenology by the Nazis) to strong (in crop and animal science, for example). The judgments made by advocates of eugenics in humans have been biased, usually racist. Eugenicists also typically have unrealistic expectations of the ability of science to control biology and to produce outcomes that are free of significant **biopsychosocial** risk. Their motivations are usually based on **racism**. Genetic changes can affect the germ line, not just an individual; they are especially ethically challenging because the future individuals affected by alteration of the germ line cannot consent. In contemporary **genethics** and **genomic ethics**, the invocation of eugenics is used to state that a proposed change in the human genome is ethically suspect, at best, or **ethically impermissible**, at worst. *See also* COSMETIC GENOMICS.

EUTHANASIA. A good death. Euthanasia names a variety of **clinical practices**. The term *euthanasia* can mean dying with as little **pain, distress,** or **suffering** as clinically possible, as **Francis Bacon** (1561–1626) proposed. More recently, the term *euthanasia,* or *euthanasie* in German, has also meant **killing** a patient without the patient's consent. This is the meaning of *euthan-*

asie undertaken by the Nazi physicians during the Third Reich and World War II. Distinctions are now made among **involuntary active euthanasia, voluntary active euthanasia, involuntary passive euthanasia,** and **voluntary passive euthanasia.** There is controversy about whether these distinctions withstand close scrutiny. *See also* LETTING DIE.

EVALUATIVE UNDERSTANDING. *See* DECISION-MAKING CAPACITY.

EVIDENCE-BASED MEDICINE. The habit of basing **clinical judgment,** treatment planning, and prognosis on the best available evidence, as an antidote to the distorting effects of **bias** in clinical practice. A nascent form of evidence-based medicine was introduced by Francis Bacon (1561–1626) who insisted that physicians base clinical practice on "experience." By *experience* Bacon did not mean a physician's personal experience in **patient care,** which is intrinsically biased and therefore unreliable for the scientific practice of medicine. Bacon understood the term *experience* to mean the carefully observed, analyzed, and reported results of natural and controlled experiments. Bacon's concept of experience was influential on the development of the **ethical concept of medicine as a profession.**

The goal of evidence-based medicine is to responsibly minimize variation in the processes and outcomes of clinical care, which is the definition of **quality** in patient care. Some physicians think that, if there are no clinical trials pertinent to the clinical management of a patient, there is no randomized **ethical obligation** to follow the discipline of evidence-based medicine. This is an error, because there are often other forms of evidence, ranging from case reports and case series reports for rare conditions to **Phase I** and **Phase II clinical trials.**

A common criticism of evidence-based medicine is that there are many aspects of **clinical practice** that have not been subjects to **Phase III clinical trials.** This is a caricature, because evidence-based medicine calls for diagnostic, therapeutic, and prognostic clinical judgment to be based on the *best available* evidence and the **critical appraisal** of that evidence. *See also* DELIBERATIVE CLINICAL JUDGMENT; ENTHUSIASM.

EVOLUTION. The process of adaption of organic life forms over time in response to different environments, resulting in variation of life forms across and within species. The mechanisms of evolution such as natural selection and adaptation have no purpose and are indifferent to human beings with their **hopes,** beliefs, and **values.** Evolution is the basis of modern biology and, therefore, of modern biomedical science and its clinical applications (e.g., the rapid adaptation of bacteria and viruses in response to exposure to medications). Those who deny evolution, so-called Creationists, do so at a very steep intellectual price: the denial of the **authority** of all modern biology and therefore all **clinical practice**.

EXECUTIVE AUTONOMY. A dimension of **autonomy** distinctive from **decisional autonomy**. Executive autonomy is self-governance in carrying out—and, as necessary, adapting—decisions. Executive autonomy is therefore a function of **executive capacity**.

EXECUTIVE CAPACITY. The ability to implement an option selected by **decision making** (i.e., the exercise of **decision-making capacity**). This includes the ability to change implementation in response to changed circumstances. Executive capacity can become impaired, to differing degrees, by **executive dysfunction** that results from frontal lobe **disorders** in the brain, which can be evaluated by neuropsychiatric examination. Executive capacity can become impaired independently of **impaired decision-making capacity** or in conjunction with impaired decision-making capacity. *See also* AUTONOMY; EXECUTIVE AUTONOMY.

EXECUTIVE DYSFUNCTION. Malfunction of brain physiology used in making, adapting, and carrying out plans, especially in response to changed or unexpected circumstances. This results in **impaired executive capacity** and, therefore, **impaired executive autonomy**. **Impaired executive capacity** can occur independently of **impaired decision-making capacity**. Impaired executive autonomy can therefore occur independently of **impaired decisional autonomy**. This means that not all **patients** who are thought to have borderline but intact **decision-making capacity** should be considered necessarily to have **executive capacity** and, therefore, **executive autonomy**.

EXPERIMENT. Clinical management where the outcome cannot be reliably predicted in **deliberative clinical judgment**. An experiment in **patient care** can be either **innovation** or **research**. Clinical management where the outcome can be reliably predicted in deliberative clinical judgment is treatment or therapy. An experiment can be performed without adherence to the intellectual **norms** of scientific method and the moral norms of **animal subjects research** or **human subjects research**. Such experiments are **ethically impermissible** in **research ethics**, and their results are scientifically and clinically worthless. Many of the **Nazi medical war crimes** involved such scientifically and ethically unacceptable experiments. It is a mistake to equate experimentation with research. All research is experimentation but not all experimentation is research.

EXPERIMENTAL PHILOSOPHY. The use of the methods of qualitative and quantitative social sciences in philosophy, including **moral philosophy**. The results of such research are incorporated into **ethical reasoning** and are also used to test the **applicability** and **adequacy** of ethical reasoning. *See also* EMPIRICAL BIOETHICS; EMPIRICAL MEDICAL ETHICS.

EXPLOITATION. A **justice**-based concept that applies to the **ethical permissibility** of outcomes in a **patient** population. Exploitation occurs when **clinical management** benefits only a very small percentage of a population while all other patients in the population experience disease-related or iatrogenic **morbidity** or **mortality**, without the opportunity for offsetting benefit. The ethical principle of justice considers such an outcome to be **ethically impermissible**. Sometimes the term *exploitation* is used to mean "use," as in the sentence "He exploited the opportunity to help others." This meaning has no special ethical significance. *See also* ETHICAL PRINCIPLE OF JUSTICE.

EXTRACORPOREAL MEMBRANE OXYGENATION (ECMO). A form of **life-sustaining treatment** that uses a pump that circulates a **patient**'s blood outside the patient's body to add oxygen to it, to support bodily organs by oxygenating them. Sometimes referred to as an "artificial lung." This is used for patients in heart or lung failure. The ethical challenges of ECMO are the same as those for other forms of life-sustaining treatment. A distinctive challenge results from uncertainty about how long patients, especially pediatric patients, can remain on ECMO and recover without major complications. *See also* END-OF-LIFE CARE.

EXTRAORDINARY MEANS. *See* EXTRAORDINARY MEDICAL TREATMENT.

EXTRAORDINARY MEDICAL TREATMENT. A concept in **Roman Catholic moral theology** that pertains to setting **ethically justified** limits on **end-of-life care**. As long as medical treatment, including **life-sustaining treatment**, continues to result in net clinical benefit for the **patient** (i.e., it continues to be a **medically reasonable alternative**), then it is **ethically obligatory** to continue provision of such treatment. This is **ordinary medical treatment**. When this is no longer the case—in other words, when continued **clinical management** is no longer a medically reasonable alternative and its risks of **morbidity, distress, pain,** and **suffering** are increasing and not offset by clinical benefit—it is **ethically permissible** to discontinue it. Such treatment has become excessively burdensome, a **beneficence**-based **clinical ethical judgment**. In addition, if continued clinical management of a gravely ill patient is so psychosocially burdensome on the family—the fundamental social unit through which the faith is sustained across generations—that it threatens the unity of the family, discontinuation is also ethically permissible. This also known as provision of medical treatment by "extraordinary means."

The distinction between ordinary medical treatment (ordinary means) and extraordinary medical treatment (extraordinary means) was made in Roman Catholic moral theology in the 16th century, long before the development of modern life-sustaining treatment, and remains remarkably durable, although it is met with skepticism in some quarters in **bioethics**. There has been recent **ethical controversy** in Roman Catholic moral theology about whether the concept of extraordinary medical treatment is applicable to the provision of **artificial nutrition** and hydration. *See also* ETHICAL AND RELIGIOUS DIRECTIVES FOR CATHOLIC HEALTH CARE SERVICES.

F

FAIRNESS. A concept that shapes the **ethical principle of justice**. Fairness can be understood in different ways. In **procedural justice**, fairness usually means equality of opportunity to pursue opportunities and human achievement. In **distributive justice**, fairness can mean equality of outcomes (**egalitarian justice**), outcomes that are the result of free choices (**libertarian justice**), outcomes that benefit the greatest number (**utilitarian justice**), or outcomes that benefit many so long as the least well off are benefited (**Rawlsian justice**).

FALSE HOPE. *See* HOPE.

FATWA. An opinion about the interpretation of Islamic law by a religious authority. It is often an *imam* responding, privately or publicly, to an inquiry by a member of the Islamic faith community. *Fatwas* display variation in interpretation of **Islamic moral theology** and provide authoritative guidance to physicians, patients, and healthcare organizations on matters of **Islamic medical ethics** and **Islamic bioethics**.

FEE-SPLITTING. The practice of a referral specialist sharing income from fees from **patients** with physicians who referred the patients. This practice also includes subsequent preferential referral to specialists who will share income from fees with the referring physician. This practice risks making the financial **self-interest** of the referring physician that physician's primary concern and motivation for the referral, which is **ethically impermissible** management of a **conflict of interest** in **professional medical ethics**. The primary concern and motivation for referral should be a **deliberative clinical judgment** about the need for referral care and the competence of the specialist to provide care consistent with the **professional virtue of integrity**. The provision against fee-splitting in the **American Medical Association** *Principles of Medical Ethics* of 1903 was an important step in the development of professional medical ethics in the United States (Baker 2009). *See also* KICKBACKS; "STARK LAW".

FEMININE BIOETHICS. Bioethics based on **feminine ethics**. *See also* FEMINIST BIOETHICS.

FEMININE ETHICS. Ethical reasoning based on **virtues** of which women are the moral exemplars (Tong 1993). The **ethics of care** is a form of feminine ethics. Feminine ethics contrasts with **feminist ethics** that emphasizes the **ethical principle of respect for autonomy** of women and the **rights** it supports, in response to patriarchy and the long history of male domination of women (Tong 1993).

FEMININE MEDICAL ETHICS. Medical ethics based on **feminine ethics**. The **professional medical ethics** of **John Gregory** (1724–1773) is based on feminine ethics in that Gregory's account of the **virtues** of **sympathy**, **tenderness**, and **steadiness**; what he called "women of learning and virtue" were the moral exemplars of these virtues (McCullough 1998). *See also* FEMINIST MEDICAL ETHICS.

FEMINIST BIOETHICS. Bioethics based on **feminist ethics**, with a strong emphasis on the **ethical principle of respect for autonomy** of women and the **rights** it supports, especially the **negative right** to be free of **medical paternalism** and **procreative rights**. For some feminist bioethicists, this right is an **absolute negative right** while for others it is a **prima facie negative right**. *See also* FEMININE BIOETHICS.

FEMINIST ETHICS. Ethical reasoning that makes central the **ethical principle of respect for autonomy** of women and the **rights** it supports, especially the **negative right** to be free of patriarchy and its long history of **paternalism** toward women. For some feminist ethicists, this right is an **absolute negative right** while for others it is a **prima facie negative right**. *See also* FEMININE ETHICS; FEMINIST MEDICAL ETHICS.

FEMINIST MEDICAL ETHICS. Medical ethics based on **feminist ethics**, with a strong emphasis on the **ethical principle of respect for autonomy** of women and the **rights** it supports, especially the **negative right** of female **patients** to be free of **medical paternalism**. For some feminist medical ethicists, this right is an **absolute negative right** while for others it is a **prima facie negative right**. *See also* FEMININE MEDICAL ETHICS.

FERTILITY CONTROL. The control of fertility, which can be achieved by preventing pregnancy using such means as sexual abstinence (which practically has very limited efficacy), **contraception**, or **sterilization**. Strictly speaking, **termination of pregnancy** is not a form of fertility control.

FETAL DEMISE. The **death** of a fetus in utero, either from natural causes or from **feticide**. Fetal demise is managed clinically by evacuating the contents of pregnancy from the woman's uterus.

FETAL PATIENT. *See* ETHICAL CONCEPT OF THE FETUS AS A PATIENT.

FETAL SURGERY. *See* MATERNAL-FETAL SURGERY.

FETAL TREATMENT. *See* MATERNAL-FETAL SURGERY; MATERNAL-FETAL TREATMENT.

FETAL VIABILITY. The ability of the fetus to exist ex utero albeit with full technologic support. The concept of fetal viability includes both biologic and technologic components. There is therefore no global gestational age at which fetal viability occurs. In developed or high-income countries, fetal viability occurs at approximately 24 weeks gestation when the fetus is not affected by **severe fetal anomalies**. Some understand the concept of viability to include only the biological capacity of an entity. In the clinical setting, this is an error. Some take the view that viability establishes the **moral status** of the fetus.

FETICIDE. The **killing** of a fetus in utero. This can be accomplished by passing a needle transabdominally into the fetal pericardium and injecting potassium chloride, which causes the fetal heart to stop, resulting in **fetal demise**. Feticide is performed as a component of **selective termination** of a multifetal pregnancy. **Ethical reasoning** about feticide focuses on whether it is **ethically permissible** or **ethically impermissible**. *See also* ABORTION; INDUCED ABORTION; TERMINATION OF PREGNANCY.

FETUS AS A PATIENT. *See* ETHICAL CONCEPT OF THE FETUS AS A PATIENT.

FIDELITY. A **virtue** that combines competence in a specific domain of human endeavor and the habit of putting first the **interests** of those on whose behalf one uses one's competence. Fidelity can therefore be understood as the habit of making the first two commitments of the **ethical concept of medicine as a profession**. A physician who practices according to the virtue of fidelity justifiably earns the **trust** of patients and, therefore, is a **fiduciary** of his or her patients.

FIDUCIARY. A social role that combines competence in a specific domain of human endeavor and the habit, or **virtue**, of putting first the **interests** of those on whose behalf one uses one's competence. A fiduciary holds these interests in **trust**. A physician becomes a fiduciary of his or her patients when the physician makes the three commitments of the **ethical concept of medicine as a profession**. **Fidelity** is therefore one of the constitutive **virtues** of being a fiduciary.

FILIAL PIETY. A core concept in the **moral philosophy** of **Confucius** (551–479 BCE). The **virtue** of filial piety requires every child to routinely follow the final decisions of their parents about how the child should behave. This does not rule out disagreement during a parent's **decision-making** process. Once a parental decision has been made, however, disagreement is to end and be replaced by obedience as a matter of strict **ethical obligation**.

"FIRST DO NO HARM". The assertion of the **ethical principle of nonmaleficence** as an **absolute ethical principle**. If nonmaleficence were an absolute ethical principle, almost everything that a physician does would become **ethically impermissible**. "First do no harm" should therefore not be used but replaced with "When at the limits of medicine to alter the course of **disability**, **disease**, **disorder**, or **injury**, proceed with caution, to prevent net clinical harm to the patient." In other words, the ethical principle of nonmaleficence should be invoked to responsibly manage the limits of the **ethical principle of beneficence**. The *Hippocratic Oath* is often cited as the source for "First do no harm," but no such language appears in the *Oath*. In *Epidemics* in the **Hippocratic Corpus**, the unknown author writes: "Declare the past, diagnose the present, foretell the future; practice these acts. As to diseases, make a habit of two things—to help or at least to do no harm." This is an invocation of the ethical principle of nonmaleficence to responsibly manage the limits of the ethical principle of beneficence.

FLETCHER, JOHN C. (1931–2004). American Episcopal priest and moral theologian. He was one of the founders of the field of **bioethics** in the United States. He served as first chief of bioethics at the Clinical Center of the United States National Institutes of Health in Bethesda, Maryland, where he developed **clinical ethics consultation** as a new field.

FLETCHER, JOSEPH (1905–1991). Protestant moral theologian and advocate of "situational ethics" (a version of act **utilitarianism**). A founder of the field of **bioethics** in the United States, he wrote *Morals and Medicine* (1954), emphasizing the patient's **rights**.

FLINT, AUSTIN (1812–1886). American physician and ethicist who defended the 1847 *Code of Medical Ethics* of the American Medical Association from its critics. He wrote *Medical Ethics and Medical Etiquette: The Code of Ethics Adopted by the American Medical Association with Commentaries by Austin Flint, M.D.* (1882). He understood **medical ethics** to constitute rules of conduct for physicians, including their deportment. For there to be a profession of medicine, these rules have to be the same for all physicians, meaning that **professional medical ethics** is not a function of the idiosyncratic **judgments** of individual physicians, a crucial feature of professional medical ethics and therefore for a national association of physicians such as the American Medical Association. *See also* CODE OF ETHICS; PILCHER, LEWIS (1845–1934); PROFESSIONAL MEDICAL ETHICS.

FLYTING. A common practice as late as the 18th century in Britain in which one physician would publicly attack another as incompetent, dangerous, drunk, and such, in a broadside that would be distributed free to passersby. **Thomas Percival (1740–1804) judged** this practice **ethically impermissible** in his *Medical Ethics* (Percival 1803). Like **John Gregory** (1724–1773), Percival argued that disagreements among physicians should be resolved on scientific grounds. In contemporary **clinical practice**, physicians can sometimes express disagreement in the patient's record, which is known as **"dueling in the chart"** and is considered ethically impermissible because it is based on **mere self-interest** and also can jeopardize the safety and quality of patient care.

FORCED CESAREAN DELIVERY. Cesarean delivery performed for maternal or fetal benefit despite the **informed refusal** of the pregnant **patient**, in violation of the **ethical principle of respect for autonomy**. This does not include performing this surgery on a physically resistant patient, because such surgery would be unsafe and therefore **ethically impermissible** on **beneficence**-based grounds. *See also* COERCED CESAREAN DELIVERY; RIGHT TO REFUSE TREATMENT.

FORCED STERILIZATION. Sterilization performed without the **informed consent** and overriding the **right to refuse** of the **patient** but without a threat. *See also* COERCED STERILIZATION; INVOLUNTARY STERILIZATION.

45 CFR 46. The United States federal regulation that is to be implemented by **Institutional Review Boards** (IRBs) in fulfilling their oversight responsibilities for **human subjects research**. Part A is referred to as the "**Common Rule**." This regulation includes definitions of key terms and requirements that must be met by clinical investigators in their protocols and implementation of protocols and for an IRB to approve and monitor research with human subjects. While all IRBs must follow 45 CFR 46, they are free to interpret its requirements as they apply locally. This results in variation in IRB processes and approvals, even across multiple IRBs that exist in healthcare organizations that conduct many clinical research studies. This variation reflects the delegation downward that is a hallmark of federalism in the United States and is therefore **health policy** and **public policy**. This variation is also a source of frustration for clinical investigators in large healthcare organizations with multiple IRBs and for investigators who participate in multi-center trials and the variation among IRBs across participating centers.

The new, expanded version of this federal regulation took effect in mid-January 2018. Major changes focus on improvements in the **informed consent process** (Menikoff, Kaneshiro, and Pritchard 2017). *See also THE BELMONT REPORT*; ETHICS OF HUMAN SUBJECTS RESEARCH; OFFICE FOR HUMAN RESEARCH PROTECTIONS; REGULATORY LAW.

"FOUR BOX" APPROACH. A method of **casuistry** that aims for comprehensive **ethical reasoning** about clinical cases by requiring in all cases identification and evaluation of "Medical Indications," "Patient Preferences," "**Quality of Life**," and "Contextual Features" (Jonsen, Siegler, and Winslade 2010).

FRAMING EFFECT. Presenting information in the **informed consent process** with the goal of influencing the **patient**'s process of **decision making** toward a specific decision. This can be done, for example, by emphasizing clinical benefit and de-emphasizing clinical harm. This is a form of **manipulation** that seeks to influence the exercise of the patient's **autonomy** without controlling the patient's decision making and thus making it involuntary. Given its potential for abuse and thus violation of the **ethical principle of respect for autonomy**, making framing effects **ethically controversial**. *See also* NUDGE.

FRANK, JOHANN PETER (1745–1821). German physician and hygienist. He wrote *System einer vollständigen medicinischen Polizei* (*A System of Complete Medical Police*, 1779). In this book, Frank called for government officials to monitor the public's health by measuring not just clinical activity (e.g., childbirth) but also social factors such as housing and prevention of accidents that can harm the public's health. His is one of the first comprehensive **public health ethics**. A distinctive component of **medical police** is the physician's primary **ethical obligation** to the state or monarch to improve public health in the interest of the monarch or state in a healthy population for such purposes as commerce and warfare, which influenced **medical ethics** in the Soviet Union (1917–1989). *See also OATH OF THE SOVIET PHYSICIAN.*

FUTILE. A general concept used to characterize **clinical management**. Its outcome is not reliably expected to occur in **deliberative clinical judgment**. *See also* FUTILITY.

FUTILITY. A general concept used to characterize **clinical management**. Its outcome is not reliably expected to occur in **deliberative clinical judgment**. This general concept has little **clinical applicability**. To make it clinically applicable, it needs to be specified with respect for "not reliably expected" and "outcome." Some set "not reliably expected" at 100 percent failure rate, which is the most demanding specification. Others set "not reliably expected" at 97–100 percent failure rate for highly morbid, low success interventions such as **cardiopulmonary resuscitation** performed on gravely ill patients.

Invoking a concept of futility without specifying the failure rate of the clinical management in question is unacceptable in **ethical analysis** because this lack of specification fails to fulfill the requirement that concepts be clearly formulated. There are seven specifications of futility: **anatomic futility**, **imminent demise futility**, **interactive capacity futility**, **physiologic futility**, **quality-of-life futility**, **qualitative futility**, and **quantitative futility**. In **clinical ethical judgment**, a form of clinical management that is judged to be futile in one or more of these seven **specifications** is not a **medically reasonable alternative**. There is, therefore, no **ethical obligation** in the **informed consent process** to offer or perform such clinical management. When such clinical management will result in iatrogenic burdens of **pain**, **distress**, or **suffering**, the physician should recommend against it.

The physician should respond respectfully to requests for futile clinical management in cases that meet one or more of these seven specifications, and the physician should explain in what sense the clinical management is judged to be futile and the evidence base for doing so, followed by a recommendation against it. Requests for clinical management are expressions of a **positive right**. Positive rights always come with limits. Because providing clinical management that is judged to be futile in one or more of these seven specifications is inconsistent with the **professional virtue of integrity**, the physician should not provide such clinical management. Organizational leaders have an ethical obligation to create and implement organizational policy that sustains and does not undermine professional integrity. *See also* END-OF-LIFE CARE.

G

GALEN (130–120). Greek physician and philosopher. His medical texts influenced the history of medicine for centuries. He wrote commentaries on ethics in the **Hippocratic Corpus** and *That the Best Physician is Also a Philosopher*. He acknowledges Hippocratic texts and then builds on them. For example, he interprets the admonition from *Epidemics*, "As to diseases, make a habit of two things—to help or at least to do no harm," to mean that the physician should think through clinically challenging cases, identifying an implication of what is now known as the **ethical principle of beneficence** for **clinical judgment**.

GENDER. The social construction of **sex** in gender identity and relationships. Gender displays wide variation and can change during an individual's lifetime. Some take the view that gender is constrained to varying degrees by human biology. Some take the view that gender is not constrained by human biology. The **biopsychosocial** view of gender accepts that there are biological constraints that currently are incompletely understood. *See also* DISORDERS OF SEXUAL DEVELOPMENT; INTERSEX CONDITION.

GENDER IDENTITY DISORDER. Also known as "gender dysphoria." This condition is a **disorder** that manifests in a persistent identification with the **gender** opposite to the **sex** of a **patient**. This condition is incompletely understood in its **biopsychosocial** dimensions (e.g., the biological origins and constraints of this condition). In adolescents, this condition can be nondurable. These factors make the process of **pediatric assent** and the **informed permission** of parents challenging.

GENE EDITING. Removing and replacing genome sequences by a new technology, Clustered Regularly Interspaced Short Palindromic Repeats (CRISPR). The use of the term *editing* suggests that this technology is precise and has the capacity to control human biology; both of these claims are dubious from the perspective of the history of medicine because such beliefs have a weak evidence base. Consequently, such beliefs should be regarded as

enthusiasm. CRISPR is also a form of germ-line engineering, raising ethical issues about unknown risk that could affect future individuals who cannot provide **informed consent** for such exposure to risk. Gene editing is new and has not been well studied in animal, much less human, models. Whether it should be considered **ethically permissible** or **ethically impermissible** is ethically uncertain. *See also* GENETIC ENGINEERING; GERM LINE GENETIC/GENOMIC ENGINEERING; SOMATIC CELL GENETIC/GENOMIC ENGINEERING.

GENERAL PROHIBITION AGAINST KILLING A PATIENT. Professional medical ethics is grounded, among other sources, in the **beneficence**-based **ethical obligation** of the physician to protect and promote the health-related interests of the **patient. Killing** a **patient** is, on its face, not compatible with this ethical obligation. This means that both **voluntary active euthanasia, involuntary active euthanasia**, and **feticide** after **viability** are **ethically controversial**. *See also* EUTHANASIA.

GENETHICS. Ethical reasoning about the science, **clinical research**, and **clinical practice** of genetics and genomics.

GENETIC COUNSELING. Providing information to a patient about a genetic diagnosis or risk assessment by a master's level counselor, a doctoral-level geneticist, or a medical geneticist (physician). The information may include diagnostic information (e.g., about a developmental disorder in a child), risk assessment (e.g., for increased risk of forms of cancer), pharmacogenomics (affecting selection and dosing of drugs), and reproductive risk. Historically, genetic counseling has been a component of **prenatal genetic diagnosis**. Because the decision to remain pregnant when a genetic fetal anomaly has been detected before the gestational age of **viability** is not a medical but personal decision about which the genetic counselor has no professional expertise, the **norm** was **non-directive counseling**. This norm, however, should not be universalized to all the results of genetic or genomic analysis, because **directive counseling** will be **ethically justified** in many cases, for example, recommending preventive measures to mitigate increased risk of disease, or recommending change in medication or dosing of an already prescribed medication. *See also* PRENATAL DIAGNOSIS.

GENETIC ENGINEERING. There are two basic forms of genetic engineering. The first is the use of genetic technologies to alter the genes of somatic cells to improve the **clinical management** and outcomes of **disability, disease, disorders**, or **injury** in an individual **patient**. This is known as **somatic cell genetic/genomic engineering**. The second is alteration of germ cells to improve the clinical management and outcomes of disability, disease, or injury in an individual patient and that patient's genetic descendants. This is known as **germ line genetic/genomic engineering**. Somatic cell engineering has the potential to reduce the burden of disability, disease, disorder, or injury for an individual patient whereas germ cell engineering has the potential to reduce this burden for a population of patients. Ethical concerns about genetic engineering include unknown short-term and long-term risk resulting from genetic material being inserted in the wrong place or functioning incorrectly. There is **ethical controversy** about germ-line engineering because future patients are not able to provide **informed consent** to being placed at risk, including potentially clinically unmanageable risk.

GENETIC INFORMATION NONDISCRIMINATION ACT. Federal **statutory law** enacted in 2008 in the United States, known as GINA. "The purpose of the act is to prohibit discrimination on the basis of genetic information with respect to health insurance and employment" (https://www.eeoc.gov/laws/statutes/gina.cfm, accessed 14 September 2017). *See also* INVIDIOUS DISCRIMINATION; JUSTICE.

GENITAL MUTILATION. Mutilation of female genitalia. In other words, it is the surgical alteration of a girl's or woman's anatomy that results in **biopsychosocial** harm, as judged in **deliberative clinical judgment**, that is not offset by biopsychosocial goods, as determined in deliberative clinical judgment or as judged from that individual's perspective, including cultural or religious perspective. The risk of harm is increased when the surgery is performed by someone not qualified to do so and without appropriate infection control. Like other forms of mutilation, genital mutilation is **ethically impermissible**.

GENOME SEQUENCING. The mapping of the genome in part (whole exome sequencing, mapping the active coding regions of the genome) or in its entirety (whole genome sequencing). The results of such sequencing include diagnoses (including unexpected diagnoses not related to the reason for ordering sequencing, known as "incidental findings"); risk assessment (including unexpected risk assessment); reproductive risk assessment; pharmacogenomics with implications for choice of medications and their dosing; and variants of currently uncertain clinical significance (i.e., previously unreported alleles of genes known or suspected to be associated with **disability** or **disease**). These results may have clinical implications for other individuals genetically related to the patient whose genome has been sequenced. These results present challenges to the **informed consent process** and to the limits of the professional **ethical obligation** of **confidentiality**, especially when the implications for the health of others are serious, far-reaching, and irreversible. Professional associations such as the American College of Medical Genetics and Genomics (http://www.acmg.net, accessed 14 September 2017) and American Society of Human Genetics (http://www.ashg.org, accessed 14 September 2017) have provided guidance for **research** and **clinical practice**. *See also* GENETHICS.

GENOMIC ETHICS. Ethical reasoning about the science, **clinical research**, and **clinical practice** of genomics. *See also* GENETHICS.

"GEORGETOWN MANTRA". This phrase is used to characterize the four-principle approach to **bioethics** and **medical ethics** that appeals to the **ethical principle of beneficence**, the **ethical principle of nonmaleficence**, the **ethical principle of respect for autonomy**, and the **ethical principle of justice**. The phrase is meant to have negative connotations for two main reasons. The four principles are deployed in a formulaic way, rather than in the disciplined approach required by **ethical reasoning**. In addition, the exclusive focus on ethical principles, resulting in omission altogether of **virtues**, is an inadequate approach.

The use of *Georgetown* in the phrase references the fact that Tom L. Beauchamp, coauthor of ***Principles of Biomedical Ethics***, made his academic career at Georgetown University in Washington, DC, in the **Kennedy Institute of Ethics** and the Department of Philosophy. The use of *mantra*, however, is a distortion of *Principles of Biomedical Ethics*. From its first edition (Beauchamp and Childress 1979) to its most current, seventh edition (Beauchamp and Childress 2013), this book has emphasized that both ethical principles and virtues must be included in ethical reasoning in bioethics and rejects formulaic application of principles and virtues to cases. *See also* PRINCIPLISM.

GERIATRIC ASSENT. Decision making with and for a geriatric (65 years of age and older) **patient** with diminished **decision-making capacity**. The patient should be asked by the **surrogate** and the healthcare team what is important to him or her, to identify his or her values, and these should be considered by the surrogate and care team. The importance of these values to the patient, especially as they bear on the patient's current and future **quality of life**, should be weighed in the context of the **prima facie ethical obligation** to protect the life and health of the patient. Both of these clinically ethically significant considerations must be taken into account and weighed against each other, to meet the **substituted judgment standard** of **surrogate decision making**. *See also* ASSENT.

GERIATRIC ETHICS. Ethical reasoning about the **professional ethics** of **clinical practice, clinical research,** and education about **patients** aged 65 and older.

GERM LINE GENETIC/GENOMIC ENGINEERING. The use of techniques to alter the portions of the genome that are thought to cause a **patient's disease** or **disorder** and that will also reduce or eliminate the risk of disease in germ cells, which will affect genetic descendants. Germ line engineering has the potential to reduce the burden of disability, disease, or injury for an individual patient and for the entire population of that patient's genetic descendants. The ethical concerns about genetic engineering include unknown short-term and long-term risk resulting from genetic material being inserted in the wrong place or functioning incorrectly. There is **ethical controversy** about germ line engineering, including its short-term and long-term safety and the inability of future individuals to consent to being placed at risk, especially unknown right. When in **deliberative clinical judgment,** such intervention is expected to result in net clinical benefit, it becomes a **medically reasonable alternative** that should be offered to the patient in the **informed consent process.** Germ line engineering undertaken as **innovation** or **research** may be offered only after it has been prospectively reviewed for its scientific, clinical, and **ethical justification;** an acceptable level of risk; and its informed consent process. *See also* GENETHICS; SOMATIC CELL GENETIC/GENOMIC ENGINEERING.

GHOST SURGERY. Performing surgery on another physician's **patient,** by agreement with that physician without the **consent** of the patient. In **professional medical ethics,** this practice is an egregious violation of the ethical **norm** of requiring **informed consent** for surgical procedures. *See also* DECEPTION.

GIFTS FROM INDUSTRY. Until the 1990s in the United States, while there were critics of physicians and trainees accepting gifts from the pharmaceutical and device manufacturers industries—including pens, clipboards, meals, textbooks (which can be very expensive); presentations from industry speakers bureaus; paid trips to attend industry-sponsored conferences—the practice was thought to be **ethically permissible** and was therefore widespread. Medical students led a national effort to stop this practice, and, as evidence mounted of system **bias** resulting from gifts ("irrational prescribing practices" was the conclusion of one study), the practice was considered to be **ethically impermissible** in **professional medical ethics.** Medical schools and teaching hospitals have adopted policies that prohibit direct gifts, and support for educational activities must be completely independent of industry control. The latter gifts must be "unrestricted educational grants" received by the organization, the course director must have complete **autonomy** over the program, the Office of Continuing Medical Education must prospectively review and approve such educational events to ensure that they will be free of bias, participants must be asked for their evaluation of presentations for industry bias (e.g., use of trade names for drugs rather than generic names), and all presenters must disclose their **conflicts of interest**. *See also* MERE SELF-INTEREST; SELF-INTEREST.

GINA. *See* GENETIC INFORMATION NONDISCRIMINATION ACT.

GISBORNE, THOMAS (1758–1846). English Anglican priest and moral theologian. His moral philosophy of role-based ethical obligations ("offices," from **Cicero**) influenced **Thomas Percival's** (1740–1804) medical ethics. He wrote *An Enquiry into the Duties of Men in the Higher and Middle Classes of Society in Great Britain Resulting from Their Respective Stations, Professions and Employment* (1794). Gisborne used the term *professions* to mean an occupation and not in the sense of **professional medical ethics**. These occupations comprised reciprocal obligations of the individual in a role (e.g., a gentleman or lord of an estate) and those subordinate to **power** that originates in that role (e.g., tenant farmers). The individual in power had a **role-related ethical obligation** to protect those subordinate to his power. This obligation used to go under the name of **paternalism**.

GOSSES. A concept from **Jewish moral theology** and **Jewish medical ethics** that refers to a **patient** who is actively **dying** (i.e., death is expected within three days). It is **ethically permissible** not to initiate or to discontinue **life-sustaining treatment** for such patients. *See also* END-OF-LIFE CARE.

GREGORY, JAMES (1753–1821). Physician and son of **John Gregory** (1724–1773). His critiques of the management of the **Royal Infirmary** of Edinburgh emphasized that the physician's primary commitment should be to patients and not the self, which is a central theme of his father's **medical ethics**. The **ethical obligation** of infirmary managers was to see to it that patients received **clinical management** supported in Baconian, **experience**-based **clinical judgment**, a nascent form of **healthcare justice**. *See also* PROFESSIONAL VIRTUE OF SELF-SACRIFICE.

GREGORY, JOHN (1724–1773). Professor of medicine (1766–1773) at the University of Edinburgh and First Physician to His Majesty the King (1765–1773); author of *Lectures on the Duties and Qualifications of a Physician* (1772), the first English-language text on **professional medical**

ethics. Gregory was born in Aberdeen, Scotland, into a family of distinguished academicians. As a student at the University of Edinburgh and Leiden in the Netherlands, he became immersed in the **philosophy of science** and **philosophy of medicine** of **Francis Bacon** (1561–1626). Bacon called for science and medicine to be based on the unbiased, carefully observed results of natural and controlled **experiments**. This was a nascent form of what is now known as **evidence-based medicine**.

When he was in medical practice in Aberdeen, he helped to found and participated actively in the Aberdeen Philosophical Society, a group of literate men in philosophy, theology, medicine, and science. In his presentations to the society, Gregory developed ideas that he incorporated into his *A Comparative View of the State and Faculties of Man with Those of the Animal World* (1765), which established him as a leading physician of the Scottish Enlightenment and helped him gain appointment in 1766 to the medical faculty of the University of Edinburgh. This group read **David Hume**'s (1711–1776) *Treatise of Human Nature*.

Hume described the *Treatise* in its subtitle as an "Attempt to Introduce the Experimental Method of Reasoning into Moral Subjects." The result was a Baconian "science of man" and "science of morals." Hume reports in the *Treatise* on his discoveries about "principles," real, constitutive processes by which human beings engage the world and each other. The principal discovery of Hume's moral science is the principle of **sympathy**: the capacity all of us have to enter directly into the lived experiences of others.

Gregory adapted Hume's principle of sympathy, wedded to Baconian scientific medicine, to create his **professional medical ethics**. While in medical practice in London in the 1760s, Gregory attended the intellectual salons for men and women sponsored by Elizabeth Montagu (1718–1800), a wealthy widow who championed the intellectual development of women at a time when women were denied formal education. Her goal was to create an environment in which men and women could be intellectually intimate without the frisson of sexual attraction. Intellectually serious women were women of learning and virtue. Such women, exemplified for Gregory by Mrs. Montagu and his own wife, a gifted mathematician, became the exemplars of the sympathetic physician described in Gregory's *Lectures on the Duties and Qualifications of a Physician* in 1772. Women of learning and virtue were exemplars of the virtues of **tenderness** and **steadiness**: the self-disciplined, affective engagement with the joys and sorrows of others. Gregory adapted these virtues as the regulators of sympathy, to prevent overreaction and underreaction to the plight of patients. This **feminine ethics**, in which women of learning and virtue are the role models for all to follow, shaped Gregory's *A Father's Legacy to His Daughters*, published posthumously in 1774 and in many subsequent editions well into the 19th century. *Lectures* can be read as his legacy to his medical students and future physicians. Gregory is regarded as an inventor, along with **Thomas Percival** (1740–1804), of professional medical ethics. *See also* ETHICAL CONCEPT OF MEDICINE AS A PROFESSION.

GRISWOLD CASE. *Griswold v. Connecticut* (381 U.S. 479), decided by the United States Supreme Court in 1965, struck down state restrictions on access to **contraception** by married couples. The majority opinion by Associate Justice William O. Douglas articulated the constitutional **right to privacy** in reproductive **decision making**. The word *privacy* does not appear in the United States Constitution or Bill of Rights and thus is not an enumerated right. It is, instead, a right inferred by sections of the Constitution. Justice Douglas described these inferences as "penumbra" (*Latin*: shadows). The inferential right to privacy in reproductive decision making was thus introduced on controversial constitutional grounds. The 1973 decisions of the United States Supreme Court in the companion cases of *Roe v. Wade* (410 U.S. 113) and *Doe v. Bolton* (410 U.S. 179) invoked the constitutional right to privacy of pregnant women to make decisions about the disposition of pregnancy with their physicians and thus inherited the controversy about the right to privacy in constitutional law. *See also* ABORTION.

GRISWOLD V. CONNECTICUT. *See* GRISWOLD CASE.

GRONINGEN PROTOCOL. A procedure proposed by two Dutch physicians for **euthanasia** of infants, with the meaning of **killing** them, or performing **involuntary active euthanasia**, when the infant has "serious disorders or deformities associated with suffering that cannot be alleviated and for whom there is no hope of improvement" (Verhagen and Sauer 2005, 959). This proposal for **ethically justified** infanticide remains **ethically controversial**. The authors elsewhere reported that the Protocol was used to perform **infanticide** on a series of patients with spina bifida, a condition that does not cause suffering that cannot be alleviated and that can be improved with surgery and physical therapy.

GUT FEELINGS. Vague, sometimes inchoate sense or feeling that a character trait or behavior is **ethically impermissible, ethically obligatory**, or **ethically permissible**. This is sometimes also known as the "yuck factor," a kind of instinctual reaction that a character trait or behavior is ethically impermissible. Gut feelings constitute an unreliable source of **ethical reasoning** in that they do not meet the criterion of **clarity** in ethical reasoning and are also at risk of reflecting nothing more than bias or even attitudes of **invidious discrimination**. The ancient Greek philosopher Plato (427–347 BCE) taught that such feelings or instinctual reactions should be rigorously

Content

examined for ethical concepts that they may be invoking. If ethical reasoning clarifies these concepts and identifies their implications, these concepts can guide ethical reasoning and the gut feeling should be put aside as **mere opinion**. If this does not turn out to be the case, the discipline of ethical reasoning requires that gut feelings be ignored.

GUY DE CHAULIAC (1290–1370). French physician. He wrote medical ethics based on the requirement that the physician be **competent**, which benefits the sick.

GYNECOLOGICAL ETHICS. Ethical reasoning about the **professional ethics** of **clinical practice, clinical research**, and education in women's health.

H

HARM PRINCIPLE. A **beneficence**-based **ethical principle** that places justified limits on the exercise of an individual's **autonomy** when the behavior of that individual is reliably predicted to result in harm to the **interests** of others. The strength of the harm principle is a function of three ethically significant dimensions of harm: whether the harm is serious (**legitimate self-interests** are put at risk), far-reaching (many forms of legitimate self-interest are put at risk), and irreversible (loss of **health** that cannot be restored to the *status quo ante*, permanent **disability**, or **death**). The stronger the reliably predicted harm is in each of these three dimensions, the stronger the **ethical justification** for the restriction on the individual's autonomy. This ethical reasoning can support the **judgment** that the behavior in question is **ethically impermissible**. *See also* ETHICAL PRINCIPLE OF NONMALEFICENCE; PRECAUTIONARY PRINCIPLE.

THE HASTINGS CENTER. Founded in 1969 as part of the Institute of Society, Ethics, and the Life Sciences (no longer used), by the philosopher Daniel Callahan and the physician Willard Gaylin, the Hastings Center is a private, nonsectarian, independent research center to support and promote interdisciplinary study in what became the field of **bioethics**. The center publishes the journals titled *Hastings Center Report* and *IRB*. *See also* KENNEDY INSTITUTE OF ETHICS.

HAYS, ISAAC (1796–1879). American physician and ethicist. He played a leading role in creating the **American Medical Association** *Code of Medical Ethics* **of 1847**. He was a social contractarian, a political philosophy that influenced the 1847 *Code*'s reasoning that the freely assumed **ethical obligations** of physicians to **patients** and to society created **rights** of physicians to expect that patients and society would do their part to enable physicians to fulfill these freely assumed ethical obligations. These derivative rights create ethical obligations of patients and society to cooperate with physicians in **patient care** and **public health**. *See also* BELL, JOHN (1796–1872); CODE OF ETHICS.

HEALTH, CONCEPT OF. Health comprises normal anatomy and physiology, including neurophysiology, as well as psychological and social well-being (Engel 1977). There is disagreement in the **philosophy of medicine** literature on whether the concept of health is value free (based on observed normal structure and function) or value laden (taking *normal* to include value judgments). The World Health Organization has put forth a concept of health that is of very wide scope: Health is "a state of complete physical, mental, and social well-being and not merely the absence of disease or infirmity" (World Health Organization 1948). One goal of this ambitious definition is to strengthen appeals to high-resource countries to support healthcare services and education in low-resource countries. *See also* CONDITION; DISABILITY; DISEASE; DISORDER; INJURY.

HEALTH INSURANCE PORTABILITY AND ACCOUNTABILITY ACT (HIPAA). Federal **statutory law** and **regulatory law** that implements the statute that provides protection for the **privacy** of protected health information. *See also* HEALTH POLICY; PUBLIC POLICY.

HEALTH LAW. Administrative law, common law, and **statutory law** applied to matters of health and healthcare, broadly understood. This scope includes regulation of **clinical practice, clinical research,** approval of new drugs and devices, and food safety. Health law has been and continues to be an important component in the development of **bioethics.** *See also* HEALTH POLICY.

HEALTH POLICY. Requirements from governments (e.g., U.S. Public Health Service) and guidance from nongovernmental organizations (e.g., American Hospital Association, Pan-American Health Organization, World Health Organization) and professional associations of physicians (e.g., American Medical Association) about **health,** healthcare practices, and **research** of individuals, healthcare organizations, businesses, and governments. In the federal system of the United States, health policy is made by city, county, state, and federal governments in the form of **common law** (e.g., **abortion** policy), **regulatory law** (e.g., approval of new drugs and devices by the U.S. Food and Drug Administration), and **statutory law** (restrictions on use of federal funds to pay for **induced abortion**). As a general rule, what is not explicitly prohibited in health policy is permissible. **Ethical reasoning** about what health policy ought to be typically appeals to the **ethical principle of justice,** to address the healthcare needs of populations of **patients.** The size of these populations and the cost of meeting their clinical needs usually outstrips the capacity of **charity care** in a community. *See also* PUBLIC POLICY.

HEALTHCARE DISPARITIES. Differences in economic status, ethnicity, gender, geography, race, religion, and sex that adversely affect **access to healthcare** and that are allowed by physicians to introduce **bias** into **clinical judgment**, resulting in uncontrolled variation in the processes and therefore outcomes of **patient care**. Uncontrolled variation in the processes and outcomes of **clinical management** is the antithesis of **quality** and is, therefore, **ethically impermissible** in **professional medical ethics** and as a matter of justice, especially **egalitarian justice, healthcare justice**, and **Rawlsian justice**. Healthcare organizations, therefore, have an **ethical obligation** to identify and eliminate, by progressively reducing the incidence of, healthcare disparities. *See also* ETHICAL PRINCIPLE OF JUSTICE; EVIDENCE-BASED MEDICINE.

HEALTHCARE ETHICS CONSULTATION. *See* CLINICAL ETHICS CONSULTATION.

HEALTHCARE JUSTICE. A **specification** of the **ethical principle of justice** for **clinical practice, clinical research**, and for the organization and financing of clinical practice and research that requires that each **patient** be provided **clinical management** supported in **deliberative clinical judgment**. Healthcare justice puts a strong emphasis on the **quality** of patient care and, therefore, the **ethical obligation** of physicians and other healthcare professionals to continuously improve the quality of **patient care**.

HEALTHCARE REFORM. A movement in **health policy** in the United States to improve access (by providing sources of payment for all), **quality** and, by improving quality, responsibly manage costs (i.e., lower the rate of inflation of healthcare services to make such increases predictable and affordable for both private and public payers). These were the three goals of the Affordable Care Act (also known as "Obama Care"), enacted by Congress and signed into law by President Obama in 2010. *See also* PUBLIC POLICY; RIGHT TO HEALTHCARE.

HEALTHCARE SYSTEM. A centrally organized, led, funded, and coordinated **clinical management** of patients in multiple settings and facilities. In the United States, Veterans Health Affairs and the Medical Corps of the armed services are healthcare systems. However, overall in the United States, there are public and private payers, public and private providers, private payers that are affiliated with faith communities and that are secular, with no central organization, leadership, funding, or coordination. Despite its everyday use, the term *healthcare system* does not apply in the United States. It does in other countries, such as the National Health Service in the United

Kingdom. The American approach reflects the deeply held suspicion of concentrated power in both the private sphere (hence antitrust law) and the public sphere (separation of powers), which results in inefficiencies but which, it is believed, protects our freedom, especially the **negative right** against interference by potentially controlling public or private **power**. *See also* HEALTH POLICY.

HELA. An immortal cell line, originating in 1951, from cervical cancer cells of an African American **patient**, Ms. Henrietta Lacks. (The acronym is taken from the first two letters of her first and last names.) This was done without her knowledge or consent, at a time that predates by more than two decades **45 CFR 46**, the federal regulations for **human subjects research**. In 2013, the genome sequence was made and published without consent of Ms. Lacks's surviving family members. There is **ethical controversy** about consent for cells and other biological materials that are banked for future research, usually without identifiers but with links to the identity of the source kept separately. There is also ethical controversy about compensating a patient or a deceased patient's heirs for cell lines that generate significant income for the laboratory whose inventiveness and labor produced the cell line. *See also* ETHICS OF HUMAN SUBJECTS RESEARCH; INFORMED CONSENT; RESEARCH.

HELSINKI DECLARATION. *See* DECLARATION OF HELSINKI.

HEMODIALYSIS. A form of **life-sustaining treatment** to support or replace kidney function. *See also* DIALYSIS; END-OF-LIFE CARE.

HENRI DE MONDEVILLE (1260–1316). French surgeon and ethicist. Wrote one of the first texts on **surgical ethics**, included in his *Chirurgia* (1306), using intellectual and moral standards based on the concept of the conscientious, competent surgeon who helps the sick by providing surgical management only when it is needed. Second-rate surgeons can be readily recognized because they cater to the wishes of the wealthy without question, anticipating **John Gregory**'s (1724–1773) view in his **professional medical ethics** that the true physician treats poor and the wealthy **patients** alike.

HERZ, MARKUS (1747–1803). German physician and philosopher. He is the probable author of the "Oath of Maimonides" and "The Daily Prayer of a Physician," attributed to **Maimonides** (1135–1204).

HETERONOMY. A state of being under controlling **power** of another individual, an organization, or the state. This means that an individual has lost his or her **autonomy**. This can occur, for example, when a **patient** is subject to a physician's **medical paternalism**. *See also* INVOLUNTARY; VOLUNTARY.

HINDU BIOETHICS. Bioethics based on **Hindu moral theology**, drawing on such sources as *Caraka Samhitā* and *Suśruta-Samhitā* (Young 2009a, 2009c), thus contributing to the pluralism of bioethics.

HINDU MEDICAL ETHICS. Medical ethics based on **Hindu moral theology**, drawing on such sources as *Caraka Samhitā* and *Suśruta-Samhitā*. Moral theology, because it is not secular, is not methodologically adequate to serve as the basis of **professional medical ethics**. One aspect of Hindu medical ethics transcends this limitation: the effort of *brāhmaṇa* practitioners to distinguish themselves from those they took to be irregulars or **quacks**. They did so by appealing to the idea of a real physician's behavior, which should be based on **virtues** such as benevolence and prudence (Young 2009a, 2009c).

HINDU MORAL THEOLOGY. Ethical reasoning drawing on such sources as *Caraka Samhitā* and *Suśruta-Samhitā*. Moral theology, because it is not secular, is not methodologically adequate to serve as the basis of **professional medical ethics**.

HIPAA. *See* HEALTH INSURANCE PORTABILITY AND ACCOUNTABILITY ACT (HIPAA).

HIPPOCRATES (460–370 BCE). Greek physician and ethicist to whom is attributed the **Hippocratic Corpus**, including the *Hippocratic Oath*, *The Art*, and *Epidemics*.

HIPPOCRATIC CORPUS. A collection of texts written from the late fifth to the early fourth centuries BCE, on clinical and ethical topics in medicine produced by multiple authors and attributed to Hippocrates. It is not known which of these texts, if any, Hippocrates himself wrote. This collection includes writings on **medical ethics**, especially the *Hippocratic Oath*, *The Art*, and *Epidemics*.

The Art is notable for its admonition not to continue treatment when disease has "overmastered" the sick individual, to avoid the "madness" of such treatment. In contemporary clinical practice, when treatment of a gravely ill patient is described as "crazy," this ancient text is invoked. *Epidemics* is mistakenly cited as the origin of the dictum **"First do no harm"** (later Latinized as ***Primum non nocere***). The text reads: "Declare the past, diagnose the present, foretell the future; practice these acts. As to diseases, make a habit of two things—to help or at least to do no harm." The primary ethical obligation of the physician to the sick individual is beneficence based, to help the patient. When reaching the limits of **clinical management** to alter the course of a disease or injury, the physician has an ethical obligation, based in the ethical principle of nonmaleficence, not to provide clinical management that results in net clinical harm to the sick individual. The clinical texts in the Hippocratic Corpus include descriptions of the natural history of **diseases** and **injuries** and the therapeutic minimalism of treatment of them, to avoid the physician being blamed for bad outcomes, including especially **death**. *See also* HIPPOCRATIC TRADITION.

HIPPOCRATIC OATH. The author is unknown, but the *Oath* is attributed to Hippocrates. The *Oath* was probably created to address the problem of a shortage of sons of the Koan School physicians and the need to bring non-kinfolk into the guild, who could not be presumed to be loyal (Jouanna 1999). The *Oath* can therefore be read as a guild oath and not an oath of **professional medical ethics**.

The *Oath* starts with a promise to uphold a "written covenant" of loyalty to teachers and to preserve the "art" (translation of *techné*) of medicine, the unchanging and unchangeable body of knowledge about the four humors and the clinical management of disease and injury. The *Oath* contains a number of prescriptions (e.g., to maintain confidentiality) and proscriptions (against the use of a pessary to induce abortion, because of its danger of causing the pregnant woman to die and not because of the moral status of the fetus) with no supporting **ethical justification** for them (von Staden 1996, 2009).

The *Oath* was sworn for centuries, with a Christian version introduced early in the Common Era. The *Oath* fell out of favor in the early centuries of the Common Era (Nutton 2009). *See also* HIPPOCRATIC TRADITION; *OATH ACCORDING TO HIPPOCRATES, IN SO FAR AS A CHRISTIAN MAY SWEAR IT.*

HIPPOCRATIC TRADITION. The view in much of the literature of **bioethics** and **medical ethics** that there is an unbroken history from ancient Greece to the 20th century of Hippocratic **beneficence** and **medical paternalism** that has been corrected by the introduction by bioethicists of the **ethical principle of respect for autonomy** and the **rights** that this principle generates. Scholars have recently shown that there is, in fact, no continuous history of reference to the **Hippocratic Corpus**, especially the ***Hippocratic***

Oath (Nutton 2009), and no continuous history of adopting medical paternalism as a **norm** (McCullough 2011). The concept of a Hippocratic Tradition should therefore be regarded as historical fiction.

HISTORY OF MEDICAL ETHICS. The scholarly study of the various literatures of **medical ethics** and **professional medical ethics** throughout history, including written and oral sources, in all cultures and nations of the world. One of the first histories of Western medical ethics appears in the *Manual of Medical Jurisprudence* (Ryan 1831) by the Irish physician Michael Ryan (1800–1840). It is noteworthy that the first edition of the *Encyclopedia of Bioethics* (Reich 1978), the major reference work for **bioethics** that consolidated the new field and propelled it forward, contains a large section, "Medical Ethics, History of." The entries covered both Western and non-Western medical ethics. This proposed a self-understanding of bioethics as including the history of medical ethics. This section has been revised and expanded in subsequent editions, including the current edition (Jennings 2014). There has recently appeared the first global history of medical ethics (Baker and McCullough 2009a). Refer to the introduction and bibliography.

HIV. *See* HUMAN IMMUNODEFICIENCY VIRUS.

HOCHE, ALFRED (1865–1943). German physician and advocate, with Karl Binding (1841–1920), of **voluntary active euthanasia** and **involuntary active euthanasia** of patients whose lives had no value for others. Their *Die Freigabe der Vernichtung lebensunwerten Lebens* (*The Release and Destruction of Life Devoid of Value*, 1920) became part of the justificatory framework for the crimes against humanity carried out in Nazi Germany during World War II. *See also* NAZI MEDICAL WAR CRIMES.

HOFFMANN, FRIEDRICH (1660–1738). German physician and ethicist in the "*medicus politicus*" tradition. This tradition provides an account of the ethics of the physician who is subordinate to the power of those who employed him, based on the virtue of **prudence**, interpreted by Hoffmann as enlightened **self-interest**. By this, he meant that the physician should incorporate into his conception of self-interest the interests of the patient (e.g., respectful, chaste relationships with female patients). Prudence-based **clinical practice** was essential because physicians were subordinate to the **power** of the well-to-do who could afford a physician's fees and to the power of government over municipal and court physicians. His *Medicus Politicus* (*The Politic Doctor*) was published in 1738.

HOMOSEXUALITY. Sexual orientation in which a man or woman is attracted to individuals of the same sex. Homosexuality was considered by the American Psychiatric Association (APA) to be a mental illness until, in 1973, the APA made the **deliberative clinical judgment** to abandon this position. Homosexuality was then removed from the APA's *Diagnostic and Statistical Manual*, on which psychiatrists and other mental health professionals based diagnosis and treatment planning. This was considered a major accomplishment in the then-emerging movement for the **rights** of homosexuals. It also created an **ethical controversy** about the concepts of **disease** and **disorder** and the **power** of those concepts in clinical discourse, **clinical management**, **health policy**, and **public policy**.

HONESTY. The **professional virtue** that creates an **ethical obligation** never to say anything false and only to say what is true to a **patient**. Discretion in timing of truthful disclosure is required, based on a **deliberative clinical judgment** that the patient would not be able to cope **biopsychosocially** with such disclosure and would therefore be harmed by it, a **beneficence**-based constraint known as **therapeutic privilege**. The risk in allowing for such discretion is that disclosure can be postponed to the point that a patient may lack **decision-making capacity** or from reasons of self-interest (i.e., avoiding the stress to the physician of giving a patient bad news). *See also* THERAPEUTIC PRIVILEGE; TRUTH-TELLING.

HOOKER, WORTHINGTON (1806–1872). American physician, educator, and ethicist. He wrote *Physician and Patient; or, A Practical View of the Mutual Duties, Relations and Interests of the Medical Profession and Community*, emphasizing the scientific practice of medicine combined with **professional virtues**. The Latinate version of "**First do no harm**," "or *Primum non Nocere*," is sometimes attributed to Hooker. *See also* ETHICAL PRINCIPLE OF NONMALEFICENCE.

HOPE. A concept with two components: (1) the desire for a future state of affairs (2) that has a probability greater than 0 and less than 1. If the probability of a future state of affairs is 1, one should expect it to occur. If the probability of a future state of affairs is 0, the desire for it becomes a false hope. The strength of the desire for a future state of affairs may be much stronger than low probability of its occurrence. It is not a false hope or a false belief for a **patient, surrogate**, or family member to desire a highly valued future state of affairs (e.g., surviving a grave, life-threatening condition, even when its probability is very, very small). Such hopes should not be taken away. Unfortunately, there is an **ethical obligation** of the physician to correct a false hope, respectfully and attentive to potential adverse **bio-**

psychosocial impact on the individual with the false hope. Hope for a very low probability state of affairs should not be considered or managed as a false belief or as irrational.

HOSPITAL. A healthcare organization that provides multiple levels of **clinical care**. The nature, risks, and complexity of its procedures require multi-specialty and multidisciplinary teams to responsibly manage patient care. Some hospitals have emergency centers, and some do not. In the United States, there are many kinds of hospitals. Hospitals can be private or public. Private hospitals can be not-for-profit (sometimes known as voluntary hospitals) or for-profit. Not-for-profit hospitals can be supported by faith communities or be nonsectarian or secular. For-profit hospitals can be owned by corporations or by physicians. There are myriad combinations of these classifications.

The not-for-profit, nonsectarian hospital is modeled on the Royal Infirmaries of the United Kingdom, which were established in the 18th century for the working sick poor and funded by annual contributions by their employers. In the 19th century, faith-community-sponsored private, not-for-private hospitals were established, partly as a matter of **moral theology** (i.e., the **ethical obligation** to care for the sick) and partly as a response to **invidious discrimination** against members of a faith community, especially physicians and nurses of faith. **James Gregory** (1753–1821), a Scottish physician who wrote a stinging critique of the management of the **Royal Infirmary** of Edinburgh, argued that the managers of the Royal Infirmary have an ethical obligation to see to it that every patient receives clinical management supported by the scientific judgments of physicians and surgeons. He thus based **organizational ethics** on **professional medical ethics**. In France, after the Revolution of 1789, hospitals replaced *Hôtel-Dieu* (**House of God**), which were sponsored by the Roman Catholic Church. A major ethical challenge for hospital leaders is to create and sustain an **organizational culture** based on **professional medical ethics**.

HOUSE OF GOD. Hospitals in France and Francophone countries that were sponsored by the Roman Catholic Church, known as *Hôtels-Dieu*. These were replaced by secular, private, not-for-profit hospitals. *Hôtel-Dieu* is the source of the title of Samuel Shem's *The House of God*, a satirical novel about interns (first-year residents) training in a major hospital in the urban Northeast of the United States (Shem 1978). This novel remains popular among American medical students and residents. *See also* HOSPITAL; ROYAL INFIRMARY.

HUFELAND, CHRISTIAN (1762–1836). German physician and ethicist. He wrote a **medical ethics** influenced by the German philosopher Immanuel Kant (1724–1804), emphasizing treating the patient as an end in himself or herself and not a mere object of experiments. Sustaining a good reputation is another basis for his medical ethic. He wrote *Enchiridion Medicum* (*Manual of the Practice of Medicine*, 1836), which influenced the development of Japanese medical ethics in the 19th century. Hufeland's medical ethics is distinctive for addressing the physician's **ethical obligation** to be aware of and control costs for the sick and for the state.

HUMAN EXPERIMENTATION. The performance of **experiments** on human beings. When experiments are well designed and conducted, with prospective oversight and approval, they should be classified as **research**. However, in the history of human experimentation, there are many examples of experiments that were not well designed and conducted or were conducted without prospective oversight, approval, or **informed consent**, including **innovations** in surgery and many of the experiments conducted by the **Nazi doctors**. Not all human experimentation is **human subjects research**. Sometimes, especially in the early period of **bioethics** in the 1970s, the terms *human experimentation* and *human subjects research* were used synonymously; this was—and remains—a conceptual error.

HUMAN GENOME PROJECT. A project funded by the U.S. National Institutes of Health to map the entire human genome. This scientific advance inaugurated the field of **genomic ethics**. *See also* ETHICAL, LEGAL, AND SOCIAL IMPLICATIONS (ELSI) RESEARCH PROGRAM; GENETHICS.

HUMAN IMMUNODEFICIENCY VIRUS. The virus that causes **acquired immune deficiency syndrome**.

HUMAN RIGHT. A **right** that all human beings possess in virtue of being human. As a consequence, human rights precede governments; their legitimacy is a function of their recognition and implementation of human rights. Human rights include **negative rights**, such as security of one's person, health, and property and freedom of expression, and **positive rights**, such the right to health and healthcare. An appeal to human rights supports a transnational, transcultural, and transreligious approach to **medical ethics** and **bioethics**. Some philosophically ground human rights in **natural rights** and others, such as the United Nations **Universal Declaration of Human Rights**, take a pragmatic approach (McKeon 1948). *See also* UNIVERSAL DECLARATION OF HUMAN RIGHTS AND BIOETHICS.

HUMAN RIGHTS BIOETHICS. Bioethics based on **human rights**. The United Nations Educational, Scientific and Cultural Organization (better known as UNESCO) published the **Universal Declaration of Human Rights and Bioethics** in 2005 (United Nations Educational, Scientific and Cultural Organization 2005). *See also* UNIVERSAL DECLARATION OF HUMAN RIGHTS.

HUMAN SUBJECTS RESEARCH. Research performed with humans, either to advance science or to improve the care of human **patients**. Human subjects research in **ethically permissible** only when it has received prospective review and approval by an **Institutional Review Board** (United States) or **Research Ethics Committee** (other countries). *See also* ETHICS OF HUMAN SUBJECTS RESEARCH.

HUMANAE VITAE (OF HUMAN LIFE). An **encyclical** issued by Pope Paul VI (1897–1978; papacy: 1963–1978) of the Roman Catholic Church in 1968, upholding the traditional prohibition in **Roman Catholic moral theology** of artificial **contraception** as contrary to **natural law**. Many members of this faith community ignored this teaching and continue to do so.

HUME, DAVID (1711–1776). Scottish moral scientist, philosopher, historian, and diplomat. In his *Treatise of Human Nature* (Hume 1739), he reports the scientific discovery and mechanism of the principle of **sympathy**, the natural capacity of all human beings to enter into the affective life of others and that motivates us to respond to the **pain, distress,** and **suffering** of others. In his moral philosophy, he identifies virtues that should regulate sympathy. Hume's **moral science** and **moral philosophy** of sympathy become the basis for the **professional medical ethics** of **John Gregory** (1724–1773). Hume also argued that **suicide** is **ethically permissible** as a way to avoid suffering at the end of life. *See also AEQUANIMITAS*; EMPATHY.

I

IACUC. *See* INSTITUTIONAL ANIMAL CARE AND USE COMMITTEE (IACUC).

IBERO-AMERICAN BIOETHICS PROGRAM. A research and teaching center for **medical humanities** founded in La Plata, Argentina, at the Institute for the Medical Humanities of the José María Mainetti Foundation, by Dr. José Alberto Mainetti.

ICSI. *See* INTRACYTOPLASMIC SPERM INJECTION (ICSI).

ICU. Intensive Care Unit. *See* CRITICAL CARE.

IDEAL. A valued goal toward which one ought to strive, knowing that sometimes one will not succeed in achieving the goal. It is not **ethically obligatory** in all cases to pursue moral ideals. This is in contrast to moral **norms,** because moral norms generate **ethical obligations**.

IMMINENT DEMISE FUTILITY. A form of clinical management is technically possible but the patient in **deliberative clinical judgment** is expected to die during the current admission and not recover interactive capacity before death occurs. The **ethical justification** for this **specification** of futility is based on the rejection of **vitalism** in **professional medical ethics**, in other words, rejection of the view that there is an ethical obligation to preserve a patient's life even when the patient has no capacity for a relationship to his or her environment. This view is not accepted in the **moral theology** of some religions, for example, Orthodox Judaism and Islam. This difference can create **ethical conflict** in **decision making** about **end-of-life care** between care teams and **surrogates**. *See also* FUTILITY.

IMMORAL. Used to characterize actions as **ethically impermissible** and individuals as having bad character (i.e., a preponderance of **vices** over **virtues**).

IMPAIRED DECISIONAL AUTONOMY. Diminished **autonomy**, or self-governance, resulting from the reduced ability to make decisions. Impaired decisional autonomy is distinct from **impaired executive autonomy**. Impaired decisional autonomy is a function of cognitive and affective **disorders**. *See also* "DECISIONAL"; IMPAIRED DECISION-MAKING CAPACITY.

IMPAIRED DECISION-MAKING CAPACITY. Reduced ability, to differing degrees, to make **decisions** (i.e., to accomplish one or more of the components of **decision-making capacity**). Some impairments are reversible. When not urgent, **decision making** should be postponed and potentially reversible impairments addressed. When this impairment is reduced significantly but not enough to fall below a threshold of acceptability, **assisted decision-making** should be attempted. When this fails or when the impairment is below an accepted threshold, a **surrogate** is required to make decisions for the patient, following the two standards for **surrogate decision making**—the **substituted judgment standard** and the **best interests standard**. *See also* "DECISIONAL"; IMPAIRED DECISIONAL AUTONOMY.

IMPAIRED EXECUTIVE AUTONOMY. Diminished self-governance resulting from the reduced ability to carry out and, as necessary, adapt decisions. Impaired executive autonomy is distinct from **impaired decisional autonomy**. Impaired executive autonomy is a function of **executive dysfunction**. *See also* EXECUTIVE AUTONOMY; EXECUTIVE CAPACITY; IMPAIRED EXECUTIVE CAPACITY.

IMPAIRED EXECUTIVE CAPACITY. Diminished self-governance resulting from reduced ability to carry out and, as necessary, adapt decisions. Impaired executive autonomy is distinct from **impaired decision-making capacity**. Impaired executive capacity is a function of **executive dysfunction**. Executive capacity can become impaired independently of impaired decision-making capacity or in conjunction with impaired decision-making capacity. *See also* EXECUTIVE AUTONOMY; EXECUTIVE CAPACITY; IMPAIRED EXECUTIVE AUTONOMY.

IMPAIRED PHYSICIAN. A physician whose ability to discharge his or her **professional responsibilities** in **clinical care**, **research**, or education is reduced to a questionable or unacceptable level by drug or alcohol abuse, mental illness, or highly disruptive life changes (e.g., suicide of a spouse or child). It is now accepted that, in an **organizational culture** based on **professional medical ethics**, there in an **ethical obligation** on the part of physicians, residents, and medical students, as part of the professional responsibility of self-regulation and the **beneficence**-based **ethical obligation** to protect patients from unsafe **clinical management**, to report such physicians to leadership of a healthcare organization. The **norm** is anonymous reporting, to prevent retaliation, and referral by leadership to confidential clinical management (e.g., an Employee Assistance Program). Refractory cases may require suspension or termination of employment. Requirements of **statutory law** and **regulatory law** to report impaired physicians to state medical licensing agencies must be fulfilled.

IN RE QUINLAN. *See* ADVANCE DIRECTIVE.

IN UTERO FETAL DEMISE. The death of a fetus in the pregnant woman's uterus. There is little or no **ethical controversy** about in utero fetal demise from natural causes. In utero fetal demise has clinical ethical significance because of the need to identify its causes by means of a postmortem examination when feasible and with **consent**. This information can be used to calculate recurrence risk and plan preventive approaches to a subsequent pregnancy; both of these issues figure prominently in counseling women who have experienced in utero fetal demise. The **medically reasonable alternatives** are inducing labor or continuing the pregnancy until spontaneous labor begins. Intrapartum management should be based on maternal indications only. There is a strong **beneficence**-based **prima facie ethical obligation** to the pregnant woman to avoid cesarean delivery. The **professional virtue** of **compassion** creates an **ethical obligation** to provide counseling and psychosocial support for women who have experienced in utero fetal demise.

IN VITRO FERTILIZATION. A form of **assisted reproduction** in which ova are obtained from a woman that are then fertilized with sperm in a laboratory. Resulting embryos are analyzed for clinical acceptability, including the use of **preimplantation genetic diagnosis**. Those considered acceptable are candidates for **embryo transfer**. There are three **beneficence**-based outcomes by which in vitro fertilization is considered to be successful: creation of viable embryos that are candidates for embryo transfer; initiation of pregnancy; and live birth. For **patients**, the most important **autonomy**-based outcome is live birth. Nonspecific statements about success are noninformative and potentially misleading (e.g., a laboratory could have a higher percentage of pregnancies initiated than the percentage of live births) in advertisements and in the **informed consent process** and are therefore **ethically impermissible**. *See also* ASSISTED REPRODUCTIVE TECHNOLOGIES (ART).

INCOMPETENCE. The absence of **competence**, or the inability to complete a specific task at a specific time. There are two components of this inability: decisional autonomy and **executive autonomy**. *Incompetence* is therefore not a synonym for *lack of decision-making capacity* but is sometimes used this way. For example, in the clinical setting, *incompetence* is often used interchangeably with *lack of decision-making capacity*.

Some take the view that the term *incompetence* should be used only in the legal context, in other words, court proceedings to determine **legal incompetence** (i.e., the loss of decision-making capacity or the loss of **executive capacity** to a degree that the individual should lose his or her **right** to control his or her own affairs). Incompetence is task-specific, for example, in the inability to manage one's own financial affairs without substantially damaging one's financial interests; the inability to make healthcare decisions without substantially putting one's health at risk; or serious, far-reaching, and irreversible loss, or putting one's life at risk.

The cognitive and affective demands of competence and incompetence are a function of the complexity of the task. A patient may be competent for simple decisions such as **simple consent** to a needle stick, while also incompetent to make complex decisions such as **informed consent** to heart catheterization to unblock coronary arteries. Incompetence is also time specific, because competence can wax or wane over time. In both **health law** and **medical ethics**, the assessment of incompetence should be guided by the **presumption of decision-making capacity**, which means that the **burden of justification** is on a court of law or physician to make a reliable **clinical judgment** that a patient is incompetent.

The clinical assessment of a **patient**'s competence starts from the presumption of decision-making capacity. This means that the burden of justification is on the physician, which is met by adhering to the discipline of **deliberative clinical judgment**. *See also* AUTONOMY.

INCOMPETENT. In the state, temporary or permanent, of having lost the **competence** to perform a specific task at a specific time, either in the **judgment** of a court of law or in the **deliberative clinical judgment** of a physician. *See also* INCOMPETENCE.

INDEPENDENT MORAL STATUS. An individual has one or more properties required to generate **moral status** independently from all other entities. There is disagreement in **moral philosophy** on what these properties are. This phrase is often used synonymously with the terms *person* and *personhood*. *See also* DEPENDENT MORAL STATUS.

INDIVIDUAL CONSCIENCE. A fundamental set of beliefs and convictions about **values** that should define who an individual is and, therefore, support a life characterized by the **virtue** of **integrity**. The individual conscience of a physician arises from moral sources other than **professional medical ethics** (e.g., **moral theology**, family upbringing, or reflection on experience). Acting in ways inconsistent with the **ethical obligations** generated by these fundamental beliefs and convictions is not compatible with integrity and is therefore **ethically impermissible** for an individual. In professional medical ethics, **individual conscience** can come into conflict with **ethical obligations** generated by professional medical ethics. The **ethical justification** of **conscientious objection** in such circumstances appeals to individual conscience. *See also* PROFESSIONAL VIRTUE OF INTEGRITY.

INDIVIDUALISM. **Ethical reasoning** that emphasizes **autonomy** and the **rights** of individuals and the **ethical principle of respect for autonomy**, especially **negative rights**. This approach to ethical reasoning strongly opposes **paternalism** by the state and **medical paternalism**. *See also* COMMUNITARIAN ETHICS; LIBERTARIAN JUSTICE.

INDUCED ABORTION. The use of medical or surgical means to evacuate the contents of the uterus before **fetal viability**. There is **ethical controversy** about induced **abortion**, resulting from different positions on the **moral status** of the fetus in **moral philosophy** and **moral theology**. There has also been resulting ethical controversy in the global history of medical ethics, complicated by clinical findings about the anatomy and physiology of the developing fetus (e.g., the gestational age at which the fetus is capable of experiencing **pain**). *See also* ABORTION; TERMINATION OF PREGNANCY.

INFANTICIDE. The **killing** of an infant; also known as **involuntary active euthanasia** of an infant. There is a long history of the practice of infanticide in many places and cultures in the world, although the practice has been **ethically controversial**. Some of the world's religions regard infanticide to be **ethically impermissible** on grounds of their **moral theology**. In **bioethics**, infanticide has been **ethically justified** on the grounds that killing an infant is not the killing of a **person**, in other words, an individual human being with **independent moral status** (Tooley 1981). *See also* GRONINGEN PROTOCOL.

INFERTILITY. The inability of either men or women to initiate a pregnancy. Infertility is a **condition** that can be understood as a **disease** or a **disability**. In the debate about whether infertility is a disease, those who argue that it is not a disease conclude that there is no **ethical obligation** to provide infertility services and, therefore, no ethical obligation of private or public payers to fund such services. This conclusion is erroneous because an argument to show that a condition is not a disease does not show that that condition is not a disability. Moreover, there are potentially serious **biopsychosocial** sequelae of infertility for some individuals and couples. Thus, even if one takes the view that infertility is not a disease, there are good reasons to classify it as either a disability or a condition that has clinically significant biopsychosocial risks (as pregnancy does), for which **clinical management** should be considered and covered by payers. *See also* ASSISTED REPRODUCTION.

INFORMED CONSENT. The authorization of a **patient** to **clinical management** or to participation in **human subjects research** on the basis of information adequate to the cognitive, evaluative, and affective complexity of the decision to provide or refuse to provide such authorization. Informed consent is **ethically obligatory** when there is clinically significant risk to the patient or when a healthcare organization requires informed consent (Whitney et al. 2004). When the clinical risk is low, **simple consent** is **ethically permissible**. *See also* ETHICAL PRINCIPLE OF RESPECT FOR AUTONOMY; INFORMED CONSENT CASES; INFORMED CONSENT PROCESS.

INFORMED CONSENT CASES. A series of cases in the common law established the legal concept of informed consent: providing the patient with enough information to complete the informed consent process meaningfully.

In *Natanson v. Kline* (354 P.2d 670 [Kan. 1960]), the Kansas Supreme Court ruled in a case in which the plaintiff provided simple consent to cobalt radiation therapy for the clinical management of breast cancer but was not informed about its risks, many of which she experienced. The Court held that simple consent was not sufficient when clinical management has significant risk and that the patient needed to be sufficiently informed before authorizing or refusing to authorize clinical management.

The **professional community standard** was rejected as adequate in *Canterbury v. Spence* (464 F.2d. 772, 782 D.C. Cir. 1972) in a case in which the patient's mother, acting as his surrogate, was not informed about the risks of laminectomy, including the risk of paralysis from a fall. On leaving his bed (apparently unattended) the patient fell and was paralyzed. The surgeon had met the professional community standard, which omitted information about such risk. The Court held that that there should be a patient-oriented standard that would be fair to both the patient, by providing sufficient information, and to the physician, by not having a standard that would allow retrospective second-guessing. The **reasonable person standard** was articulated: providing a patient what *any patient* in that patient's clinical circumstances needed to know.

INFORMED CONSENT PROCESS. A process of **decision making** engaged in by the patient and the patient's physician or other clinician in which the goal is an informed and **voluntary** decision by the patient to authorize or refuse to authorize clinical management. This process implements the **ethical principle of respect for autonomy**.

The role of the physician in achieving the goal of an informed decision comprises five **ethical obligations**: (1) to describe the patient's diagnosis; (2) to present to the patient all the **medically reasonable alternatives** for managing the patient's **condition, disease, disability, disorder**, or **injury** with their clinical benefits and risks; (3) to make a reasonable effort to ensure that the patient understands each medically reasonable alternative; (4) to support the patient's evaluation of the medically reasonable alternatives on the basis of the patient's **values** and beliefs; and (5) to elicit the patient's authorization or refusal of authorization. The role of the physician in achieving the goal of a voluntary decision by the patient comprises the ethical obligation to make a reasonable effort to ensure that the patient's decision-making process and final decision are free of controlling internal and external influences.

The **common law** and **statutory law** of informed consent focus on the physician's **legal obligation** to disclose information to the patient about his or her **condition** and its clinical management. There are two legal standards, which developed in American common law during the middle decades of the 20th century in both state and federal courts. The first, which applies in the majority of the states in the United States, is the **reasonable person standard**. The second is the **professional community standard**. In the above account of the components of the informed consent process, the second component meets the reasonable person standard. In the common law, a "rough understanding" of disclosed information by the patient is sufficient. The informed consent process described here aims for more: replication in lay terms by the patient of the physician's **clinical judgment**.

For all adult patients, there is a **presumption of decision-making capacity**. Fulfilling the second ethical obligation for an informed decision should meet the **reasonable person standard** in applicable common and statutory law for disclosure of information to the patient. Fulfilling the fourth obligation for an informed decision satisfies the **substituted judgment standard** for **surrogate decision making**. Decision making for minor patients by parents occurs under the ethical constraint of the **best interests of the child**, which creates a **beneficence**-based ethical obligation of parents to authorize clinical management that is expected to protect the life or health of their child. The concept of **parental permission** or **informed permission** governs decision making by parents for pediatric patients.

When an adult patient with **decision-making capacity** or the **surrogate** of a patient who lacks decision-making capacity refuses to authorize clinical management that has been offered or recommended, there is a strict legal obligation to meet the requirements of **informed refusal**. Physicians have a parallel **ethical obligation** to meet this requirement, based on the **ethical principle of respect for patient autonomy**. Physicians also have the professional ethical obligation to protect the healthcare organization from unnecessary exposure to liability, and the protection of the **legitimate self-interest** in preventing exposure to litigation for **professional liability**. *See also* ASSENT; INFORMED CONSENT CASES.

INFORMED PERMISSION. Decision making by parents or guardians of a pediatric patient under the ethical constraint of the **best interests of the child standard** and a component of **pediatric ethics**; also known as **parental permission**. This ethical standard creates an **ethical obligation** of parents and guardians to authorize **clinical management** that is reliably expected in **deliberative clinical judgment** to protect and promote the pediatric patient's health-related interests. The concept of parental permission reflects **ethical reasoning** about the **parent-child relationship** as based primarily on **parental responsibility** to protect children and not primarily **parental rights**; the authority and strength of parental rights are a function of parents fulfilling parental responsibility. The concept of parental permission has been endorsed by the American Academy of Pediatrics (1995, 2016). Parental responsibility places **ethically justified** limits on parental **autonomy**, which distinguished informed permission from **informed consent** of an adult patient for his or her medical care. *See also* INFORMED PERMISSION PROCESS.

INFORMED PERMISSION PROCESS. Decision making by parents or a guardian about authorizing **clinical management** that is reliably expected in **deliberative clinical judgment** to protect and promote the health-related interests of the pediatric patient. The components of this process include informing the patient in a developmentally appropriate way about his or her **condition, disability, disease, disorder,** or **injury**; describing the **medically reasonable alternatives** for clinical management for the condition and the clinical benefits and risks of each such alternative; eliciting the patient's preference; and taking that preference into account by both pediatric healthcare professionals and parents or guardians and giving that preference weight commensurate with the maturity of the patient's decision-making process.

There is **ethical controversy** about how much weight should be given to the patient's preferences. *See also* BEST INTERESTS OF THE CHILD STANDARD; PARENTAL PERMISSION; PARENTAL RESPONSIBILITY; PARENTAL RIGHTS; PARENT-CHILD RELATIONSHIP; PEDIATRIC ETHICS.

INFORMED REFUSAL. The **absolute legal obligation** (in the United States) and **absolute ethical obligation** to inform a **patient** who refuses to authorize offered or recommended **clinical management** in the **informed consent process** about the clinical risks that the patient is taking as a consequence of not receiving such clinical management. *Truman v. Thomas* (27 Cal.3d 285) from 1980, the **common law** case that established informed refusal, involved a physician who recommended a PAP smear to the patient, who refused. The physician did not inform her of the risk of not detecting presymptomatic cervical cancer, which was detected only at Stage IV, when treatment could not prevent her death. This disclosure should be documented in the patient's record in detail.

The **ethical obligation** of the physician in **professional medical ethics** goes further, especially in cases of refusal that have risks of potentially serious, far-reaching, and irreversible harm to the patient, and calls for a **preventive ethics** approach that includes exploring the patient's reasoning on the assumption that the patient has a good reason from his or her perspective; identifying the **medically reasonable alternatives** for clinical management supported by **values** the patient expresses and pointing this out to the patient along with a recommendation of that clinical management; expressing concern for the clinical risks that the patient is taking; asking the patient to reconsider; and following up with the patient to ask the patient to reconsider. *See also* INFORMED CONSENT; INFORMED REFUSAL CASE; RIGHT TO REFUSE TREATMENT.

INFORMED REFUSAL CASE. The landmark case for **informed refusal** is from California in 1980, *Truman v. Thomas* (611 P. 2d 902, 27 Cal. 3d 285, 165 Cal. Rptr). The **patient**, Mrs. Truman, had received obstetric care from Dr. Thomas, who recommended that Mrs. Truman should have a PAP smear, which can detect preclinical cellular changes in the cervix, including pre-cancerous and cancerous changes. The patient refused but Dr. Thomas did not explain to the patient the risks that she was taking by refusing. She subsequently died from cervical cancer at the age of 30 that an earlier PAP smear might have prevented. The California Supreme Court ruled that there is a **legal obligation** in **common law** of the physician to inform the patient about the clinical risks that the patient takes when he or she refuses to authorize **clinical management** that has been recommended by the physician. Dr. Thomas had testified that mitigating the risk of undiagnosed cervical **disease** was clinically important. This supports a general rule in the **informed consent process** that the **reasonable person standard** is satisfied when the physician provides the patient with clinically salient information about the benefits and risks of clinical management, because such risks shape **deliberative clinical judgment**.

INJURY. Abnormal anatomy resulting from a cause or causes external (such as trauma) or internal (such as bone fracture resulting from severe osteoporosis) to an individual's body. Abnormal physiology may also result. *See also* CONDITION; DISABILITY; DISEASE; DISORDER.

INNOVATION. A clinical **experiment** undertaken to benefit an individual patient. In 2008, the Society of University Surgeons recommended that planned innovation should be subjected to prospective review for its scientific and clinical justification and that the **informed consent process** make clear to the patient that the proposed **clinical management** is not a **medically reasonable alternative** and that the patient is therefore free to refuse to authorize the innovation (Biffl et al. 2008). Innovation can also be understood as pre-**research**, to gather data for the plausibility of a hypothesis to be tested in a **clinical trial**.

INSTITUTE OF SOCIETY, ETHICS AND THE LIFE SCIENCES. *See* THE HASTINGS CENTER.

INSTITUTIONAL ANIMAL CARE AND USE COMMITTEE (IACUC). The committee of an organization that sponsors **animal subjects research** charged by federal law with the responsibility to provide prospective review and approval of research with animals. The committee has an **absolute ethical obligation** to assess research protocols for their scientific merit and the prevention and responsible **clinical management** of the **pain** and **distress** of the animal subjects. *See also* ANIMAL WELFARE ACT; ETHICS OF ANIMAL SUBJECTS RESEARCH.

INSTITUTIONAL ETHICS COMMITTEE. *See* CLINICAL ETHICS COMMITTEE; ETHICS COMMITTEE.

INSTITUTIONAL REVIEW BOARD (IRB). A permanent committee of a healthcare organization that conducts **human subjects research** that is required by law in the United States to provide prospective oversight and approval and prospective monitoring of the scientific and ethical quality of such research and the **informed consent process** for enrollment in a **clinical**

trial. The board is also known by its acronym, IRB. An Institutional Review Board is usually located in an Office of Research but has **autonomy** from the organization's leadership, which means that the decisions of the board cannot be appealed to the organization's leadership. The board is expected to apply **45 CFR 46** to protocols, as well as guidances issued by the **Office for Human Research Protections** of the United States Department of Health and Human Services. The statutory authority for IRBs is the 1974 National Research Act (Public Law 93-348), which was enacted after a series of scandals of abuse of human subjects research in the United States in the post–World War II period (1945–). In other countries, the name for these oversight committees is **Research Ethics Committee**. *See also THE BELMONT REPORT*; ETHICS OF HUMAN SUBJECTS RESEARCH; SCIENTIFIC INTEGRITY.

INSURANCE. A form of payment for healthcare services that manages the risk of the small percentage of patients who need such services at any given time by spreading the cost over a large population. The larger the population, the lower the insurance premiums. The typical health insurance plan includes deductibles (the amount an insured individual has to pay out-of-pocket before payment by the insurance plan begins) and co-payments (the amount that the patient pays along with the insurance company). When deductibles and/or co-payments are very high, individuals of modest income may not be able to afford them, a circumstance known as underinsurance. Access to affordable insurance (total cost of premiums, deductibles, and co-payments) is an essential component of implementing the **right to healthcare**. In **public policy**, health insurance paid by one's employer is not taxed as income, and premiums are also tax deductible (subject to limitations). *See also* HEALTH POLICY.

INTEGRITY. A **virtue** that requires adherence to standards of intellectual and moral excellence and the integration of one's life that results from sustained adherence to standards of intellectual and moral excellence. *See also* PROFESSIONAL VIRTUE OF INTEGRITY; SCIENTIFIC INTEGRITY.

INTELLECTUAL PROPERTY. An invention of a process or product that is unique and to which one has **rights** that can be secured by such measures as copyright, patent, and trademarks. The right to intellectual property is one of the drivers of **innovation** in the biomedical sciences. Patents, however, also create economic barriers to the use of intellectual property by others, especially in low-income countries. There is **ethical controversy** about modifying patents or violating them in such countries in order to make new medications affordable and thus more effectively achieve public health goals. *See also* PUBLIC POLICY.

INTERACTIVE CAPACITY FUTILITY. A form **of clinical management** is technically possible but the patient in **deliberative clinical judgment** is expected to survive but not ever to recover interactive capacity. The **ethical justification** for this specification of futility is based on the rejection of **vitalism** in **professional medical ethics**, rejection of the view that there is an ethical obligation to preserve a patient's life even when the patient has no physiologic capacity for a relationship to his or her environment. This view is not accepted in the **moral theology** of some religions, for example, Orthodox Judaism and Islam. This difference can create **ethical conflict** in **decision making** about **end-of-life care** between care teams and **surrogates**. *See also* FUTILITY; PERMANENT VEGETATIVE STATE.

INTEREST. A stake that an individual has in the past (in how the past is interpreted, including one's past behavior), the present, and the future. Interest can be a function of an individual's **moral status**, preferences, or social role. Moral status creates an interest in having others fulfill **ethical obligations** to an individual; the strength of these obligations varies according to the strength of the individual's moral status. Preferences create interests that vary in strength as a function of the importance of a preference to an individual and to others who are expected to act on that preference. Social roles create interests in the goals or purposes of a social role and vary in strength according to the importance of the social role. In virtue of being a **patient**, an individual human being has an interest in the protection and promotion of his or health and life. Interests that generate justified claims to be treated in a specified way become the basis of an individual's **rights**. Health-related interests may generate a **right to healthcare**. *See also* CONFLICT OF INTEREST; LEGITIMATE SELF-INTEREST; MERE SELF-INTEREST; SELF-INTEREST.

INTERPROFESSIONAL RELATIONSHIPS. *See* BOUNDARY ISSUES; MEDICAL ETHICS.

INTERSEX CONDITION. A phrase for classifying individuals who are not unambiguously one **sex** or the other, usually on the basis of anatomy thought to be definitive of female or male sex. The suspicion of an intersex condition in a neonate can be triggered by abnormal appearance of the external genitalia, discordance between chromosomal sex identified in prenatal testing of the fetus and the anatomic sex of the infant, or results of neonatal screening for conditions such as congenital adrenal hyperplasia. Current science no longer supports the view that sex is bifurcated into male and female. Like all biological traits, sex displays biological variation. In pediatric discourse, the term *intersex condition* has been replaced by the term ***disorders of sexual development***. *See also* GENDER; GENDER IDENTITY DISORDER.

INTRACYTOPLASMIC SPERM INJECTION (ICSI). A variant of **in vitro fertilization** in which, under a microscope, a single sperm is injected into an ovum. This technique is used in cases of defective sperm function, regarded as the most common form of male **infertility**. There have been **beneficence**-based concerns about possible increased risk of congenital problems in children conceived in this way. This technique is a component of **assisted reproductive medicine**. *See also* ASSISTED REPRODUCTIVE TECHNOLOGIES (ART).

INTRAPROFESSIONAL RELATIONSHIPS. *See* BOUNDARY ISSUES; MEDICAL ETHICS.

INTRINSIC WORTH. The idea that a human being has **value** for himself or herself and also for others on the basis of constitutive properties of the individual. Intrinsic worth is also another way to express the concept of **independent moral status**. *See also* DIGNITY; PERSONALISM.

INTUITION. A term frequently used in **moral philosophy** with variable meaning (Audi 2015), ranging from an initial **judgment** that must be tested in a deliberative process (Brody 2003) to a nondiscursive, immediate, and therefore error-free intellectual taking up of truths in the world. The English philosopher **Richard Price** (1723–1791) used *intuition* with this latter meaning, resulting in a form of **moral realism**. Price's method of moral realism influenced **Thomas Percival**'s (1740–1804) **medical ethics**.

INVIDIOUS DISCRIMINATION. Making and acting on **ethically impermissible** distinctions among individuals or groups, because the distinctions attach moral significance to morally irrelevant traits of individuals or groups, which violates the **ethical principle of justice**, especially **egalitarian justice**. Many forms of invidious discrimination are outlawed, for example, denying patients access to medical care based on race. *Discrimination* is often used as a synonym for *invidious discrimination*. However, there is an ethically neutral use of *discrimination* to mean making distinctions among things, as in a discriminating taste for wine or fine food.

INVOLUNTARY. A **patient**'s decision or implementation of a decision is involuntary when it is subject to internal controlling influences, such as extreme pain or unreasoning fear, or external controlling influences, such as **coercion**. An important form of external controlling influence is an intrinsically coercive environment (e.g., prison). There is **ethical controversy** about whether individuals in such coercive environments can provide **consent** that is **voluntary**, even though they may be able to provide **informed consent**. *See also* AUTONOMY.

INVOLUNTARY ACTIVE EUTHANASIA. Killing a **patient** without the patient's authorization in the **informed consent process**. This is **ethically impermissible** in **professional medical ethics** but is legally permitted in the Netherlands. *See also* ALKMAAR CASE; GRONINGEN PROTOCOL; REMMLINK REPORT (1990).

INVOLUNTARY COMMITMENT. The **power** of a court of law to order a **patient** to be admitted without the patient's **consent** and overriding his or her **right to refuse** treatment because the patient is legally **incompetent** or poses reliably predictable danger of serious, far-reaching, and irreversible harm to himself or herself or others. There was a long history in the United States of abuse of the power of involuntary commitment. As a result, courts have put the **burden of justification** on the state to establish grounds for involuntary commitment and have protected the right to refuse treatment of the involuntarily committed. Physicians who are assigned by the court the task of evaluating individuals have the **professional obligation** to be clear with the patient that the physician is acting as an agent of the court and to meet professional **norms** for performing such evaluation and testifying in court proceedings. *See also* AUTONOMY; QUARANTINE.

INVOLUNTARY EUTHANASIA. Euthanasia undertaken without the authorization of the **patient** in the **informed consent process**. **Active euthanasia** (i.e., **killing** a patient) is **ethically impermissible** in **professional medical ethics** because it violates **professional integrity**. Involuntary active euthanasia is *a fortiori* ethically impermissible. Involuntary **passive euthanasia** is **ethically permissible** when the patient's wishes are unknown and discontinuing **life-sustaining treatment** is based on the **best interests standard** of **surrogate decision making**. *See also* LETTING DIE; VOLUNTARY ACTIVE EUTHANASIA; VOLUNTARY EUTHANASIA; VOLUNTARY PASSIVE EUTHANASIA.

INVOLUNTARY PASSIVE EUTHANASIA. Discontinuing **life-sustaining treatment** to achieve the **letting die** of the **patient**, without the patient's **consent**. Involuntary **passive euthanasia** is **ethically permissible** when the **surrogate** authorizes discontinuation of life-sustaining treatment based on the **substituted judgment standard** and, when the patient's wishes are unknown, discontinuing life-sustaining treatment is based on the **best interests standard** of **surrogate decision making**. *See also* VOLUNTARY EUTHANASIA; VOLUNTARY PASSIVE EUTHANASIA.

INVOLUNTARY STERILIZATION. **Sterilization** without the **informed consent** of the **patient** with a threat (**coerced sterilization**) or without a threat (**forced sterilization**). There is a long history of **involuntary** surgical procedures that result in **sterilization** of women in the United States. This practice sometimes occurred as the result of physicians' decisions to perform sterilization of women of color, including African American and Mexican American women, as well as low-income women and women with intellectual disabilities (then known as mental retardation). Sterilization was also performed under court order. In both cases, **invidious discrimination** played a role.

This use of state power was challenged in the federal courts, resulting in a ruling from the United States Supreme Court that endorsed this use of state power in an opinion written by Justice Oliver Wendell Holmes (*Buck v. Bell* 274 U.S. 200 [1927]). A single sentence from Holmes is often quoted: "Three generations of idiots is enough." The Supreme Court has not reversed this opinion. Federal and state **common law**, **regulatory law**, and **statutory law** now protect the **right** of both female and male patients to provide informed consent for sterilization, which includes the **right to refuse** sterilization. To protect the exercise of this right from undue influence and **coercion**, there is a mandatory waiting period after the patient has provided informed consent for sterilization. *See also* COERCION.

IRB. *See* INSTITUTIONAL REVIEW BOARD (IRB).

IRREVERSIBLE CONDITION. A condition that is defined in applicable **advance directive** legislation and, when it has been diagnosed by the patient's attending physician, creates a legal permission to discontinue **life-sustaining treatment**. An irreversible condition differs from a **terminal condition** in that a patient with an irreversible condition is not expected to die in the near future. Instead, the patient is expected to survive for some indeterminate time but to have permanently lost awareness and therefore interactive capacity. The invocation of this concept in **clinical ethical rea-**

soning rejects **vitalism** and appeals to **interactive capacity futility**. *See also* PERMANENT VEGETATIVE STATE; PERSISTENT VEGETATIVE STATE.

ISLAMIC BIOETHICS. Bioethics based on the **moral theology** of Islam, drawing on such resources as the *Qur'an*, the revealed word of God to the prophet Mohammed, and *Haddiths*, the collection of the sayings of the prophet Mohammed, as well as *fatwas*, contributing to the pluralism of bioethics (Ilkilic 2009). *See also* ISLAMIC MEDICAL ETHICS; ISLAMIC MORAL THEOLOGY.

ISLAMIC MEDICAL ETHICS. Medical ethics based on **Islamic moral theology**, drawing on such resources as the *Qur'an*, the revealed word of God to the prophet Mohammed, and *Haddiths*, the collection of the sayings of the prophet Mohammed, as well as *fatwas* (Ilkilic 2009). **Moral theology**, because it is not secular, is not methodologically adequate to serve as the basis of **professional medical ethics**. *See also* ISLAMIC BIOETHICS.

ISLAMIC MORAL THEOLOGY. Ethical reasoning based on such resources as the *Qur'an*, the revealed word of God to the prophet Mohammed, and *Haddiths*, the collection of the sayings of the prophet Mohammed, as well as *fatwas* (Ilkilic 2009). Moral theology, because it is not secular, is not methodologically adequate to serve as the basis of **professional medical ethics**. *See also* ISLAMIC BIOETHICS; ISLAMIC MEDICAL ETHICS.

IVF. *See* IN VITRO FERTILIZATION.

IVY, ANDREW C. (1893–1978). American physician and physiologist who served as representative of the American Medical Association and gave testimony in *United States of America v. Karl Brandt et al.* (1946–1947). *See also* NAZI MEDICAL WAR CRIMES.

J

JACOBOVITZ, IMMANUEL (1921–1999). Jewish rabbi and scholar. He is the author of *A Comparative and Historical Study of the Jewish Religious Attitude to Medicine and Its Practice* (1959), a broad examination of topics in **medical ethics** from the perspective of **Jewish moral theology** (Zohar 2009). *See also* JEWISH BIOETHICS; JEWISH MEDICAL ETHICS.

JANER, FÉLIX (1771–1865). Spanish physician and ethicist. His *Elementos de moral médica* (*Treatise on Medical Morality*, 1831) acknowledges the influence of **John Gregory**'s (1724–1773) **medical ethics**. Janer endorsed Gregory's account of **truth-telling** as an **ethical obligation** to those with serious illnesses.

JAPANESE MEDICAL WAR CRIMES. Biological warfare programs, such as **Unit 731**, conducted by the Imperial Japanese Army from 1939 to 1945, that conducted unethical experiments using human subjects, comparable to the crimes against humanity of the Nazi doctors but with no prosecution by Allied countries after the end of World War II in the Pacific. *See also* NAZI MEDICAL WAR CRIMES.

JEHOVAH'S WITNESSES. A Christian faith community, many of whose members are people of color. Jehovah's Witnesses consider themselves to have an **ethical obligation** originating in their **moral theology** of blood and blood products not to accept blood transfusion and prohibited blood products, even when necessary to prevent death, based on their interpretation of Holy Scripture. This commitment is an expression of the more general, core commitment of people of faith: if required by circumstances not of their own making to make a choice between obedience to the word of God or continuing to live, they are without hesitation to obey the word of God as a matter of religious **conscience**.

Every person of faith, indeed every person, should be able to understand this commitment. It is important to be clear that a Jehovah's Witness who refuses death-preventing treatment does not wish to die. It is also important to be clear that it is very well established in **pediatric ethics** and **health law** that Jehovah's Witnesses are not ethically or legally free to refuse life-saving use of blood or blood products for their child who is a **patient**. Finally, physicians have no **authority** to engage in disputes about the interpretation of Scripture; this is the work of theologians. *See also* ETHICAL PRINCIPLE OF RESPECT FOR AUTONOMY; RIGHT TO REFUSE TREATMENT.

JEWISH BIOETHICS. Bioethics based on **Jewish moral theology**, drawing on such resources as the Torah and the rabbinic ethical literature (Steinberg 2003; Zohar 2009), contributing to the pluralism of bioethics. *See also* JEWISH MEDICAL ETHICS.

JEWISH MEDICAL ETHICS. Medical ethics based on **Jewish moral theology**, drawing on such resources as the Torah and the rabbinic ethical literature. Moral theology, because it is not secular, is not methodologically adequate to serve as the basis of **professional medical ethics** (Steinberg 2003; Zohar 2009). *See also* JEWISH BIOETHICS.

JEWISH MORAL THEOLOGY. Moral theology drawing on resources of Judaism. Such resources include the Torah and the rabbinic ethical literature. *See also* JEWISH BIOETHICS; JEWISH MEDICAL ETHICS.

JUDGMENT. The disciplined classification of items of interest into appropriate categories based on criteria for inclusion into the category and sometimes also criteria for exclusion from the category. Clinical judgment seeks to assign a **patient**'s **condition** into a diagnostic category, based on professional interpretation of criteria that include signs and symptoms, as well as imaging and laboratory analysis. Ethical judgment seeks to assign behavior, personal characteristics, practices, and policies into one of three categories: **ethically permissible, ethically obligatory**, and **ethically prohibited**. *See also* DELIBERATIVE CLINICAL JUDGMENT; EVIDENCE-BASED MEDICINE.

JUST. A behavior, **health policy, public policy**, or practice that is supported by the **ethical principle of justice** in at least one of its **specifications**. *See also* UNJUST.

JUSTICE. *See* ETHICAL PRINCIPLE OF JUSTICE.

JUSTIFICATION. Ethical analysis and **ethical argument** that provides an account of the character formation or behavior that is either **ethically permissible** or **ethically obligatory**. *See also* ETHICAL REASONING.

K

KAIBARA EKIKEN (1630–1714). Japanese physician and Confucian scholar. He wrote *Yojokun* (*Teaching and Care of Life*, 1713), which emphasizes a multifaceted concept of health that physicians should support and restore when lost. He held the view that moderation in all things played a central role in sustaining one's health. This is known as *Yojo*, or "care for life." Kaibara provided instruction on how to follow the self-discipline at the heart of "care for life."

KAPPA LAMBDA SOCIETY OF HIPPOCRATES. Also known as Secret Kappa Lambda Society of Hippocrates. It was founded in 1819 by Dr. Samuel Brown (1796–1830), a professor at the University of Transylvania medical school in Lexington, Kentucky. The society privately published "extracts" of the *Medical Ethics* (Kappa Lambda Society 1823) of **Thomas Percival** (1740–1804) that became the conduit through which passages from *Medical Ethics* were included in the **American Medical Association** *Code of Medical Ethics* **of 1847**. Two authors of the 1847 *Code*, Dr. **John Bell** (1796–1872) and Dr. **Isaac Hays** (1796–1879), were members of the Kappa Lambda Society (Baker 2013). *See also* CODE OF ETHICS.

KELLY, FATHER GERALD, SJ (1902–1964). American Jesuit priest of the Roman Catholic Church. He wrote a **Roman Catholic moral theology** of medicine titled *Medico-Moral Problems* (1949–1954). *See also* MORAL THEOLOGY.

KENNEDY INSTITUTE OF ETHICS. Founded in 1971 at Georgetown University in Washington, DC, by the Dutch physician and ethicist André Hellegers (1926–1979), with the support of the Joseph P. Kennedy Jr. Foundation. Also known as the Kennedy Institute, it is dedicated to scholarly work in the field of **bioethics**. The institute also houses the Bioethics Research Library (https://bioethics.georgetown.edu/, accessed 14 September 2017), the largest bioethics research library in the world. The institute also publishes the *Kennedy Institute of Ethics Journal* (https://www.press.jhu.edu/journals/kennedy-institute-ethics-journal, accessed 14 September 2017).

KEVORKIAN, DR. JACK (1928–2011). An American pathologist who gained notoriety for his advocacy of **physician-assisted suicide** and **voluntary active euthanasia**. After a number of attempts at prosecution, he was tried and convicted in Michigan for second-degree homicide after publicly engaging in voluntary active euthanasia. When he went public with cases in which he engaged in voluntary active euthanasia and made himself open to prosecution, he met criteria for **civil disobedience**. *See also* VOLUNTARY ACTIVE EUTHANASIA.

KICKBACKS. A form of **fee-splitting** in which a referral specialist or healthcare facility shares a portion of income with physicians who make referrals. Because this practice makes the physician's **self-interest** the physician's primary motivation, kickbacks constitute **conflicts of interest** that are **ethically impermissible** in **professional medical ethics**. This position has been adopted by the American Medical Association (http://journalofethics.ama-assn.org/2010/12/coet1-1012.html, accessed 14 September 2017). It is a criminal act to exchange items of value, especially money, for referral of federal healthcare business (42 U.S.C. § 1320a-7b.). *See also* "STARK LAW".

KILLING. The introduction into the living body of an individual human being of a life-taking pathological process that is not disrupted and therefore causes death. There is a general prohibition in **professional medical ethics** against physicians killing **patients**. There is **ethical controversy** about whether **voluntary active euthanasia, involuntary active euthanasia**, and **physician-assisted suicide** are **ethically permissible** in professional medical ethics and **health law**. There is also ethical controversy about whether killing can be distinguished clearly from **letting die**. *See also* ACTIVE EUTHANASIA; KILLING/LETTING DIE DISTINCTION.

KILLING/LETTING DIE DISTINCTION. In **professional medical ethics, killing** is distinct from **letting die**, especially with respect to the cause of the **death** of the **patient**. Moreover, there is a general prohibition in professional medical ethics against killing, whereas letting a patient with a **terminal condition** or an **irreversible condition** die is **ethically permissible**. Rachels (1975) has argued that the "bare difference between killing and letting die" is not decisive in **ethical reasoning** about what is ethically permissible and **ethically impermissible** in **end-of-life care**; other morally relevant considerations, such as the physician's motivation, play the decisive role. There is ongoing **ethical controversy** about whether there is any ethically significant difference between killing and letting die (Rachels 1975).

L

LACKS, HENRIETTA. *See* HELA.

LEAKE, CHAUNCEY (1896–1978). American biomedical scientist and leader in academic medicine. His 1927 edition of Thomas Percival's (1740–1804) *Medical Ethics* (1803) made this landmark text in the history of **medical ethics** readily available for physicians, medical educators, scholars, and students. Leake considered Percival's **professional medical ethics** to be concerned with **medical etiquette,** which for Leake meant the intraprofessional concerns of physicians. This interpretation remains influential in the **bioethics** literature but has been challenged in recent scholarship on Percival (Baker 2013). *See also* ETIQUETTE.

LECTURES ON THE DUTIES AND QUALIFICATIONS OF A PHYSICIAN **(1772).** Six lectures on **professional medical ethics** by the Scottish physician-ethicist **John Gregory** (1724–1773). They were preceded by *Observations on the Duties and Qualifications of a Physician, and on the Method of Prosecuting Enquiries in Philosophy* (1770). Following a then-common practice, Gregory first published the lectures anonymously, to test public reception of them. The reception was positive, prompting Gregory to revise *Observations* and publish them under his name as *Lectures*. Gregory, perhaps the most prominent physician of the **Scottish Enlightenment**, gave these lectures to his medical students at the University of Edinburgh in the 1760s, as they transitioned from the lecture hall to bedside learning in the **Royal Infirmary** of Edinburgh.

Gregory appealed to a **philosophy of medicine** and to **moral science.** He appealed explicitly to the **philosophy of science** and philosophy of medicine of **Francis Bacon** (1561–1626). Bacon called for medicine to be based on "experience": the carefully observed results of natural and controlled experiments. The goal of doing so was to establish the clinical competence of medicine as a scientifically based profession.

Gregory also appealed to the **moral science** of **David Hume** (1711–1776) and its principle of **sympathy**: the capacity we all have to enter into the lives of others and experience it as they do. Sympathy requires regulation by two professional virtues. The first is **tenderness**: the direct engagement with the affective dimensions of the patient's experience of illness. The second is **steadiness**: managing one's own response to the plight of the **patient** by not becoming hard-hearted and not losing control of one's emotions. The moral exemplars of tenderness and steadiness were, for Gregory, "women of learning and virtue," resulting in a **feminine medical ethics**.

The result of these two appeals was the creation of the first professional medical ethics based on the **ethical concept of medicine as a profession**. **Thomas Percival** (1740–1804) added to this account in significant ways.

Gregory then provides a sympathy-based account of a variety of clinical ethical topics, including **confidentiality**, especially of female patients; temperance (an important consideration at a time when water was not potable and physicians seeing well-to-do patients in their homes were offered a "cordial," i.e., spirit beverage); respect for the **right** of the patient to speak "where his own life and health are concerned," one of the earliest occurrences of the discourse of rights in the history of medical ethics; the "governance" of the patient (i.e., attempting to control the patient completely), which he rejects as implausible; the obligation not to abandon incurable, dying patients, which reversed a standard that was adopted in the **Hippocratic Corpus**; the obligation to attend to and address the **pain** and **suffering** of the **dying** patient, what he called "smoothing the avenues of death"; and the need for "**candor**," the intellectual virtue of being open to "conviction" (i.e., changing one's scientific beliefs and clinical practice on the basis of new evidence).

Gregory addresses the relationship between medicine and religion at length, in response to the then-popular phrase "*Ubi tres medici, ibi duo atheii*," or "Where there are three physicians there are two atheists." Gregory argues that, while medicine is based on science, there is no necessary incompatibility between scientific medicine and religion. The result of this argument was to establish that professional medical ethics is secular. The term *secular* has two components. First, no appeal to divinity or revelation or sacred books is required for professional medical ethics because it is based on biological science and moral science. Second, there is no necessary conflict between professional medical ethics and religion. Gregory intended the secular nature of professional medical ethics to make it transreligious, transcultural, and transnational. *Lectures* was translated into German (1778), French (1787), Italian (1791), and Spanish (1803). An edition was published in the United States in 1817. Gregory's *Lectures* was acknowledged as an important source of influence by the framers of the new **American Medical Association *Code of Medical Ethics* of 1847**.

LEGAL INCOMPETENCE. The determination by a civil court that an individual lacks **competence** or the inability to complete a specific task at a specific time.

LEGAL OBLIGATION. An action that is required by law. That one has a moral or **ethical obligation** does not by itself establish that one also has a legal obligation, because the justification of a legal obligation appeals to additional considerations, such as feasibility (Is a proposed new legal obligation permitted under constitutional law and compatible with other legal obligations?), urgency (Is there a compelling public interest in creating a new legal obligation?), effectiveness (Are people reasonably expected to routinely fulfill a new legal obligation?), and enforceability (Can the new legal obligation be enforced fairly?). Not being able to establish that an ethical or moral obligation should become a new legal obligation does not count against the justification of the ethical or moral obligation. *See also* DUTY; OBLIGATION.

LEGAL RIGHT. A **right** of individuals grounded in sources of the law, including the constitutions of the states and federal government, **administrative law**, **common law**, **regulatory law**, and **statutory law**. Not all **moral rights** are legal rights. Most legal rights have their origins in moral rights. *See also* RIGHT.

LEGITIMATE SELF-INTEREST. Forms of **self-interest** that are based in past, present, or future states of affairs that are highly valued by an individual (e.g., activities or relationships that an individual regards as definitive of his or her personal identity), and the necessary conditions for protecting and promoting such interests. Legitimate self-interest also includes the necessary conditions for having and acting on interests of any kind (e.g., health, life, and personal security). There is **ethical controversy** about whether legitimate self-interests are to be sacrificed without limits (i.e., in every case in which they conflict with **ethical obligations**). *See also* INTEREST; MERE SELF-INTEREST.

LETTING DIE. The discontinuation of **life-sustaining treatment**, resulting in the **patient**'s already existing life-taking condition causing the patient's death. In **professional medical ethics**, there is a **prima facie ethical obligation** of a physician to initiate and provide life-sustaining treatment, thus placing the **burden of justification** on its discontinuation. It is therefore a mistake to believe that in professional medical ethics the claim that a physician let a patient die is *by itself* an excusing condition. Letting die is not **killing**, because when life-sustaining treatment is discontinued the cause of the resulting death of the patient is an already existing life-taking pathology, not a life-taking pathology that the physician has introduced into the patient's body. There is ongoing **ethical controversy** about whether there is any ethically significant difference between killing and letting die (Rachels 1975). *See also* KILLING/LETTING DIE DISTINCTION.

LETTING DIE/KILLING DISTINCTION. *See* KILLING/LETTING DIE DISTINCTION.

LIBERTARIAN JUSTICE. A **specification** of the **ethical principle of justice** that focuses on **distributive justice** and calls for resources to be allotted by price and the ability to pay. This interpretation assumes that an individual's wealth and capacity to pay has been earned without violating the liberty-based **rights** of others. Libertarian justice strongly supports market solutions in **health policy** as a **procedural justice**–based response to the challenges of access to healthcare and cost control. Libertarian justice does not address the **quality** of **clinical care**. *See also* EGALITARIAN JUSTICE; HEALTHCARE JUSTICE; RAWLSIAN JUSTICE; UTILITARIAN JUSTICE.

LICENSURE. The formal granting by the responsible government of permission to practice medicine or one of the other healthcare professions. The word *licensure* comes from the Latin *licet*, meaning "allow" or "permit." In the federal system of the United States, licensure is done by the states, commonwealths, and territories. In the United Kingdom, the Royal Colleges, bishops, and, later, medical and surgical corporations chartered by the monarch controlled licensure, as a tool to limit entry into the small, crowded market for the private practice of medicine in the homes of the wealthy. The state took over this function as a result of the Medical Act of 1858 by creating a licensing agency, which is now known as the General Medical Council. *See also* HEALTH POLICY; PUBLIC POLICY.

LIE. Representing as true what one knows to be false. Lying is **ethically impermissible** in the **informed consent process** because it is a form of **deception**. *See also* TRUTH-TELLING.

LIFE. A **cluster concept** that includes the following capacities: to take in sources of nutrition, process them (metabolism), and excrete waste; to maintain biological stability (homeostasis); to grow and develop; to adapt to the environment; to respond to stimuli; and to reproduce. Not all are required in every case. For example, a male **patient** with aspermia or a postmenopausal female patient is not able to reproduce autonomously, but each is surely alive. A critically ill patient requiring **life-sustaining treatment** may not be able to maintain homeostasis without such support, but is surely alive. There are also borderline cases, including viruses, which are parasitic on host cells for reproduction, and prions, proteinaceous infectious particles, which can replicate but not reproduce. These and other borderline cases should be expected for the cluster concept of life because borderline cases should be expected for all cluster concepts. How many capacities must be present for an entity to be considered to be alive is a vexed matter known as the sorites problem or sorites paradox. *See also* DEATH.

LIFE CYCLE. The pattern of human existence from conception through birth, infancy through childhood, adolescence through adulthood, and aging, infirmity, dying, and death. If there is a universal experience for human beings, it is this pattern with its rhythms. The world's religions attempt to give **meaning** to this pattern, often in **moral theology**. The world's philosophies do the same, often in **moral philosophy**. Medicine engages human life at every stage of the life cycle, creating intersections with moral theology and moral philosophy. This reality helps to explain why both moral theology and moral philosophy contribute to **bioethics** and **medical ethics**.

LIFE SUPPORT. *See* LIFE-SUSTAINING TREATMENT.

LIFE UNWORTHY OF LIFE. From the German, *lebensunwerten Lebens*, a concept put forth by **Karl Binding** (1841–1920) and **Alfred Hoche** (1865–1943). This concept was used to classify patients as having no **value** to others, which became part of the justificatory framework for the crimes against humanity carried out by Nazi Germany during World War II. *See also* NAZI MEDICAL WAR CRIMES.

LIFE-SUSTAINING TREATMENT. The use of mechanical, pharmaceutical, and other interventions to supplant or replace the function of organs when the organ's malfunction is considered life-threatening in **deliberative clinical judgment**. Life-sustaining treatment has two goals: (1) prevention of imminent death; and (2) survival with at least some interactive capacity. The second goal rejects *vitalism*, which is countenanced in some moral theologies. *See also* ADVANCE DIRECTIVE; END-OF-LIFE CARE; FUTILITY.

LIGUORI, ALPHONSUS (1696–1787). Italian Roman Catholic bishop. His **moral theology** addresses both the **ethical obligations** and sins of physicians. He systematized **casuistry**, or **analogical reasoning**, from **paradigm cases** of right or wrong conduct or good and bad character to new cases to analyze behavior or character in the new case to reach a **judgment** about whether it is **ethically impermissible, ethically obligatory**, or **ethically permissible**. One goal of such systemization is to minimize the risk that physicians might encounter a case that is *sui generis*, which would mean that there was no paradigm case to guide **ethical reasoning**, thus increasing the chances of erroneous **judgment**.

LIMITED RIGHT. *See* PRIMA FACIE RIGHT.

LIVING WILL. An **advance directive** completed by a **patient** or, where permitted by law, a patient's **surrogate**, that refuses initiation and continuation of **life-sustaining treatment** when a patient has (a) lost **decision-making capacity** and (b) a **terminal condition** or an **irreversible condition** as defined in applicable advance directive legislation. Some jurisdictions allow both written and oral living wills. *See also* DIRECTIVE TO PHYSICIANS; DURABLE POWER OF ATTORNEY FOR HEALTHCARE; MEDICAL POWER OF ATTORNEY.

LONG-TERM CARE. The provision of **biopsychosocial** support and services to **patients** with diminished capacity for independent living, especially patients with reduced capacity for the activities of daily living and the activities of independent living. A major challenge in **ethical reasoning** about long-term care planning is balancing the **values** of independence and safety. It has been argued in this reasoning that safety should not be reduced to biological (i.e., physical or bodily) safety but should also include psychological and social safety. Protecting the latter two dimensions of safety may provide the basis of an **ethical justification** of increased physical risk.

Most long-term care services are provided by family members, usually female family members, known as "informal" caregivers. The increasing biopsychosocial burdens of care raise challenges for these women of the limits of the **virtue** of **self-sacrifice**. When these limits are reached, individuals and families turn to "formal" caregivers, healthcare professionals and personal aides, who provide paid services in the home or in assisted-care and long-term care facilities.

Long-term care services are paid for by individuals and their families from net income and savings, by private long-term care insurance (which can be very expensive), and by **Medicaid** for those who qualify by income and savings. Individuals and families of color use Medicaid as a source of payment less often than do white individuals and families. The increasing cost of institutional long-term care (nursing homes) paid by Medicaid has become a major financial challenge for many state governments. *See also* ETHICS OF CARE; GERIATRIC ETHICS.

M

MAIMONIDES (MOSES BEN MAIMON, 1135–1204 CE). Spanish Talmudist and physician. His **Jewish medical ethics** emphasizes the primacy of the capacity to heal in the care of the sick even on the Sabbath. He opposed what he characterized as irrational treatments, which are inconsistent with this emphasis. Maimonides remains an important source of influence on **Jewish bioethics**. "Oath of Maimonides" and "The Daily Prayer of a Physician" are attributed to him but were probably written by **Markus Herz** (1747–1803).

MALPRACTICE INSURANCE. *See* PROFESSIONAL LIABILITY.

MANIPULATION. The use of psychological, communication, and other tools to strongly influence **decision making** by a **patient**. Manipulation is understood not to involve **coercion** or other measures that would result in a decision-making process that is not **voluntary**. However, because manipulation aims to strongly influence the decision-making process and therefore poses a threat to the patient's **autonomy**. From the perspective of the **ethical principle of respect for autonomy**, manipulation bears the **burden of justification**. *See also* BEHAVIORAL PSYCHOLOGY; NUDGE.

MARX, KARL FRIEDRICH HEINRICH (1796–1877). German physician. He took the view that "medicine is a part of ethics" and that physicians were justified in sometimes not accepting some wishes of patients. **Medical ethics** should be based, he held, on the physician's honor, a form of self-regard.

MATERNAL-FETAL MEDICINE. A subspecialty of obstetrics and gynecology, focusing on high-risk pregnancy and the obstetric management of fetal anomalies, for the benefit of maternal, fetal, and neonatal **patients**. The **professional medical ethics** of maternal-fetal medicine appeals to the **ethical concept of the fetus as a patient**.

MATERNAL-FETAL SURGERY. Surgery performed for the benefit of the fetal **patient** and **neonatal patient**. This surgery, whether open or minimal access (e.g., via fetoscopy), creates clinical risk for both the pregnant and fetal patients, from the procedure itself and for the current and future pregnancy. These risks must be disclosed in the **informed consent process**. The **professional medical ethics** of maternal-fetal surgery, therefore, require the identification and balancing of three **ethical obligations**: beneficence-based and **autonomy**-based ethical obligations to the pregnant patient, and beneficence-based obligations to the fetal patient. Some accounts treat respect for autonomy of the pregnant woman and, therefore, autonomy-based ethical obligations to her as **absolute ethical obligations**. Other accounts treat the **ethical principle of beneficence** and the **ethical principle of respect for autonomy** as prima facie and therefore the ethical obligations that they generate as prima facie. *See also* ETHICAL CONCEPT OF THE FETUS AS A PATIENT.

MATERNAL-FETAL TREATMENT. Invasive medical (e.g., use of medication) or surgical **clinical management** performed for the benefit of the fetal **patient** and **neonatal patient**. Such clinical management treatment creates clinical risk for both the pregnant and fetal patients, from the treatment itself and for the current and future pregnancy; these risks must be disclosed in the **informed consent process**. The **professional medical ethics** of maternal-fetal surgery, therefore, requires the identification and balancing of three **ethical obligations**: beneficence-based and **autonomy**-based ethical obligations to the pregnant patient; and beneficence-based obligations to the fetal patient. Some accounts treat respect for the autonomy of the pregnant woman and, therefore, autonomy-based ethical obligations to her to be **absolute ethical obligations**. Other accounts treat the **ethical principle of beneficence** and the **ethical principle of respect for autonomy** as prima facie and, therefore, the ethical obligations that they generate as prima facie. *See also* ETHICAL CONCEPT OF THE FETUS AS A PATIENT.

MATHER, COTTON (1663–1728). New England Puritan minister. His teachings include the view that being a physician and being a cleric is an "angelic conjunction," at a time when it was not uncommon to be both. Such a physician-clergyman is in a position to treat both disease and spiritual problems, anticipating the importance of the spiritual dimensions of **patient care** for both **patients** and physicians.

MAXIMIN JUSTICE. *See* RAWLSIAN JUSTICE.

MAXIMIN PRINCIPLE OF JUSTICE. *See* RAWLSIAN JUSTICE.

McCORMICK, RICHARD A., SJ (1922–2000). Roman Catholic Jesuit priest and moral theologian. He was one of the founders of the field of **bioethics** in the United States. His annual "Notes on Moral Theology" in *Theological Studies* were widely read and influential on **moral theology**, especially **Christian moral theology** and **Roman Catholic moral theology**. He served as the Rose F. Kennedy Professor of Christian Ethics in the Kennedy Institute of Ethics at Georgetown University in Washington, DC, from 1974 to 1986.

MECHANICAL CIRCULATORY DEVICE. *See* MECHANICAL CIRCULATORY SUPPORT.

MECHANICAL CIRCULATORY SUPPORT. The use of implantable devices, such as the left-ventricular device or Impella device, to support circulation, or external devices, such as extracorporeal membrane oxygenation, to support circulation and provide oxygen to the blood. Mechanical circulatory support is a form of **life-sustaining treatment**, which means that **ethical reasoning** about such support is the same as that about life-sustaining treatment. Phrases such as *destination therapy* and *bridge to transplantation* should not be used because they fail to classify such support accurately in **professional medical ethics**. *See also* END-OF-LIFE CARE; FUTILITY.

MEDIATION. A technique of negotiation developed in the law and brought into **clinical ethics consultation**, especially in cases in which a **patient** or a **surrogate** or other family member has made a request for **clinical management** that the physician and care team has refused to implement. The goal is to find some common ground to serve as the basis for resolving the **ethical conflict**.

A problem for mediation arises when the physician and care team are **ethically justified** in their **judgment** that implementing the request would violate the **professional virtue of integrity**. In such a case, there is no potential for common ground. The conflict needs to be resolved by the ethically justified and legally permissible exercise of **power** exerted by the healthcare organization to protect the professional integrity of its professional staff and avoid the exercise of **raw power**. **Advance Directives Acts** in some jurisdictions allow for the exercise of such ethically justified power in **end-of-life care**. *See also* FUTILITY; RIGHT TO REFUSE TREATMENT.

MEDICAID. In the United States, a program of payment for healthcare costs for those determined to be medically indigent. Funding is shared by the states and federal government, with the states determining eligibility requirements. About 40 percent of children are covered by this program and about half of births. Payment levels are usually lower than **Medicare** and private insurance. The program was enacted in 1965 (https://www.medicaid.gov/, accessed 14 September 2017). *See also* HEALTH POLICY; PUBLIC POLICY.

MEDICAL EMERGENCY. A **condition** of a **patient** that can cause **death** or serious, far-reaching, and irreversible **disability** or **disease** unless **clinical management** begins immediately, which means that there is no time for either the **informed consent process** or **informed refusal**. This clinical reality creates an **ethically justified** exception to the **ethical obligation** to obtain **consent** from the patient. There is a **prima facie ethical obligation** to initiate clinical management immediately, based on the **ethical principle of beneficence** and **presumed consent**, unless there is valid refusal of it, in the form of an **advance directive** or the informed refusal of a **surrogate** for patients with an **irreversible condition** or a **terminal condition**. *See also* INFORMED CONSENT PROCESS.

MEDICAL ERROR. Medical error can occur in one of two ways: (1) the process of **clinical judgment** supported in **deliberative clinical judgment** is implemented incorrectly (doing the right thing the wrong way, e.g., administering the wrong dose of a drug that was correctly prescribed); or (2) the wrong process of clinical management is provided, in other words, clinical management that is not compatible with deliberative clinical judgment (doing the wrong thing, e.g., administering a contraindicated drug).

During the late 1990s, there emerged strong **consensus** among professional associations of physicians about the professionally responsible management of medical errors. Such rapid consensus formation is unusual in the history of **professional medical ethics**. When a medical error results in an adverse outcome for the **patient**, the patient should be informed by the responsible physician because such disclosure is **ethically obligatory** by the **reasonable person standard** of the **informed consent process**. For the same reason, there is an ethical obligation to inform the patient about medical errors that have been addressed but remain clinically significant because of the risks they have created. In both cases and for the same reason, the patient should also be informed about the plan of correction and provide **informed consent** to it. As a matter of **professional integrity**, the case should be reviewed in organizational processes to improve patient safety and **quality**. There is also agreement that medical errors that have been corrected in the course of clinical management such that they are not clinically significant do not create an **ethical obligation** to inform the patient because such disclosure is not required by the reasonable person standard of the informed consent process.

MEDICAL ETHICS. The disciplined study of morality—what is **ethically permissible**, **ethically impermissible**, and **ethically obligatory**—in the practice of medicine; the decisions and behavior of patients; physician leadership; the policies and practices of healthcare organizations, both public and private (such as private clinics and hospitals, public clinics and hospitals, and private and public hospital systems) as they influence physicians and patients; physicians engaged in **innovation** and **research** with animal and human subjects; in medical education; and the role of physicians and patients in **health policy** and **public policy** formulated and implemented by the executive, judicial, legislative, and regulatory branches of government at all levels (e.g., in the United States, at the local, regional, state, and federal levels). There is a global history of medical ethics, written by both physicians and nonphysicians dating to the ancient world (Baker and McCullough, 2005). **Professional medical ethics** becomes part of the history of medical ethics during the 18th-century enlightenments in Scotland and England. Professional medical ethics has become a global discipline that aims to be transcultural, transnational, and transreligious. Refer to the introduction and *see also* BIOETHICS; BIOMEDICAL ETHICS.

MEDICAL ETHICS; OR, A CODE OF INSTITUTES AND PRECEPTS. Probably the first book with this title in English in the global history of medical ethics, by the English physician and ethicist **Thomas Percival** (1740–1804). The full title is *Medical Ethics; or, A Code of Institutes and Precepts, Adapted to the Professional Conduct of Physicians and Surgeons* (Percival 1804). The title reveals that Percival meant this to be a book about **professional medical ethics** and to unite physicians and surgeons into one profession, ending centuries of separation into rival groups and guilds. The word *institutes* at that time meant physiology, including mental physiology, or the basic science of medicine. In professional medical ethics, the word *institutes* means **moral science** or moral physiology, or how **judgments** should be made. *Precepts* means practical guides based on moral science.

Percival drew on the moral science of **David Hume** (1711–1776) and **Richard Price** (1723–1791). Percival preceded *Medical Ethics* with his *Medical Jurisprudence* (Percival 1794), which he distributed to friends and scholars for their comments. He was asked by the trustees of the **Royal Infirmary** of Manchester to write a guidebook to help with the transition from a healthcare organization that had been controlled by a small number of families of physicians into a large, comprehensive hospital. The hospital's staff was to be open to men (there were no women physicians or surgeons at this time in England) of talent. Instead of an ethics of loyalty to family, an **ethics of cooperation** was needed (Baker 2009).

Medical Ethics comprises four chapters: "Of Professional Conduct Relative to Hospital or Other Medical Charities"; "Of Professional Conduct in Private, or General Practice"; "Of the Conduct of Physicians to Apothecaries"; and "Of Professional Duties in Certain Cases Which Require a Knowledge of Law." *Medical Ethics* is an acknowledged source of the **American Medical Association** *Code of Medical Ethics* **of 1847**; the *Code* includes many verbatim passages from Percival's book.

Percival adopts **John Gregory**'s (1724–1773) account of the **ethical concept of medicine as a profession**. Percival makes the important contribution of conceiving medicine as a "public trust" and not a self-interested merchant guild. The third commitment of the ethical concept of medicine as a profession is therefore formulated as the commitment to sustain medicine as a public trust rather than a **self-interested** merchant guild, which medicine had been for centuries in Britain.

MEDICAL ETIQUETTE. The proper manners of physicians toward their **patients** and each other. There has been a tendency in the literature of **bioethics** and **medical ethics** to dismiss medical etiquette as self-serving or mere manners, and thus devoid of ethical significance.

This skepticism reflects the crisis of manners and **etiquette** in the 18th century, created by the loss of confidence that one could infer from good manners to good character. For ethicists such as **John Gregory** (1724–1773), this posed a challenge, which he addressed by identifying what should count as the etiquette in **professional medical ethics**. The professional physician is never to be ostentatious, calling attention to his many sacrifices. Moreover, the physician's professional demeanor should not change with the social class of the patient or, in contemporary parlance, with the source of payment for the patient. Gregory can be read as attempting to restore confidence in the inference from true professional etiquette of a physician to professional character and the **professional virtues**. In the context of professional medical ethics, medical etiquette is, therefore, not mere etiquette but of considerable ethical significance, because professional behavior and demeanor show **respect** for patients, their families, and professional colleagues.

Some, such as **Chauncey Leake** (1896–1978), dismiss medical etiquette as mere rules of behavior among physicians or between physicians and other healthcare professionals. This is a mistake, because there are ethically significant **boundary issues** when physicians interact with other physicians and healthcare professionals, especially when they compete for patients. These boundary issues should be managed on the basis of the commitment to **competence** in **patient care**.

MEDICAL HUMANITIES. Scholarly work and teaching on **clinical practice**, **research**, and **health policy** from the disciplinary perspectives of the humanities (art history, history, literature, narrative, and the qualitative social sciences) and the deployment of this scholarship in teaching and **patient care**. While philosophy is a humanities discipline, the use of the term *medical humanities* is meant to distinguish this field of inquiry from **medical ethics** and **philosophy of medicine**. *See also* PERSONALISM.

MEDICAL JURISPRUDENCE. Generally understood to mean the application of law to medicine, including **clinical practice** and **research**. However, in the 18th century, the scope of medical jurisprudence included **medical ethics**. For example, **Thomas Percival**'s (1740–1804) *Medical Jurisprudence* (Percival 1794) includes sections on medical ethics for hospital practice and medical ethics for private practice, as well as "Of the Knowledge of Law Requisite for Physicians and Surgeons." By the early 19th century, medical ethics was not included in the scope of medical jurisprudence, for example, in **Theodoric Romeyn Beck**'s (1791–1855) *Elements of Medical Jurisprudence* (Beck 1823). *See also MEDICAL ETHICS; OR, A CODE OF INSTITUTES AND PRECEPTS.*

MEDICAL JURISPRUDENCE **BY THOMAS PERCIVAL.** A privately published and circulated text of 1794 by **Thomas Percival** (1740–1804). Percival drafted this text in response to a request from the trustees of the **Royal Infirmary** of Manchester, in England, because of the lack of cooperation among two families of physicians who controlled appointments to the "faculty," or professional staff, and among physicians, surgeons, and apothecaries. *Medical jurisprudence*, as then used, included **medical ethics** as well as matters of law that physicians needed to know. The text, therefore, addresses medical ethics for hospital practice and medical ethics for private practice and also includes a section titled "Of the Knowledge of Law Requisite for Physicians and Surgeons." This text became the basis for Percival's 1803 *Medical Ethics*. *See also* MEDICAL JURISPRUDENCE.

MEDICAL MORALITY. This phrase has two meanings. The first is as a synonym for **medical ethics**. The second use is to refer to the actual beliefs and practices of physicians about good character and proper behavior. These can be described using the methods of **empirical bioethics** and **empirical medical ethics**. This sets the stage for improving medical morality using the methods of **ethical reasoning** of **normative bioethics** and **normative medical ethics**. *See also* BIOETHICS; ETHICS; PROFESSIONAL MEDICAL ETHICS.

MEDICAL PATERNALISM. Paternalism practiced by a physician, in other words, interference by a physician with the **autonomy** of the **patient** justified by appeal to **beneficence**-based clinical ethical judgment to protect the patient from harm. The objections to medical paternalism appeal mainly to the **ethical principle of respect for autonomy**. This ethical principle grounds the **negative right** to noninterference with an individual's decisions and judgments and behavior based on them.

Some take the view that this is an **absolute negative right**, where medical paternalism is always **ethically impermissible**. Some take the view that this is a **limited negative right** or **prima facie negative right**, where medical paternalism is sometimes **ethically permissible**. Some bioethicists also object to medical paternalism on the grounds that physicians and other healthcare professionals do not have the intellectual **authority** to make judgments for patients about what is in their interests, which reflects a thoroughgoing skepticism of **beneficence-based clinical judgment** and **deliberative clinical judgment**.

Many bioethicists understand the field to be a response to the long history of medical paternalism as an accepted practice in the history of medical ethics, even though the textual evidence does not support this interpretation of the history of medical ethics (McCullough 2011). *See also* PATERNALISTIC.

MEDICAL POLICE. This phrase has two meanings: (1) a system of **public health** and a **medical ethics** in which the physician's primary **ethical obligation** is to the state, a concept introduced into the histories of medical ethics, medicine, and public health by **Johann Peter Frank** (1745–1821) in 1799; (2) a **code of medical ethics** for the self-government of physicians in various states of the United States in the early 19th century (Baker 2013). *See also* SYSTEM OF MEDICAL ETHICS.

MEDICAL POWER OF ATTORNEY. An **advance directive** by which a **patient** names and authorizes a **surrogate** to make decisions for the patient when the patient is determined to have lost **decision-making capacity**. The patient does not have to have an **irreversible condition** or a **terminal condition**. Usually, it is legally required that a Medical Power of Attorney is written, in a form prescribed in law, and witnessed. *See also* DURABLE POWER OF ATTORNEY FOR HEALTHCARE.

MEDICAL TOURISM. The practice of **patients** traveling to other countries for medical or surgical care, at a lower cost than they would pay in the United States, even with travel expenses. In some countries, the physicians offering these services are certified by specialty boards in the United States.

There is no **ethical controversy** about the **right** of patients to engage in this practice. Objections to medical tourism appear to arise from the **self-interest** of physicians in avoiding lower-priced competition. Should a patient who has traveled abroad for medical or surgical care experience complications, he or she often turns to local physicians for the management of these complications. In **professional medical ethics**, once these individuals present for care, they become patients and should receive **clinical management** based on **deliberative clinical judgment**. The **professional virtue of self-efface-ment** creates an **ethical obligation** of physicians not to express or be **biased** by their own personal views about the **prudence** of medical tourism.

MEDICALLY INDICATED. A term of art used in medical discourse to refer to a form of clinical management that is expected to benefit a **patient** clinically. This is, therefore, a **beneficence**-based concept. The strength of the term *medically indicated* is a function of the evidence base for expected clinical benefit. That a form of **clinical management** is medically indicated (i.e., a **medically reasonable alternative**), does not mean that the physician has an **ethical justification** to implement it without the patient's **informed consent**, except in **medical emergencies**.

MEDICALLY REASONABLE ALTERNATIVE. A form of **clinical management** that satisfies two conditions: it is technically possible, and it is supported in **deliberative clinical judgment** and **beneficence**-based clinical judgment and is, therefore, reliably expected to benefit the patient clinically. In the **informed consent process**, the physician leading the process has an **ethical obligation** to present all of the medically reasonable alternatives to the patient—or to the patient's **surrogate**—for consideration of authorization. There is no ethical obligation to offer clinical management that is not technically possible. There is no ethical obligation to offer a form of clinical management that is technically possible but not supported in deliberative and beneficence-based clinical judgment. Nor is there a **legal obligation** to do so. *See also* ETHICAL PRINCIPLE OF BENEFICENCE.

MEDICARE. In the United States, a program of payment funded by the federal government for the healthcare costs of the elderly (more than 65 years of age), the disabled, and those with end-stage renal disease. Part A covers hospital care, Part B covers physician fees, and Part D covers pre-scription drugs. Part C is managed care provided by private insurance com-panies that are paid by Medicare. Medicare does not cover all healthcare costs. "Medigap" insurance is offered by private insurance companies to address this problem. The program was enacted in 1965 (https://www.ssa.gov/medicare/, accessed 14 September 2017). *See also* HEALTH POLICY; PUBLIC POLICY.

MEDICUS POLTICUS. The concept of the "politic physician" (sometimes mistranslated and misunderstood as the "political physician"). The word *politic* has its origins in the power structure of royal courts, in which everyone is subject to the power of the sovereign. "Politic" **ethics** addresses how one ought to comport oneself when one is in a relationship of asymmetrical power (i.e., when one is relatively less powerful, sometimes much less powerful). The politic courtier acts on the **virtue** of **prudence**, which schools one in the discipline of identifying one's **legitimate self-interests** and acting to protect and promote them. In **medical ethics**, the politic physician, employed in a royal court or by a municipality in the 17th and 18th centuries, was subordinate to royal or mayoral power and was therefore at risk of being dismissed from employment and confronting poverty. (This was a time when there was no economic security for physicians, a phenomenon that dates only from the end of World War II.)

Physician-ethicists such as **Rodrigo de Castro** (1550–1627) and **Friedrich Hoffmann** (1660–1738) wrote texts to guide the **ethical reasoning** of physicians in this position of asymmetrical power relationships, titled *Medicus Politicus*, based on the virtue of prudence. Hoffmann's distinctive contribution was to interpret the physician's legitimate self-interests on the basis of the **interests** of the **patient**, known as enlightened self-interest. The concept of *medicus politicus* and its ethical reasoning based on the virtue of prudence have current application to the asymmetrical power relationships of physicians to organizational leaders, private and public payers, and to government authorities.

MENTAL HEALTH DIRECTIVE. An **advance directive** that a **patient** with mental illness or disorder can complete, when he or she has **decision-making capacity**, to provide advance **informed consent** or **informed refusal** of psychiatric care at a time when the patient, in the psychiatrist's **deliberative clinical judgment**, needs such treatment but has lost decision-making capacity. Applicable law may restrict the scope of treatment that can be addressed in a mental health directive. *See also* DIRECTIVE TO PHYSICIANS; LIVING WILL.

MERCY KILLING. Killing a **patient**, with or without authorization in the **informed consent process**, in order to relieve **distress, pain**, and **suffering**. In **professional medical ethics**, mercy killing with or without the authorization of the patient is **ethically impermissible**. Given the capacities of palliative care to provide symptom relief and effective management of **distress, pain,** and **suffering,** mercy killing is also considered to be clinically unnecessary in professional medical ethics. *See also* EUTHANASIA.

MERE OPINION. A **judgment** that is held without argument (i.e., without supporting reasons in the form of implications of relevant ethical concepts that have been clarified and used consistently). In many places in the *Dialogues*, Plato (427–347 BCE) has Socrates, correctly, dismiss mere opinion as having no intellectual **authority** in **ethical reasoning**.

MERE SELF-INTEREST. Forms of **self-interest** that are not based in past, present, or future states of affairs that are highly valued, or should be highly valued, by an individual, as are **legitimate self-interests**. Mere self-interests are transitory or only weakly valued. They are therefore justifiably sacrificed when in conflict with **ethical obligations**. *See also* INTEREST.

METAETHICS. Ethical theory. Ethical theory includes elaboration of general, abstract accounts of the meaning of the concepts, such as an **ethical principle** and a **virtue**, and methods, such as transcendental reasoning deployed by the German philosopher Immanuel Kant (1724–1804 CE), of **ethical reasoning**. Ethical theory also aims to show how these concepts join together and thus display **coherence** and **applicability**. *See also* ETHICS.

MILITARY MEDICAL ETHICS. *See* PROFESSIONAL MILITARY MEDICAL ETHICS.

MINIMALLY CONSCIOUS STATE. A **clinical judgment** that a patient's awareness has been greatly but not completely diminished. This awareness is not manifested in the patient's behavior but is claimed to be detected by changes in brain function identified by functional magnetic resonance imaging. Given that the determination that a patient is in a **persistent vegetative state** or a **permanent vegetative state** is also a clinical judgment, the boundaries between a minimally conscious state and a vegetative state should not be taken to be sharp but blurred. This has raised issues about the reliability of a **clinical ethical judgment** that a patient in a permanent vegetative state has an **irreversible condition**, as defined in an applicable **Advance Directives Act**. There is **ethical controversy** about the **moral status** of individuals diagnosed to be in a minimally conscious state. *See also* PERSON; PERSONHOOD.

MOLL, ALBERT (1862–1939). German physician. His *Ärtzliche Ethik* (*Doctor's Ethics*, 1902) is comprehensive and includes **ethics of research with human subjects**, arguing that written **consent** is required for research with significant risks. This text was translated into Russian in the late 19th century and provoked a critical response there. Moll's **medical ethics** is based on the role of the physician as healer, and his approach was practical, taking the form of a handbook.

MONOPOLY POWER. A monopoly exists when there is a single provider of a good or service in the marketplace that gains **power** over market exchanges. This can occur in healthcare when a healthcare organization such as a large, multihospital system gains such a large market of **patients** that insurance companies must include the system in order to market their plans. The result is that the hospital system may decide to use its market power to pursue revenue streams as its primary concern and motivation. This can create an **organizational culture** that is incompatible with the **ethical concept of medicine as a profession**. Physician leaders in such healthcare organizations have an **ethical obligation** to their professional colleagues and the organization's patients to protect and sustain the **professional virtue of integrity** and an **organizational culture** based on the ethical concept of medicine as a profession (Chervenak and McCullough 2005).

MONOPSONY POWER. A monopsony exists when there is a single purchaser of goods or services in the marketplace that gains **power** over market exchanges. This can occur in healthcare when an insurance company gains such a large market of **patients** that physicians and healthcare organizations must accept contracts from the insurance company if they hope to sustain their business models. It is essential that they do so, a reality captured in the management dictum "No margin, no mission." Physicians and healthcare organizations find themselves in a position of inferior power to the monopsony payer. The concept of *medicus politicus* or the politic physician, applies in this case. The **ethical concept of medicine as a profession** creates an **ethical obligation** to the healthcare organization's physicians, other healthcare professionals, and patients, when accepting what is analyzed to be an economically disadvantageous contract, to protect and sustain the **professional virtue of integrity** and an **organizational culture** based on the ethical concept of medicine as a profession (Chervenak and McCullough 2005).

MONSTER. A word used in the past to refer to infants with what are now called congenital anomalies and were once called birth defects. The meaning is taken from the Latin *monster*, meaning a sign or portent sent from the gods for transgressing against them. In Christian traditions, this word is taken over and means a sign or portent sent from God to punish women for the sins of intercourse. There were two such sins: sexual intercourse with animals (producing "wolf boys," or extreme hirsutism); and sexual intercourse during menstruation (the "unclean period"). The remedy for the woman was to be shriven of her sin. The remedy for the infant might include **infanticide**, placement in a foundling home where the mortality rate from neglect was very high, abandonment with the expectation of death, or survival. There was **ethical controversy** about this practice, originating in different accounts of the **moral status** of such infants. *See also* CHILD; SEVERE FETAL ANOMALY.

MORAL. Ambiguous between actions that are **ethically obligatory** and **ethically permissible** and individuals as having good character (i.e., a preponderance of **virtues** over **vices**). *See also* ETHICAL; IMMORAL; UNETHICAL.

MORAL DISTRESS. The experience of **distress** for a healthcare professional when he or she is not able to provide **clinical management** that is supported in **deliberative clinical judgment**. This distress is ethically significant because it originates in challenges to, threats to, and violations of the **professional virtue of integrity** (Thomas and McCullough 2015).

MORAL JUDGMENT. A **judgment** about whether behavior is **ethically impermissible, ethically obligatory, ethically permissible, ethically controversial**, or ethically uncertain or about good and bad **character**, using the tools of **ethical reasoning**.

MORAL NORM. A **norm** or standard for correct behavior or character formation that generates an **ethical obligation** to conform to that standard. *See also* ETHICAL REASONING.

MORAL OBLIGATION. *See* ETHICAL OBLIGATION. *See also* OBLIGATION.

MORAL PHILOSOPHY. Ethical reasoning using concepts and methods from philosophical **ethics**. *See also* ETHICS.

MORAL PLURALISM. The histories of **ethics, bioethics**, and **medical ethics** provide indisputable evidence that there are competing approaches to **ethical reasoning**. These approaches include **moral theology** and **moral philosophy**. Given the large number and theological diversity of the world's religions, moral theology displays marked variation across and within faith communities and traditions. Given the large number and diversity of the world's philosophical methods, schools, and traditions, moral philosophy displays marked diversity. This double diversity defines moral pluralism.

Moral pluralism does not entail **ethical controversy** on all topics, because there can be agreement on the outcome of ethical reasoning that starts from diverse conceptual origins (Beauchamp and Childress 2013), for example, that murder (the intentional **killing** of an innocent other) is **ethically impermissible**, that there are **human rights** that must be acknowledged and protected by governments in order for them to be considered ethically and politically legitimate, and that adult **patients** with intact **decision-making capacity** should provide **informed consent** for invasive, clinically risky procedures. The diverse approaches of moral theology and moral philosophy can also display **complementarity**: none alone is sufficient to capture the full range of moral concern, but each contributes to comprehensive ethical reasoning. This is the basis for **pluralistic casuistry**.

MORAL PSYCHOLOGY. A field of inquiry deploying methods of both **moral philosophy** and psychology. Moral psychology can also be classified as a form of **experimental ethics**. *See also* MORAL REALISM; MORAL SCIENCE.

MORAL REALISM. A method for **moral philosophy** in which **judgments** about what is **ethically impermissible**, **ethically permissible**, or **ethically obligatory** are justified by appeal to the moral properties of things in the world. This method allows for **moral judgments** to be true or false. Moral realism was deployed by **Richard Price** (1723–1791), whose moral philosophy was a major influence on **Thomas Percival**'s (1740–1804) **professional medical ethics**. *See also* ETHICAL REASONING; MORAL SCIENCE.

MORAL RIGHT. A **right** established by **ethical reasoning**, typically by appealing to **metaethics**, or ethical theories. *See also* LEGAL RIGHT.

MORAL SCIENCE. A method of investigating "principles" (constitutive causal process in an entity) that generate valued attitudes and behavior toward others. This method was based on the scientific method set out by **Francis Bacon** (1561–1626) and used by such figures as the Scottish moralist **David Hume** (1711–1776) and the Scottish physician-ethicist Dr. **John Gregory** (1724–1773). Moral science predates contemporary **moral psychology** by more than two centuries. *See also* ETHICAL REASONING.

MORAL STATUS. An entity is such that others have an **ethical obligation** to protect and promote the **interests** of that entity. An entity may have **independent moral status** that it generates on its own or **dependent moral status** that is generated by a social role occupied by the entity. *See also* PERSON; PERSONHOOD.

MORAL THEOLOGY. Ethical reasoning that appeals to sources of moral **authority** in a specific faith community. Moral theology contributes to the pluralism of **bioethics** and **medical ethics**. Moral theology, because it is not secular, is not methodologically adequate to serve as the basis of **professional medical ethics**.

MORAL TRUTH. The concept that **ethical reasoning** can be true, because the concepts invoked in **ethical analysis** describe moral facts: realities in the world that are independent of individuals engaged in ethical reasoning. There is disagreement in contemporary **moral philosophy** about the ground and limitation of moral truth. The method of **ethical reasoning** appealing to moral truths is known as **moral realism**.

MORALITY. The actual beliefs of individuals or groups about good and bad **character** and right and wrong behavior. These are investigated using the methods of **descriptive medical ethics** and **descriptive bioethics**. **Ethical reasoning** seeks to improve morality. Sometimes, the terms *morality* and *ethics* are used interchangeably, which can be confusing and therefore should be avoided.

MORBIDITY. A general term of art in medical discourse to refer to the presence of a **condition, disability, disease, disorder**, or **injury** in a **patient** or population of patients.

MORE, SAINT THOMAS (1478–1535). English lawyer, philosopher, and statesman. A Roman Catholic, he opposed King Henry VIII's separation from the Roman Catholic Church and was executed for treason. In his *Utopia* (1516), he considered the permissibility of **suicide** and **euthanasia** (in the sense of a death with minimized pain).

MORTALITY. A term of art in medical discourse to refer to the **death** of a **patient**.

MUTILATION. Surgical alteration of an individual's anatomy that results in **biopsychosocial** harm, as judged in **deliberative clinical judgment**, that is not offset by biopsychosocial goods, as judged from that individual's perspective, including a cultural or religious perspective. This distinguishes mutilation from **cosmetic surgery**. Because mutilation results in net harm to a **patient** it is incompatible with the **ethical principle of beneficence** and the **ethical principle of nonmaleficence**. Mutilation is therefore **ethically impermissible** in **bioethics, medical ethics**, and **professional medical ethics**. *See also* GENITAL MUTILATION.

N

NARRATIVE ETHICS. The use of such genres of writing as autobiography, biography, diary writing or journaling, novels, poetry, short stories, and plays to explore topics in **bioethics**, **medical ethics**, and **professional medical ethics**. These techniques of imagination help increase insight into the experiences of being a **patient**, family member, or healthcare professional, especially the affective dimensions of such experience that are not captured in **ethical reasoning** based on **moral philosophy**. An important advantage claimed for narrative ethics is "thick description" of cases (i.e., richness of detail and context) in contrast to brief case summaries that are used in teaching and scholarship. *See also* MEDICAL HUMANITIES.

NATIONAL CATHOLIC BIOETHICS CENTER. Founded in 1972, this center "conducts research, consultation, publishing and education to promote human dignity in health care and the life sciences, and derives its message directly from the teachings of the Catholic Church" (https://www.ncbcenter.org/, accessed 14 September 2017). *See also* MORAL THEOLOGY; ROMAN CATHOLIC MORAL THEOLOGY.

NATIONAL COMMISSION. *See* PRESIDENTIAL COMMITTEE.

NATIONAL HEALTH INSURANCE. The provision of health insurance for all, known as universal coverage, by the government. Advocates for national health insurance invoke competing accounts of the **ethical principle of justice** and the **right to healthcare**. Critics point out that, in the United States, national health insurance would concentrate too much **power** in the government. Concern about concentrated power in both the public and private sectors has a long history in the United States. This concern explains why, despite the considerable inefficiencies that result, the United States Constitution divides the power to govern among three co-equal branches of government and why there are five branches of the armed services. *See also* HEALTH POLICY; PUBLIC POLICY.

NATIONAL MEDICAL ASSOCIATION (NMA). The national association of African American physicians in the United States, which was founded in 1895 in response to the **racist** exclusion policies and practice of the medical societies in the southern states during the era of legal segregation. In 2008, the **American Medical Association** issued a formal apology for the wrong done to African American physicians (Baker 2013). The NMA is a party to the **American Medical Association** *Principles of Medical Ethics*.

NATURAL DEATH. A process of **dying** without **life-sustaining treatment** and in a **hospital** that aims to preserve **dignity** and is based on the **ethical principle of respect for persons**. This concept came to prominence in the United States and other developed countries in the 1970s in response to what was perceived as the dehumanization of **patients** in **critical care** units, epitomized in the **Quinlan Case**. The concept of a natural death played a major role in the first **Natural Death Acts** that were enacted in the late 1970s that authorized **living wills**. The preambles (an opening statement in **statutory laws** in which the legislature states the purpose of legislation) of these statutes often expressed rejection of a dehumanized dying process. *See also* EUTHANASIA.

NATURAL DEATH ACT. Legislation in the wake of *In re Quinlan* in the late 1970s and 1980s in the United States to authorize preparation and implementation of **living wills**. This genre of **statutory law** also provides civil and criminal immunities for physicians and other healthcare professionals who implement a patient's living will. California enacted the first such statute in 1976. *See also* ADVANCE DIRECTIVE; ADVANCE DIRECTIVES ACT.

NATURAL EXPERIMENT. Carefully observing and reporting a previously unknown or unreported **disability, disease,** or **injury** in a **patient,** to learn more about its course and thus forming hypotheses about how **clinical management** of it might be improved. *See also* BACON, FRANCIS (1561–1626); EVIDENCE-BASED MEDICINE.

NATURAL LAW. A concept of deist metaphysics in which a creator god (not the God of religions, which distinguishes **deism** from **theism**) creates all of physical reality, which is ordered in patterns caused by the laws of nature. This order of nature is oriented to human good. Natural law metaphysics thus provides the foundation for **natural rights**. The protection and exercise of these rights are oriented to human good. After the introduction of **evolution** and its core concept of variation in the 19th century by Charles Darwin (1809–1882) was introduced into the history of biology, the concept that the natural world has an orientation—a direction or purpose—toward human good collapses. This conceptual change undermines the foundations of natural law because the patterns of nature do not require appeal to natural law for their explanation and because the patterns of nature have no purpose or aim.

NATURAL RIGHT. A **right** that an individual has in virtue of being a creature of a creator god. A natural right precedes all states and, therefore, all **legal rights**. The state is therefore accountable to natural rights, not vice versa. This means that a state that does not recognize and enforce natural rights is illegitimate. Natural rights are thought to originate in a creator god, rather than the God of revealed religions. This is a **deist** approach to natural rights, which is also taken to **natural law**, the metaphysical foundation of natural rights. As such, natural rights are transnational, providing a basis for international law.

NAZI DOCTORS. Physicians who supported *Nationalsozialismus* (German: National Socialism and the origin of the term *Nazi*) of Adolf Hitler in Germany in the 1930s through 1945 (when Germany surrendered to the Allied powers unconditionally and the Nazi Party was abolished). Many of them committed crimes against humanity, and some of these physicians were put on trial in Nuremberg for crimes against humanity. *See also* NAZI MEDICAL WAR CRIMES.

NAZI MEDICAL WAR CRIMES. War crimes and crimes against humanity, including unethical experimentation and mass murder, conducted by physicians during the Third Reich in Germany (1933–1945). The physician leaders were prosecuted in *United States of America v. Karl Brandt et al.*, a trial conducted under the auspices of the War Tribunal in Nuremberg, West Germany. Seven were executed, including Karl Brandt (1904–1948), Adolf Hitler's (1889–1945) personal physician. This trial produced the **Nuremberg Code**. *See also* JAPANESE MEDICAL WAR CRIMES.

NEGATIVE ABSOLUTE RIGHT. A justified claim of an individual against other individuals, organizations, or the state to noninterference in thought and action, especially in the pursuit of one's **interests** and the fulfillment of one's **ethical obligations**. An absolute **negative right** creates **absolute ethical obligation** of noninterference. *See also* ABSOLUTE RIGHT; NEGATIVE PRIMA FACIE RIGHT.

NEGATIVE EUGENICS. A subset of **eugenics** that uses techniques of breeding, genetics, or genomics to mitigate or remove traits that are considered undesirable. Negative eugenics has a long history of being racist. *See also* POSITIVE EUGENICS.

NEGATIVE PRIMA FACIE RIGHT. A justified claim of an individual against other individuals, organizations, or the state to noninterference in thought and action, especially in the pursuit of one's **interests** and the fulfillment of one's **ethical obligations**. A prima facie **negative right** creates **prima facie ethical obligation** of noninterference. *See also* NEGATIVE ABSOLUTE RIGHT; PRIMA FACIE RIGHT; RIGHT.

NEGATIVE RIGHT. A justified claim of an individual against other individuals, organizations, or the state to noninterference in thought and action, especially in the pursuit of one's **interests** and the fulfillment of one's ethical obligations. A negative **right** creates the **ethical obligation** of noninterference. A negative right can create either an **absolute ethical obligation** or a **prima facie ethical obligation**. An adequate justification for a negative right will establish criteria to guide **judgment** about whether the negative right is prima facie or absolute. *See also* POSITIVE RIGHT.

NEONATAL CRITICAL CARE. Also known as neonatal intensive care. The provision of **critical care** to **neonatal patients** (up to one year of age). Ethical issues in neonatal intensive care concern the **ethical justification** of initiating clinical intervention for infants near **viability** or infants with major anomalies and of setting **ethically justified** limits on **life-sustaining treatment**. *See also* END-OF-LIFE CARE; LIFE-SUSTAINING TREATMENT.

NEONATAL INTENSIVE CARE. *See* NEONATAL CRITICAL CARE.

NEONATAL PATIENT. A **patient** from birth through the end of the first year of life. Neonatal intensive care units are designed for the **clinical management** of such patients who need **life-sustaining treatment** in response to such conditions as prematurity and congenital anomalies. *See also* CHILD; NEONATAL CRITICAL CARE; PEDIATRIC ETHICS.

NEUROETHICS. **Ethical reasoning** about care of patients with neurological **disability, disease, disorder**, or **injury**, and **innovation** and **research** to improve the **clinical management** of such patients.

NICU. Neonatal intensive care unit. *See* NEONATAL CRITICAL CARE.

NIPT. *See* NONINVASIVE PRENATAL TESTING.

NO MORE THAN MINIMAL RISK. A concept used in **research ethics** on pediatric **subjects** and in **45 CFR 46**, the federal regulation of such research. In general, no more than minimal risk is risk that is no greater than that experienced by a child in everyday life. There is **ethical controversy** about how to interpret this concept. On the one hand, the reference set could be healthy children. On the other, the reference set could be children with the same diagnosis as children to be included in a clinical trial. The latter interpretation makes good clinical sense, but permits higher levels of risk as acceptable in a study design than the former interpretation would. *See also* ETHICAL PRINCIPLE OF NONMALEFICENCE; HARM PRINCIPLE; PRECAUTIONARY PRINCIPLE.

NONAGGRESSIVE NEONATAL MANAGEMENT. Foregoing **neonatal critical care** for palliative care for a live-born infant for whom it is **ethically justified** not to initiate **life-sustaining treatment**. Nonaggressive neonatal management is ethically justified when **beneficence**-based obligations to the fetal or neonatal patient have reached their limits or ceased to exist, based on a clinical evaluation of the fetus's or neonate's condition. *See also* PALLIATIVE CARE.

NONAGGRESSIVE OBSTETRIC MANAGEMENT. Foregoing **aggressive obstetric management** for planned vaginal delivery with two outcomes: stillbirth; or live birth followed by **nonaggressive neonatal management**. Nonaggressive obstetric management is **ethically justified** when **beneficence**-based obligations to the fetal and **neonatal patient** have reached their limits or ceased to exist, based on a clinical evaluation of the fetus's **condition**. *See also* PALLIATIVE CARE.

NON-DIRECTIVE COUNSELING. In the **informed consent process**, the physician offers all **medically reasonable alternatives** but makes no recommendation of any one of them, leaving this **decision** to the **patient**. This is the strict meaning of **shared decision making**. *See also* DIRECTIVE COUNSELING.

NONINVASIVE PRENATAL TESTING. *See* PRENATAL DIAGNOSIS.

NONMALEFICENCE. *See* ETHICAL PRINCIPLE OF NONMALEFICENCE.

NON-PATERNITY. A **biopsychosocial** condition in which the husband or male partner of a woman is not the biological father of her child. The husband or partner is assumed to be unaware of this fact. Non-paternity can be discovered by thorough history-taking of the woman or by genetic analysis of the woman and child who has become a **patient**. Informing the man that he is not the child's biological father is not compatible with the **ethical obligation** of **confidentiality** when the wife is a patient.

There are clinical circumstances in which non-paternity needs to be disclosed in the **informed consent process**, for example, for the **clinical management** of a **neonatal patient** or **pediatric patient** with a genetic **disorder** or **disease** that cannot be explained without disclosing the clinical finding of non-paternity. In the absence of such disclosure, the informed consent process will be defective because it is incomplete, which is **ethically impermissible** in **professional medical ethics**. Such disclosure may also be clinically significant for the man and the couple, for example, the reproductive risk of recurrence of the child's genetic disorder or disease for future pregnancies that the couple may initiate. *See also* ETHICAL PRINCIPLE OF NONMALEFICENCE; PRIVACY; RIGHT TO PRIVACY.

NONTHERAPEUTIC/THERAPEUTIC RESEARCH DISTINCTION. *See* THERAPEUTIC/NONTHERAPEUTIC RESEARCH DISTINCTION.

NORM. A standard for character formation or behavior to which an individual is expected to conform. Norms originate in **ethical principles** and **ethical reasoning**. Norms create **ethical obligations**. *See also* IDEAL; OBLIGATION.

NORMATIVE BIOETHICS. Ethical reasoning about what is **ethically permissible, ethically impermissible**, and **ethically obligatory** in the practice of the healthcare professions (including allied health, dentistry, medicine, nursing); the decisions and behavior of patients; the policies and practices of healthcare organizations, both public and private (such as private clinics and hospitals, public clinics and hospitals, private and public hospital systems); biomedical **innovation** and **research** with animal and human subjects; and health and environmental policy formulated and implemented by the executive judicial, legislative, and regulatory branches of government at all levels (e.g., in the United States, at the local, regional, state, and federal levels). *See also* EMPIRICAL BIOETHICS; ETHICAL REASONING.

NORMATIVE MEDICAL ETHICS. Ethical reasoning about what is **ethically permissible, ethically impermissible**, and **ethically obligatory** in the practice of medicine, the decisions and behavior of patients, physician leadership, the policies and practices of healthcare organizations, both public and private (such as private clinics and hospitals, public clinics and hospitals, private and public hospital systems) as they influence physicians and patients; physicians engaged in **innovation** and **research** with animal and human subjects; and the role of physicians and patients in health and environmental policy formulated and implemented by the executive judicial, legislative, and regulatory branches of government at all levels (e.g., in the United States, at the local, regional, state, and federal levels). *See also* BIOETHICS; EMPIRICAL MEDICAL ETHICS; MEDICAL ETHICS; PROFESSIONAL MEDICAL ETHICS.

NOSTRUMS. Also known as "secret nostrums" and "secrets." These were secret medications, usually compounds and often containing opium derivatives, that were concocted by physicians and sold to their **patients** and the public before the creation of agencies such as the U.S. Food and Drug Administration prohibited this practice. Physicians and other practitioners, including irregulars or **quacks**, could become rich from selling their secret remedies and, therefore, had an economic **self-interest** in the success of their secret remedies. **John Gregory** (1724–1773) argued that, while an air of mystery promotes compliance with regimen, nostrums are problematic because their causal mechanisms are unknown and because they can be unacceptably risky. They also violate his call to "lay medicine open" or to make medicine transparent and accountable to scientifically and clinically knowledgeable lay persons. *See also* DECEPTION; SELF-INTEREST.

NUDGE. Based on findings of behavioral psychology that our processes of **decision making** are biased and at risk of inaccuracy, it has been proposed that the architecture of decision making be altered to enhance the exercise of **autonomy** by **patients**. This is known as "libertarian paternalism" (Thaler and Sunstein 2009). The tools of nudging patients include providing incentives for healthy behavior (e.g., employers reduce cost of health insurance to employees who document healthy behavior) and defaults (e.g., putting healthy food first in a cafeteria line, because we are more likely to select the first dishes we see when in line). Individuals can be aware of some nudges (an employer incentivizing healthy behavior) and not aware of others (the placement of healthy dishes at the beginning of the cafeteria line) (Blumenthal-Barby and Burroughs 2012). Nudges are **ethically controversial**, especially to the extent that patients are unaware of them and the risk of eliding from **manipulation** to control of the patient's decision-making process. *See also* BEHAVIORAL PSYCHOLOGY; BIAS; FRAMING EFFECT; MANIPULATION.

NUFFIELD COUNCIL ON BIOETHICS. Founded in 1991 in London, England, by the Nuffield Foundation. The council has become a leading center for informing public debate and **public policy** formation on ethical issues in biomedicine, not only in the United Kingdom but also in other countries. *See also* HEALTH POLICY.

NUREMBERG CODE. Promulgated by the War Tribunal in Nuremberg, West Germany, in 1947. The first **code** of **research ethics**, includes requirements that consent always be obtained from human **subjects** of **research** and that standards of intellectual excellence in scientific investigation be followed without exception (https://history.nih.gov/research/downloads/nuremberg.pdf, accessed September 14, 2017). *See also* CODE OF ETHICS; ETHICS OF HUMAN SUBJECTS RESEARCH; NAZI MEDICAL WAR CRIMES.

O

OATH. A solemn vow or promise to fulfill a set of commitments that are taken to be definitive of what it means to live and act as a physician. The format of an oath typically does not permit **ethical justification** for the commitments that are made, a major shortcoming of oaths as sources of **ethical reasoning** in **professional medical ethics**. Oaths often contain a statement of their basis. For example, the *Hippocratic Oath* is based on the **ethical obligations** of regard for one's teachers, the protection of *techné*, and a **self-interest** in reputation. The **Declaration of Geneva**, also known as the *Physician's Oath*, is based on the "honor" of the oath-taker. In medical schools around the world, graduating medical students swear an oath, usually the Hippocratic Oath or a modernized version of it. *See also* CODE OF ETHICS.

OATH ACCORDING TO HIPPOCRATES, IN SO FAR AS A CHRISTIAN MAY SWEAR IT. A version of the *Hippocratic Oath* from the early Christian era (first several centuries of the Common Era) and sometimes presents in cruciform format. Distinctive for prohibiting inducing abortion from "above"—by elixir to cause uterine contractions—or "below"—by inserting a pessary into the pregnant woman's cervix, to cause it to dilate, resulting in uterine contractions. This prohibition appears to reflect a commitment to the moral status of the fetus, which is absent from the *Hippocratic Oath. See also* OATH; *OATH OF THE SOVIET PHYSICIAN.*

OATH OF THE SOVIET PHYSICIAN. Adopted in 1971 by the Presidium of the Supreme Soviet, to be taken by all graduates and physicians in the Union of Soviet Socialist Republics, which was dissolved 26 December 1991. The *Oath* emphasizes the physician's **ethical obligations** to the state, an approach to **medical ethics** with historical roots in **Johann Peter Frank**'s (1745–1821) concept of **medical police**. Scholars have questioned whether the *Oath's* takers did not take its provisions seriously and lived in a "bifurcated world of 'official' versus 'underground' ideologies" (Gefanis 2009, 496). *See also HIPPOCRATIC OATH;* OATH.

OBLIGATION. An action that one should complete because one has good reason to do so. When the **justification** for an obligation appeals to an **ethical principle**, a **virtue**, or a **right**, the obligation is an **ethical obligation** or moral obligation. When one fulfills one's ethical obligation, one is acting rightly. When one fails to fulfill one's obligation without support in **ethical reasoning**, one is acting wrongly. When the justification appeals to **administrative law**, **common law**, **regulatory law**, or **statutory law**, the obligation is a **legal obligation**. The term *obligation* is often used interchangeably with the term *duty*.

OBSERVATIONS ON THE DUTIES AND OFFICES OF A PHYSICIAN. A set of lectures on **professional medical ethics** by **John Gregory** (1724–1773), based on ethics lectures that he presented to medical students at the University of Edinburgh as they transitioned from the lecture hall to the **Royal Infirmary** of Edinburgh for their clinical training. As was then common, Gregory published his text on professional medical ethics to test public reception of his ideas. The book was well received, so he followed it with ***Lectures on the Duties and Qualifications of a Physician*** in 1772.

OBSTETRIC ETHICS. Ethical reasoning about the **professional ethics** of **clinical practice**, **clinical research**, and education in obstetrics and reproductive medicine.

OCCUPATIONAL MEDICINE. Clinical care of **patients** who are employees and paid for by their employers. This includes both private and government employers, thus including the Medical Corps of the United States armed services. Occupational medicine physicians thus have the **professional responsibility** to manage the resulting **conflict of commitment**: **ethical obligations** to their patients under **professional medical ethics**; and ethical obligations to employers for employee health and fitness for work or duty assignments. Of particular concern is the ethical obligation of **confidentiality**. There is agreement that the **informed consent process** requires that patients be informed about the physician's **conflict of commitment** (sometimes also called "double loyalty") and the limits on the physician's fulfillment of confidentiality.

One approach is to establish policies that provide nonspecific information that an employer needs, for example, what reasonable accommodations of the workplace need to be made to meet the requirements of the **Americans with Disabilities Act**, without providing the employer protected health information. The American College of Occupational and Environmental Medicine (http://www.acoem.org/, accessed 14 September 2017) provides guidance on such ethical challenges.

OFFICE FOR HUMAN RESEARCH PROTECTIONS. Created in 2000, "the Office for Human Research Protections (OHRP) provides leadership in the protection of the rights, welfare, and wellbeing of human subjects involved in research conducted or supported by the U.S. Department of Health and Human Services (DHHS). OHRP is part of the Office of the Assistant Secretary for Health in the Office of the Secretary of HHS. OHRP provides clarification and guidance, develops educational programs and materials, maintains regulatory oversight, and provides advice on ethical and regulatory issues in biomedical and behavioral research. OHRP also supports the Secretary's Advisory Committee on Human Research Protections (SACHRP), which advises the DHHS Secretary on issues related to protecting human subjects in research" (https://www.hhs.gov/ohrp/, accessed 14 September 2017). OHRP has the responsibility for writing and interpreting **45 CFR 46** or the **Common Rule**, adhering to **administrative law** in doing so. *See also* ETHICS OF HUMAN SUBJECTS RESEARCH; HUMAN SUBJECTS RESEARCH; RESEARCH.

OFFICE FOR THE PROTECTION FROM RESEARCH RISKS (OPRR). A federal agency that had the responsibility to implement **45 CFR 46**, better known as the **Common Rule**, the federal regulation that **Institutional Review Boards** are to implement to provide prospective review, approval, and oversight of **human subjects research**. OPRR was the predecessor agency to the **Office for Human Research Protections**. *See also* ETHICS OF HUMAN SUBJECTS RESEARCH; RESEARCH.

OHRP. Office for Human Research Protections. Usually pronounced "O-harp." *See* OFFICE FOR HUMAN RESEARCH PROTECTIONS.

OOH-DNR. *See* OUT-OF-HOSPITAL DO-NOT-RESUSCITATE ORDER.

OPEN-LABEL CLINICAL TRIAL. A **clinical trial** in which the medication being tested is labeled, so that both clinical investigators and **research subjects** know what medication is being administered. This method increases the risk of bias for both investigators and subjects, a risk that must be responsibly managed. *See also* BLINDING.

OPINIONS OF THE AMERICAN MEDICAL ASSOCIATION. A component of the **American Medical Association** *Code of Medical Ethics* in which the **American Medical Association** *Principles of Medical Ethics* are applied to a wide range of topics in **professional medical ethics** to provide **ethically justified**, practical guidance to physicians in such areas as **clinical**

practice, relationships with the pharmaceutical and device-manufacturer industries, and **research** (American Medical Association 2016). *See also* CODE OF ETHICS.

OPPORTUNITY COST. An opportunity cost occurs in the clinical setting when the use of a limited clinical resource, such as a **critical care** bed or an operating theater, is being used by a **patient**, thus blocking access to that resource by another patient. In general, an opportunity cost is **ethically justified**, or an acceptable opportunity cost, when the use of that limited resource is based on a **deliberative clinical judgment** that the patient is expected to benefit clinically, a **beneficence**-based ethical justification. When in deliberative clinical judgment the patient is not expected to benefit clinically from the use of a limited resource and there is another patient who is expected to benefit clinically from accessing that limited resource, an unacceptable opportunity cost occurs. An unacceptable opportunity is **ethically impermissible** in beneficence-based **clinical judgment** and clinical judgment based on the **ethical principle of justice**.

ORDINARY MEANS. *See* ORDINARY MEDICAL TREATMENT.

ORDINARY MEDICAL TREATMENT. A concept in **Roman Catholic moral theology** that pertains to setting **ethically justified** limits on **end-of-life care**. As long as medical treatment, including **life-sustaining** treatment, continues to result in net clinical benefit for the **patient** (i.e., it continues to be a **medically reasonable alternative**), then it is **ethically obligatory** to continue provision of such treatment. This also known as provision of medical treatment by "ordinary" means. *See also* END-OF-LIFE CARE; ETHICAL AND RELIGIOUS DIRECTIVES FOR CATHOLIC HEALTH CARE SERVICES; EXTRAORDINARY MEDICAL TREATMENT; LIFE-SUSTAINING TREATMENT.

ORGAN ALLOCATION. Policies of healthcare organizations, governments, and nongovernmental organizations about the characteristics of patients who should have priority for **organ transplantation** and evaluation of organs for transplantation. The need for such policies originates in the shortage of organs available for **organ procurement**. **Ethical reasoning** about organ allocation appeals to the **ethical principle of justice**. *See also* ORGAN DONATION; UNITED NETWORK FOR ORGAN SHARING (UNOS).

ORGAN DONATION. Policies of healthcare organizations, governments, and nongovernmental organizations about **consent** and **informed consent** by **patients** or **surrogates** to **organ procurement** for the purpose of **organ transplantation**. The **ethical obligation** to obtain consent or informed consent originates in the **ethical principle of respect for autonomy**. Consent to organ procurement can be indicated on one's driver's license. Informed consent is obtained from living donors or from the family members of patients in extremis or who have just died. *See also* ORGAN ALLOCATION.

ORGAN PROCUREMENT. Policies of healthcare organizations, governments, and nongovernmental organizations about the characteristics of **patients** who should be considered candidates for organ removal for the purpose of **organ transplantation**. The need for such policies originates in the shortage of organs available for organ procurement and the subsequent need to maximize clinical utility of removed organs. **Ethical reasoning** about organ procurement appeals to the **ethical principle of beneficence**, the **ethical principle of respect for autonomy**, and the **ethical principle of justice**. Currently, there is research to genetically modify animals to increase the efficacy of **xenografts** by reducing the immune response of the patient to an organ from an animal. This development will also create **ethical controversy** about the use of such animal models as sources of organs and whether **moral status** should be considered different from other nonhuman animals because they do not occur in nature but only in the laboratory. *See also* DEAD DONOR RULE; DONATION AFTER CARDIAC DEATH; ORGAN ALLOCATION; ORGAN DONATION; XENOTRANSPLANTATION.

ORGAN TRANSPLANTATION. Policies of healthcare organizations, governments, and nongovernmental organizations about the characteristics of patients who should be considered candidates for transplantation of organs. The need for such policies originates in the shortage of organs available for **organ procurement** and the subsequent need to maximize clinical utility of removed organs. **Ethical reasoning** about organ allocation appeals to the **ethical principle of beneficence**, the **ethical principle of respect for autonomy**, and the **ethical principle of justice**. *See also* DEAD DONOR RULE; ORGAN ALLOCATION; ORGAN DONATION; ORGAN PROCUREMENT.

ORGANIZATIONAL CULTURE. The values, policies, and practices, as well as actions and inactions, of leaders of an organization that communicate to those who work in or for the organization about its expectations for attitudes and behavior. Organizational culture is essential for maintaining **pro-**

fessional integrity. Dysfunctional organizational cultures can challenge, threaten, or undermine an organizational culture of **professionalism** (Chervenak and McCullough 2005).

ORGANIZATIONAL ETHICS. Ethical reasoning about the **obligations** of a healthcare organization, such as a multispecialty clinic or a hospital, to its patients, employees, suppliers, payers, and private and public oversight entities such as accreditation groups or a state department of health and human services. There is philosophical controversy about whether it is meaningful to speak of the **virtues** of organizations. *See also* ETHICS OF HUMAN SUBJECTS RESEARCH; ETHICS OF PATIENT CARE.

OSLER, SIR WILLIAM (1849–1919). Canadian physician and cofounder of the Johns Hopkins University medical school in Baltimore, Maryland. Osler wrote on *aequanimitas* (1889) or equanimity of physicians in patient care: the physician should in all circumstances appear "imperturbable." This is the opposite of the concept of sympathy in the **professional medical ethics** of **John Gregory** (1724–1773). Osler is revered by many physicians as the **ideal** physician. *See also* EMPATHY; SYMPATHY.

OUT-OF-HOSPITAL DO-NOT-RESUSCITATE ORDER. An **advance directive** prepared by a physician with the consent of the **patient** or a patient's **surrogate** for a patient with a **terminal condition** or an **irreversible condition** that instructs emergency medical technicians not to perform **cardiopulmonary resuscitation**, which will almost certainly result in the patient's **death**, and providing for them the same civil and criminal immunities provided for physicians and other healthcare professionals who implement a patient's advance directive. *See also* LETTING DIE.

OVUM DONATION. A component of assisted reproductive medicine. *See* ASSISTED REPRODUCTION; ASSISTED REPRODUCTIVE TECHNOLOGIES (ART); DONOR EGG.

P

PAIN. Tissue damage—or, in some accounts, threat of tissue damage—accompanied by awareness. Pain, especially acute, severe pain, can cause **distress** but can occur in the absence of distress. Pain, especially chronic pain or the anticipation of the recurrence of acute, severe pain, can cause **suffering**, but pain can occur in the absence of suffering. The term *pain* is therefore not synonymous with the terms *distress* or *suffering*. The phrase *mental pain* is imprecise but usually has the same meaning as *distress* or *suffering*. In such cases, the terms *distress* or *suffering* should be used as appropriate. There can be physiologic changes associated with pain (e.g., increased heart rate) in **patients** who have lost the capacity for awareness (e.g., patients in a **vegetative state**), and who therefore cannot be in pain. In **professional medical ethics**, there is an **ethical obligation** to prevent pain and to manage pain effectively when it occurs. This obligation, which has been recognized throughout the history of professional medical ethics, is based on the **ethical principle of beneficence** and the **professional virtue of compassion**. *See also* EMPATHY; SYMPATHY.

PALLIATIVE CARE. The provision of **clinical care** with a **biopsychosocial** approach to symptom management and to the management of **distress**, **pain**, and **suffering**, especially, but not limited to, **patients** with a **terminal condition** or **irreversible condition**. High doses of medication that would be life-threatening for patients without such conditions are not life-threatening for patients with such conditions because of changes in physiology. Thus, in the **ethics** of palliative care, aggressive pharmaceutical management of distress, pain, and suffering is **ethically permissible**, including **terminal sedation**. Palliative care has now become an essential component of **end-of-life care**.

PARADIGM CASE. In **casuistry**, a case in which **ethical reasoning** has already established what is **ethically impermissible**, **ethically obligatory**, and **ethically permissible**. Ethical reasoning about new cases is conducted in two steps: (1) determining whether the new case is similar in all ethically

219

relevant respects to the paradigm case; and (2) applying the ethical reasoning in the paradigm case to the new case. This is called **analogical reasoning**. If there is just one ethically relevant respect in which the new case is dissimilar from the paradigm case, then analogical reasoning cannot be used.

PARENTAL CONSENT. In **statutory law** and **common law**, parents are asked to provide authorization for **clinical management** of their child who is a **patient**. One limit on this **right** of parents is the **ethical obligation** and **legal obligation** to authorize clinical management necessary to save the life of a child who does not have an **irreversible condition** or a **terminal condition**. Healthcare organizations also require parents to sign forms authorizing surgery, invasive procedures, and risky procedures. However, in **pediatric ethics**, parents are not asked to consent; they are asked to provide **informed permission**. It is well established in common law that parents have an enforceable legal obligation to consent to effective, life-saving treatment. *See also* PARENTAL PERMISSION.

PARENTAL PERMISSION. One of the components of **pediatric ethics**, based on two ethical considerations: the **parent-child relationship** is one of a **beneficence**-based **ethical obligation** to protect and promote the **child**'s health-related **interests**; and the pediatrician has a **professional responsibility** to the child who is a **patient** based on the **best interests of the child standard**. It follows that parental **autonomy** in **decision making** about their child's **clinical management** is limited, resulting in justifiably limited **parental rights**. Parents therefore should not be asked for their **informed consent**, which implies an unlimited right to refuse. Instead, they should be asked for their **informed permission**. *See also* PARENTAL RESPONSIBILITY.

PARENTAL RESPONSIBILITY. The **ethical obligation** of parents of a child to protect and promote the **interests** and **rights** of their child. This reflects **ethical reasoning** that the **parent-child relationship** is primarily one of **obligation** and not rights. To the extent that parents fulfill their ethical obligations to their child, their exercise of rights over their child is **ethically justified**. This ethical reasoning is implicit in the **legal obligation** of parents not to neglect or abuse their child (as neglect and abuse are defined in applicable **statutory law** and their interpretation in **common law** and **regulatory law**). *See also* PARENTAL PERMISSION; PARENTAL RIGHTS.

PARENTAL RIGHTS. The **rights** of parents, especially in **statutory law** and **common law**. In **pediatric ethics**, however, the **parent-child relationship** is not understood primarily in terms of the rights of parents but in terms of their **ethical obligation** to protect and promote their child's health-related **interests**. For example, in the law, parents are asked for **informed consent** for the **clinical management** of their child who is a **patient**. In pediatric ethics, parents asked for their **informed permission**. *See also* PARENTAL PERMISSION; PARENTAL RESPONSIBILITY.

PARENT-CHILD RELATIONSHIP. The parent-child relationship is based primarily on **parental responsibility** to protect the **interests** of their children and not primarily **parental rights**. The **authority** and strength of these parental rights are a function of parents fulfilling parental responsibility. Specifically, the less that parents fulfill their **ethical obligation** to protect their children, the weaker their rights over their children. This **ethical reasoning** about the parent-child relationship provides the **ethical justification** for two of the three components of **pediatric ethics**: the **best interests of the child standard** and **informed permission**. This ethical reasoning about the parent-child relationship also differs sharply from the historical understanding of that relationship in which children were chattel, or movable property (in contrast to fixed property like land), over which parents had the **natural right** of property, one of the four natural rights enunciated by John Locke (1632–1704). When slavery was legal, slaves were classified as chattel. *See also* CHILD; PARENTAL PERMISSION; PARENTAL RESPONSIBILITY; PARENTAL RIGHTS.

PASSIVE EUTHANASIA. Discontinuing **life-sustaining treatment** of a **patient** with a **terminal condition** or an **irreversible condition** (i.e., engaging in **letting die**). This can be done with the patient's authorization in the **informed consent process**, which is known as **voluntary passive euthanasia**. This can be done without such authorization, which is known as **involuntary passive euthanasia**. *See also* ACTIVE EUTHANASIA; EUTHANASIA.

PASSIVE INVOLUNTARY EUTHANASIA. *See* INVOLUNTARY PASSIVE EUTHANASIA.

PASSIVE VOLUNTARY EUTHANASIA. *See* VOLUNTARY PASSIVE EUTHANASIA.

PATERNALISM. Interference by an individual, an organization, or the state with the autonomy of an individual justified by appeal to **beneficence**-based ethical judgment about the protection and promotion of that individual's **interests**. The objections to paternalism appeal mainly to the **ethical**

principle of respect for autonomy. This ethical principle grounds the **negative right** to noninterference with an individual's decisions, judgments, and behavior based on them.

Some take the view that this is an **absolute negative right**, on which view medical paternalism is always **ethically impermissible**. Some take the view that this is a **limited negative right** or **prima facie negative right**, on which view medical paternalism is sometimes **ethically permissible**. An important second line of justification appeals to skepticism about the intellectual **authority** of any individual, organization, and especially the state to claim to know what is in the interest of an individual. This view reflects a thoroughgoing skepticism of beneficence-based ethical judgment.

In the literature of **medical ethics** and **bioethics**, it is assumed that **medical paternalism** was an accepted **norm** in the **history of medical ethics** and that the field of bioethics was created, in part, to end the history of medical paternalism. It has been shown that this reading of the history of medical ethics lacks textual support (McCullough 2011). It is very important to distinguish the behavior named by the term *paternalism* from attitudes characterized as **paternalistic**, which names an attitude of authority and trustworthiness. This sense of the term *paternalistic* reflects the older meaning of *paternalism*, a medieval idea that persisted into the 18th century that an individual with power over others has an **ethical obligation** to protect these subordinates by using that power in their interests and protecting them from **raw power**. This medieval idea has its roots in Plato's (427–347 BCE) concept of the philosopher-king, whose only interests were the interests of those whom he governed.

PATERNALISTIC. The claim by an individual with **power** over another individual to possess superior **judgment** or **authority** about the **interests** of the latter individual and how best to protect and promote them. The word *paternalistic* derives from *pater*, Latin for "father." Traditionally, fathers are thought to have such superior judgment about the interests of their children and therefore have justified **authority** over their children.

It is important in **bioethics**, **medical ethics**, and **professional medical ethics** to distinguish *paternalistic* from *paternalism*. *Paternalism* names a behavior: interfering with an individual's **autonomy** for his or her own good. *Paternalistic* names an attitude, which may or may not lead to the behavior named by *paternalism*. This means that a physician's paternalistic **clinical judgment** may be justified by training and experience, which, by themselves, do not justify **medical paternalism**, because an attitude is not a behavior, much less a behavior of interference with the autonomy of a **patient**. *Paternalistic* is correctly used to characterize the **virtue** of **authority** in the **professional medical ethics** of **Thomas Percival** (1740–1804).

PATIENT. A living human being presented to a physician (or other health-care professional) for whom there are forms of **clinical management** that are expected to benefit clinically. This concept is **beneficence**-based. Consent to be presented is not required. Infants, unconscious individuals, and individuals with advanced dementia can become patients simply by being presented for care. The ethical concept of being a patient is therefore not **autonomy** based.

Presentation can also be at a distance. In the 18th century, for example, individuals would write letters to a famous doctor, describing their health problem and requesting a treatment regimen. They thus presented themselves and became patients. Telemedicine has replaced such letters. An individual can also be presented to a physician via images, tissue samples, and blood drawn for laboratory analysis. There always exist beneficial forms of clinical management, because it is always possible to attempt to comfort and support patients.

The ethical concept of being a patient replaced the concept of the sick individual (*aegrotus* in the Latin texts in Western medical ethics) who contracts with a physician, surgeon, or other practitioner for services. The concept of a **contractual relationship** between a sick individual and a practitioner is autonomy-based. A contractual relationship is based on the pursuit of self-interest by both parties, with caveat emptor (let the buyer beware) guiding the sick individual. This is not a relationship based on trust but self-protection. In sharp contrast, in a **professional relationship** based on the **ethical concept of medicine as a profession**, the patient is under the protection of the physician and therefore is justified in trusting the physician to be scientifically and clinically competent and to put the patient's health-related interests first. *See also* PROFESSIONAL MEDICAL ETHICS.

PATIENT AS PERSON. This concept has been advocated as an antidote to reducing the moral significance of being a patient to the **ethical principle of respect for autonomy** or to the **rights** of **patients**. This reduction results in an unacceptably abstract account of what it means to be a patient. From the perspective of **moral philosophy**, the **ethical principle of respect for persons** is considered to be a superior basis for being a patient. From the perspective of **moral theology**, the concept of being a person in the sense of being made in the image of God (*imago dei*) from **Christian moral theology** is considered to be a superior basis for being a patient (Ramsey 1973).

PATIENT CARE. The **clinical management** of a **patient's condition, disability, disease, disorder,** or **injury**.

PATIENT-PHYSICIAN RELATIONSHIP. Used to refer to the relationship between physicians and patients. Used in this order, the phrase emphasizes the **ethical principle of respect for autonomy** and can also signify a **contractual relationship**. *See also* PHYSICIAN-PATIENT RELATIONSHIP; PROFESSIONAL MEDICAL ETHICS.

PATIENTS' REQUESTS. The exercise of a **positive right** by a **patient** to ask for **clinical management**. When such requests are consistent with **deliberative clinical judgment** and are therefore expected to result in net clinical benefit for the patient, it is **ethically permissible** in **beneficence**-based clinical judgment to implement the request. When the request is ineffective but not clinically harmful, it is also ethically permissible in beneficence-based clinical judgment to implement, but the physician has an **autonomy**-based **ethical obligation** in the **informed consent process** to inform the patient that the requested plan of care is not expected to be clinically beneficial or harmful. When the request is for clinical management that in deliberative clinical judgment is net clinically harmful, implementing it is **ethically impermissible** in **professional medical ethics**. The physician should explain this **clinical judgment** in the informed consent process, explain why the request should not be implemented for the patient's clinical good, and recommend against it. Like all positive rights, patient's requests are not **absolute positive rights**. This approach was first described by **John Gregory** (1724–1773) in his professional medical ethics. *See also* RIGHT TO TRY.

PATIENTS' RIGHTS. The **rights** of **patients**, including the rights to **informed consent, informed refusal, right to privacy**, and the **right to try**. The **ethical justification** of these rights appeals to the **ethical principle of respect for autonomy**. The American Hospital Association has formalized the rights of patients and their **ethical obligations** in its *The Patient Care Partnership* (http://www.aha.org/content/00-10/pcp_english_030730.pdf, accessed 14 September 2017), which in 2003 replaced the association's *Patient's Bill of Rights*, first issued in 1973 and revised in 1992. *See also* AUTONOMY.

PEDIATRIC ASSENT. Assent of pediatric patients to **clinical management** and to participation in **clinical research**, one of the core components of **pediatric ethics**. The components of this process for clinical management and clinical research include informing the patient in a developmentally appropriate way about his or her **condition, disability, disease, disorder**, or **injury** and clinical management for it and eliciting the patient's preference.

Then both pediatric healthcare professionals and parents or guardians take that preference into account and give that preference weight commensurate with the maturity of the patient's decision-making process.

There is **ethical controversy** about how much weight should be given to the patient's preferences in clinical decision making. Pediatric assent is required by federal regulations that govern **human subjects research** that require the agreement of the pediatric patient to be enrolled in the clinical research protocols. This concept has been endorsed by the American Academy of Pediatrics (1995, 2016). *See also* PARENTAL PERMISSION.

PEDIATRIC ETHICS. Professional medical ethics about the clinical care of and research with patients who are minor children (less than 18 years of age). The core components of pediatric ethics are the **best interests of the child standard, parental permission**, and **pediatric assent** (American Academy of Pediatrics 1995, 2016). The first two components reflect **ethical reasoning** about the **parent-child relationship** as based primarily on **parental responsibility** to protect children and not primarily **parental rights**. The authority and strength of these parental rights are a function of parents fulfilling parental responsibility.

PEDIATRIC INTENSIVE CARE UNIT (PICU). A clinical service that provides **critical care** to pediatric **patients** (i.e., children under the age of 18). Patients over the age of 18, whose condition—usually a chronic or recurring disease—began when they were children and that has required PICU admission in the past are sometimes admitted to the PICU because there are few physicians in adult medicine who provide care for such patients. This problem is being addressed by programs that transition such children from pediatricians to specialized centers that provide multidisciplinary care for such patients. Another ethical challenge in the PICU is setting **ethically justified** limits on **life-sustaining treatment**. *See also* FUTILITY.

PEDIATRIC PATIENT. A patient between birth and the age of 18 or attainment of legal majority under provisions of applicable **common law** and **statutory law**. Decision making with the pediatric patient is guided by the concept of **pediatric assent**. As the **child** approaches the age of legal majority, pediatricians need to prepare the patient and the patient's parents for the assumption of **rights** to make decisions in the **informed consent process** and, as is the case for all adults, assumption of responsibility for the consequences of decisions and behavior in the lives of others. There is also a **professional responsibility** to arrange for transition of care of pediatric patients with chronic disease to the care of physicians specializing in the care of adult patients, when the scope of the specialist physician's practice includes taking on young adults. When such specialists are not available, pediatricians face the ethical challenges of providing clinical management for adult patients, which pediatricians are typically not qualified to do. The ethical challenge is that exceeding the limits of the pediatrician's fund of knowledge and clinical skills is not compatible with the first commitment—to competent **clinical practice**—in the **ethical concept of medicine as a profession**. *See also* BEST INTERESTS OF THE CHILD STANDARD; PEDIATRIC ETHICS.

PELLEGRINO, EDMUND D. (1920–2013). American physician, educator, and ethicist, a founder of the field of **bioethics**, and founding editor of the *Journal of Medicine and Philosophy*. Dr. Pellegrino was founding dean at two medical schools (University of Tennessee Health Science Center at Memphis; State University of New York at Stonybrook) where he started programs in the **medical humanities**. He also served as president of the Catholic University of America (1978–1982), in Washington, DC, and the director of the **Kennedy Institute of Ethics** (1983–1991) at Georgetown University, in Washington, DC. His public service included the post of chairman of the President's Council on Bioethics (2005–2009); he was appointed to this distinguished leadership position by President George W. Bush. *See also* BIOETHICS; PRESIDENTIAL COMMITTEE.

PERMANENT VEGETATIVE STATE. A **vegetative state** considered to be irreversible in **deliberative clinical judgment**, based on criteria set out by the American Academy of Neurology. The concept of **interactive capacity futility** applies to continued provision of **life-sustaining treatment** when this diagnosis has been made. *See also* ADVANCE DIRECTIVE; IRREVERSIBLE CONDITION; MINIMALLY CONSCIOUS STATE; PERSISTENT VEGETATIVE STATE.

PERSISTENT VEGETATIVE STATE. A neurological **condition** characterized by potentially reversible loss of awareness, sleep-wake cycles, and other criteria defined by the American Academy of Neurology. The diagnosis of a persistent vegetative state is a matter of **deliberative clinical judgment**. The concept of **interactive capacity futility** does *not* apply to continued provision of **life-sustaining treatment** when this diagnosis has been made, because the condition is potentially reversible. For the same reason, the concept of an **irreversible condition** in **Advance Directives Acts** does not apply. *See also* PERMANENT VEGETATIVE STATE.

PERSON. Used with at least three meanings, including (1) an entity that possesses **independent moral status** or a moral person as a function of having intrinsic characteristic(s) that generate such moral status or being a person in the philosophical sense; (2) an individual under the protection of the U.S. Constitution or a legal person; or (3) a unique individual with **dignity** and self-worth who should be valued as such. When used in its first meaning, many human beings who are **patients** are not included, such as fetuses that have achieved **viability**, neonates, pediatric patients with profound or severe cognitive disability, patients in a **permanent vegetative state**, and patients with advanced dementias.

There is disagreement in metaphysics and **moral philosophy** about which characteristics generate independent moral status and when those characteristics come into being in the early stages of human life and when they are lost in later stages of human life. The first and second meanings are sometimes conflated, for example, when being a legal person becomes a point of reference for being a person in the philosophical sense. The third meaning undergirds the **ethical principle of respect for persons**, while the first meaning undergirds the **ethical principle of respect for autonomy**. *See also* AUTONOMY; PERSONHOOD.

PERSONALISM. A method of philosophical reasoning and **ethical reasoning** that makes an individual's person the primary focus of concern. This is not the use of the term *person* as autonomous or in a Kantian sense, but the use of the term *person* connoting dignity, unique value, and inviolability. Personalism is thus closer to the **ethical principle of respect for persons** than it is to the **ethical principle of respect for autonomy**. Personalism has been prominent in **Roman Catholic moral theology** and in philosophical theology.

PERSONALIZED MEDICINE. The application of scientific and clinical information of genetics and genomics to tailor **clinical management** to the unique clinical circumstances of an individual patient. There is a major problem with this concept: patients are managed according to their **diagnosis**, which sorts the patient into a class of patients that exhibit recognizable patterns of signs, symptoms, pathology, and responses to clinical management. Genetic and genomic information will permit sorting patients into subcategories of their initial diagnosis or a changed diagnosis. This is better known as **precision medicine**, which has become the more commonly used phrase. The phrase *personalized medicine* is potentially misleading and should not be used. *See also* BIG DATA; EVIDENCE-BASED MEDICINE.

PERSONHOOD. The quality of being a **person** in its philosophical sense. An individual generates this quality when he or she has the characteristic(s) that generate **independent moral status** and therefore the **rights** of personhood. *See also* AUTONOMY; ETHICAL PRINCIPLE OF RESPECT FOR AUTONOMY; INDEPENDENT MORAL STATUS.

PGD. Ambiguous between **preimplantation genetic diagnosis** and **prenatal genetic diagnosis**. Most often used to mean the former.

PHARMACOGENOMICS. The clinical application of the results of **genome sequencing** to refine pharmacologic **clinical management** of the patient's **condition, disability, disorder,** or **disease**. Pharmacogenomics permits more reliability in the selection of medication and in dosing schedules. The clinical application of pharmacogenomics is supported by the **ethical principle of beneficence**. *See also* GENETHICS.

PHASE I CLINICAL TRIAL. The first stage of **clinical research with human subjects** in which a drug is tested for its toxicity and efficacy in slowing or arresting (even if only for a short period of time) the progress of **disease**. In such trials, subjects enrolled in the later stages of the trial may receive more clinical benefit from slowing or arresting the progress of disease, a clinical benefit that early enrollees might not experience. Clinical risk of toxicity may also increase. These potential outcomes should be made clear in the **informed consent process** for enrollment in Phase I clinical trials (Brody 1998). *See also* CLINICAL TRIAL; ETHICS OF HUMAN SUBJECTS RESEARCH; HUMAN SUBJECTS RESEARCH; PHASE II CLINICAL TRIAL; PHASE III CLINICAL TRIAL; PHASE IV CLINICAL TRIAL; RESEARCH.

PHASE II CLINICAL TRIAL. If a **Phase I clinical trial** results indicate that a drug has clinically acceptable toxicity levels and may be efficacious in its effects on a **disease**, it is then tested in a patient population to measure its effects and continue to assess its toxicity. *See also* CLINICAL TRIAL; ETHICS OF HUMAN SUBJECTS RESEARCH; HUMAN SUBJECTS RESEARCH; PHASE III CLINICAL TRIAL; PHASE IV CLINICAL TRIAL; RESEARCH.

PHASE III CLINICAL TRIAL. A randomized, **controlled clinical trial** conducted when the results of a **Phase II clinical trial** show efficacy, the drug or device is in a class in which there are other **medically reasonable alternatives,** and the condition of **equipoise** is satisfied. The research question becomes whether the new drug or device is clinically equivalent or superior to existing devices or drugs. The **informed consent process** should make clear that some aspects of such trials—randomization, blinding—have been chosen for scientific, methodological reasons and therefore have not been chosen based on a **deliberative clinical judgment** about clinical benefit for the patient. The goal of such disclosure is to prevent **therapeutic misconception**. Phase III **clinical trials** can be **unblinded** or **blinded**. They can also be **placebo-controlled clinical trials**. *See also* ETHICS OF HUMAN SUBJECTS RESEARCH; HUMAN SUBJECTS RESEARCH; PHASE I CLINICAL TRIAL; PHASE IV CLINICAL TRIAL; RESEARCH.

PHASE IV CLINICAL TRIAL. A **clinical trial** undertaken to investigate the long-term effects of new drugs and devices, which outcomes are typically not investigated in Phase I, II, or III trials and are **ethically justified** because such long-term effects could be significant in **deliberative clinical judgment**. *See also* ETHICS OF HUMAN SUBJECTS RESEARCH; HUMAN SUBJECTS RESEARCH; PHASE I CLINICAL TRIAL; PHASE II CLINICAL TRIAL; PHASE III CLINICAL TRIAL; RESEARCH.

PHILOSOPHY OF MEDICINE. Philosophical investigation of medicine, including analysis of key concepts (e.g., **disability**, **death**, **disease**), medical epistemology (What is the status of diagnosis or prognosis as claims to knowledge about the **condition** of a **patient**?), and the ontology of disease (What kind of entity is a disease?). Philosophy of medicine is a subfield of **philosophy of science** and also contributes in many ways to **bioethics** and **medical ethics**. A prominent venue for scholarship in the philosophy of medicine is the *Journal of Medicine and Philosophy*.

PHILOSOPHY OF SCIENCE. Philosophical investigation of the biological and physical sciences and of mathematics, including analysis of key concepts (e.g., causation), epistemology (What is the status of evidence-based prognosis as claims to knowledge about the world?), and ontology (Is a person alive?).

PHYSICIAN AS GENERAL. A concept in the history of Chinese medicine and medical ethics according to which the **patient** is the king who chooses a physician to function as a "general to marshal medical forces against disease" (Nie 2009, 341). This indicates that the patient has **power** over the physician and not vice versa. This concept is incompatible with **medical paternalism**. *See also MEDICUS POLTICUS*; PATERNALISM; PATERNALISTIC.

PHYSICIAN-ASSISTED DYING. A phrase used with four meanings: **involuntary active euthanasia, involuntary passive euthanasia, voluntary active euthanasia,** and **voluntary passive euthanasia.** Failure to identify which meaning is being invoked violates the requirement of **clarity** in **ethical reasoning.** Resulting equivocation risks violating the requirement of **consistency.** *See also* EUTHANASIA; KILLING; SUICIDE.

PHYSICIAN-ASSISTED SUICIDE. The physician provides the means, usually a prescription for medication to **kill** a **patient** with a **terminal condition** who has **decision-making capacity** to self-administer, which is **suicide.** This is **ethically controversial** and legally permitted in some states in the United States and in other countries. **Voluntary active euthanasia** is another form of physician-assisted suicide, where, with the authorization of the patient in the **informed consent process,** the physician administers a medication or other substance that kills the patient. This is ethically controversial and illegal in all states in the United States. It is practiced in the Netherlands. *See also* END-OF-LIFE CARE.

PHYSICIAN-PATIENT RELATIONSHIP. Used to refer to the relationship between physicians and patients. When used in this order, the phrase emphasizes the **ethical principle of beneficence** and expresses a **professional relationship** between the physician and patient. *See also* PATIENT-PHYSICIAN RELATIONSHIP; PROFESSIONAL MEDICAL ETHICS.

PHYSICIAN'S OATH. See DECLARATION OF GENEVA.

PHYSIOLOGIC FUTILITY. There is no reasonable expectation that the expected functional outcome of a form of clinical management will occur. There are two **ethical justifications** for this **specification** of futility. The first derives from the accepted concept in **ethical reasoning** that *ought* implies *can.* By *modus tolens* (If a, then b; not b; therefore, not a), there is no **ethical obligation** to undertake **clinical management** that is impossible. For example, cardiopulmonary resuscitation of a patient with total decapitation cannot restore spontaneous circulation. The second appeals to the **professional virtue of compassion** and the **ethical principle of nonmaleficence;** both of these prohibit providing clinical management that in **deliberative clinical judgment** is expected to result in net clinical harm to the patient. *See also* FUTILITY.

PICU. *See* PEDIATRIC INTENSIVE CARE UNIT (PICU).

PILCHER, LEWIS (1845–1934). American physician and ethicist. He became a fierce critic of the **American Medical Association** *Code of Medical Ethics* **of 1847**, because requiring adherence to it violated the sovereignty of individual conscience, in an essay "Code of Medical Ethics" (1883). Reflecting the **ethical reasoning** of **libertarian justice** and a commitment to the **autonomy** of physicians, Pilcher resisted the encroachment on the **rights** of physicians of the **power** of the American Medical Association as it sought to enforce the 1847 *Code*. *See also* CODE OF ETHICS; FLINT, AUSTIN (1812–1886).

PIUS XII, POPE (1876–1958; PAPACY: 1939–1958). Pope of the Roman Catholic Church. In an address, he stated that **Roman Catholic moral theology** supports aggressive palliation for a dying patient, provided that the physician does not intend to cause the patient's death. *See also* DOUBLE EFFECT, PRINCIPLE OF; END-OF-LIFE CARE; PALLIATIVE CARE.

PLACEBO. From the Latin, "I shall please." An inert substance administered to a **patient** as part of **clinical management** without the consent of the patient or to a **research subject** in a **clinical trial** with consent. In **clinical practice**, a placebo is used without being identified as such to determine if patients in **pain** experience relief, which some do. This is called a "placebo effect." There is uncertainty about whether this effect is from the inert substance or the increased level of attention from the physician and healthcare team.

Inasmuch as the patient is not informed that the pill or injection is not an active substance and is therefore given to believe falsely that it is a medication for pain, the use of placebo is a **deception**, which is not consistent with **professional responsibility** in the **informed consent process**. The use of a placebo in the clinical setting, therefore, bears a steep **burden of justification**.

In **clinical research**, a placebo is used in the control group in a **Phase III clinical trial**. This is **ethically permissible** when the risk has been managed to an accepted minimum and there is no other way to conduct the clinical trial (Brody 1998). These conditions might be met when there is no accepted medication against which a new medication can be tested or when there are doubts about the efficacy of a surgical procedure. In the informed consent process, the patient must be informed about the use of a placebo control and consent to it and being **blinded** about which arm of the trial the patients will be assigned randomly.

PLACEBO EFFECT. *See* PLACEBO.

PLACEBO-CONTROLLED CLINICAL TRIAL. The use of a **placebo** as the control arm of a **randomized clinical trial** (RCT). The **ethical justification** of an RCT requires **evidence-based** equipoise between the two arms. The use of a placebo control bears the **burden of justification**. Brody has identified some elements of that justification: "The more serious the disease process and the less likely that the established therapy will produce bad side effects, the more problematic is a placebo-controlled trial" (Brody 1998, 150). In order to meet the requirements of sound scientific design and **informed consent**, such studies of drugs should be designed as **double-blind clinical trials**. Potential **research subjects** should be informed that they might receive a placebo and that both they and the investigators will not know whether this is the case. In placebo-controlled surgical trials, only the subjects can be blinded. In such a **single-blinded clinical trial**, potential **research subjects** should be informed that they might receive a placebo and that, while the investigators will know whether this is the case, subjects will not. *See also* DECEPTION.

PLANNED PARENTHOOD CASE. A 1992 decision of the United States Supreme Court (*Planned Parenthood of Southeastern Pa. v. Casey* [505 US 833]) about the permissibility of a Pennsylvania **statutory law** in creating barriers to **induced abortion** and **termination of pregnancy** before **viability**. In her opinion for the Court, Associate Justice Sandra Day O'Connor changed the conceptual framework for the **constitutional law** of induced abortion and termination of pregnancy in the United States. In *Roe v. Wade* (410 U.S. 113) and *Doe v. Bolton* (410 U.S. 179) in 1973, the Supreme Court, in a majority opinion by Associate Justice Harry Blackmun, the conceptual framework was based on the constitutional **legal right** to **privacy**. This **negative right** creates a zone of decision making between a physician and patient and action based on such decision making from interference by the state, in the absence of a compelling state's **interest**, a vague concept that includes preventing unacceptable social threats, including threats to constitutional protections, public safety, or national security.

Associate Justice Sandra Day O'Connor replaced the conceptual framework based on privacy with a new conceptual framework based on a "liberty interest." This concept responds to a criticism of *Roe* that privacy is not explicitly included in the United States Constitution by grounding noninterference in the physician-patient relationship in the 14th Amendment, which explicitly includes liberty. Justice O'Connor changed the basis of this noninterference from a right to an "interest." In United States constitutional law, the state may restrict the pursuit of an interest, provided it does not create an "undue burden" on that pursuit. What should count as an undue burden becomes a matter for courts to decide, an aspect of Justice O'Connor's opinion to which Associate Justice Antonin Scalia (1936–2016; term on court:

1986–2016) vigorously objected. The Supreme Court recently clarified this concept to mean that the effect of the barrier on reproductive health services is to deny access to them. Justice O'Connor's opinion emphasized that *Casey* should not be understood as overturning *Roe*. Justice Blackmun concurred in Justice O'Connor's opinion. *See also* ABORTION; HEALTH POLICY; PUBLIC POLICY.

PLATO (427–347 BCE). Greek philosopher. He is the author of the *Dialogues*, in which he elaborates on metaphysics and **moral philosophy**. His quest for certainty (Gracia 2010) has intellectual descendants such as Immanuel Kant (1724–1804), who influenced **medical ethics** in the 19th century, for example, in the work of **Christian Hufeland** (1762–1836).

"PLAYING GOD". A phrase used, disapprovingly, to describe physicians who have overwhelming confidence in their own clinical judgment and practice, thus ignoring evidence-based limits of **beneficence**-based **clinical judgment**, and who also knows what is best for patients who do not know this for themselves, thus ignoring **autonomy**-based clinical judgment and the **informed consent process**. **Arnald of Villanova** (1240–1331) invoked this concept implicitly when he argued that physicians should not guarantee outcomes, because the control over nature that makes this possible belongs only to God. These physicians are often not the best physicians, even though they think that they are, as **John Gregory** (1724–1773) noted in his **professional medical ethics**.

PLURALISTIC CASUISTRY. Case-based **ethical reasoning** that starts with initial **intuitions**, in the sense of an initial, spontaneous **judgment** about what should be done in a particular case. There is no restriction on the sources of these initial judgments in that they can be drawn from diverse **metaethics** or ethical theories. These intuitions are then tested in similar cases, to make the transition from an initial judgment to a well-reasoned and clearly expressed judgment. The **ethical justification** for such considered judgments should be such that any reasonable person can understand it. These considered judgments can then be used to guide ethical reasoning about similar cases in the future (Brody 2003). *See also* CASUISTRY.

POPULATION CONTROL. The use of incentives or requirements of **contraception, abortion,** and **sterilization** to limit population growth. There is **ethical controversy** about whether population control is necessary, given alternatives such as increased educational and employment opportunities for women, which can lower reproductive rates, and increasing the supply of potable water and safe food, which can adequately meet the needs of a growing population. There are also concerns about the growth of the economy and an aging population of a nation in which the replacement rate results in no population growth or a decrease in population.

The **ethical justification** of incentives to have fewer children appeals to the **ethical principle of respect for autonomy**, which requires **voluntary** and **informed consent**, and the **ethical principle of justice**, which requires that incentives are directed to both men and women and not only to women. **Coercive** measures, because they are **involuntary**, face a very steep **burden of justification**. Historically, access to **induced abortion** has been used by states to increase their population (e.g., restricting access to abortion during times of war) so the population **killed** in war can be replaced, then relaxing those restrictions after a war ends. *See also* HEALTH POLICY; PUBLIC POLICY.

POSITIVE EUGENICS. The use of breeding and laboratory techniques to improve the genetics of a species, especially humans, by **enhancing** or adding what are considered as traits or genes that improve genetics (such as increased intelligence). *See also* EUGENICS.

POSITIVE RIGHT. A justified claim of an individual against other individuals, organizations, or the state to his, her, or its time, energy, and resources, in order to protect and promote that individual's **interests**. A **right** creates an **ethical obligation**. A positive right always creates a **prima facie ethical obligation**. An adequate justification for a positive right will establish criteria to guide **judgment** about limits on the positive right. The assertion of a positive right as an **absolute right** should be regarded with profound skepticism, since an unlimited obligation of others to protect and promote one's interests is impossible to establish because of the unacceptable burdens on others of fulfilling an **absolute ethical obligation**.

POTTER, VAN RENSSELAER (1911–2001). American biochemist and cancer researcher. He became one of the founders of the field of **bioethics** and perhaps the first to use the word *bioethics* in 1970. Potter's conception of the field was **biopsychosocial** and ecological, for example, to include the relationship between humans and nature in specific locales and globally. With a very short period of time, this broad conception of the field narrowed by omitting **ethical reasoning** about the environment and its relationship to biomedicine. More recently, there have been efforts to recover Potter's vision for the field by restoring **environmental ethics** as a component of bioethics.

POWER. Power has two related components: **decision making** and executing decisions. Power thus includes **decisional autonomy** and **executive autonomy**. More simply, power is the ability to form one's will and then effect it, directly or through others. *See also* RAW POWER.

PRAGMATISM. A distinctively American set of philosophical methods championed by such philosophers as John Dewey (1859–1952), William James (1842–1910), George Herbert Mead (1863–1931), and Charles Sanders Pierce (1839–1914). They eschewed a metaphysical approach to the meaning of truth, emphasizing that truth is found in the function of things in the world. In particular, James took the view that truths are made true. In this respect, the ethical concept of medicine, expressed in the commitments of physicians to the three components of the concept, is made true or real by physicians making and sustaining these commitments. To the extent that it is the case that enough physicians do so, it is true that there exists a profession of medicine. To the extent that this is not the case, it is not true that there exists a profession of medicine. Put another way, the profession of medicine is not some reality that exists independently of the beliefs and behaviors of physicians and healthcare organizations with an **organizational culture** that supports the **ethical concept of medicine as a profession**. *See also* ETHICAL REASONING; PROFESSIONAL MEDICAL ETHICS.

"PRAYER OF MAIMONIDES". Also known as the "Daily Prayer of Maimonides" and the "Oath of Maimonides," attributed to **Maimonides** (1135–1204), a Spanish Talmudist and physician, but written by **Markus Herz** (1747–1803). The prayer is to "Almighty God" in thanks for His gifts, including the gift of medicine. The prayer concludes: "Thou has chosen me in Thy mercy to watch over the life and death of Thy creatures. I now apply myself to my profession. Support me in this great task so that it may benefit mankind, for without Thy help not even the least thing will succeed" (https://www.ncbi.nlm.nih.gov/pmc/articles/PMC1593332/pdf/calstatejmed00063-0059a.pdf, accessed 14 September 2017).

PRECAUTIONARY PRINCIPLE. A **beneficence**-based and **prudence**-based **ethical principle** that guides **judgment** about whether risk is **ethically permissible** to take. In general, this principle holds that, when there is net expected risk from a form of **clinical management**, **health policy**, or **public policy**, then that clinical management or policy always faces a **burden of justification**. The purpose of the precautionary principle is to take risk into account, including both short-term and long-term risk. The estimate of risk, especially long-term risk, can have a weak evidence base. Such risk estimation is allowed in the application of the precautionary principle. Risk may be speculative (i.e., the risk lacks an evidence base) but concern outcomes that are serious, far-reaching, and irreversible. Such risk estimation is also allowed in the application of the precautionary principle. The precautionary principle is often invoked in **public health** and **public health ethics**. *See also* ETHICAL PRINCIPLE OF NONMALEFICENCE; HARM PRINCIPLE.

PRECISION MEDICINE. The use of information from genetics and genomics to refine the **diagnosis** of a **patient** into clinically more meaningful subcategories of the patient's diagnosis or a new diagnosis. For example, genomic differences can result in different responses to medications or their dosing schedules. This is known as **pharmacogenomics**. The development and clinical application of precision medicine is supported by the **ethical principle of beneficence**. *See also* BIG DATA; EVIDENCE-BASED MEDICINE; PERSONALIZED MEDICINE.

PREGNANCY. A **condition** that exists after implantation of the embryo in the uterine wall that can result in a spontaneous **abortion, in utero fetal demise**, an **induced abortion**, or a live birth. Pregnancy is neither a **disease**, nor a **disorder**, nor a **disability**. However, it is a condition that can increase **biopsychosocial** risks, including **morbidity, mortality**, disruption of schooling or employment (especially for adolescents), and intrapersonal and interpersonal stress for the pregnant woman as well as risks of morbidity and mortality for the fetus(es). *See also* OBSTETRIC ETHICS; PROFESSIONAL MEDICAL ETHICS.

PREIMPLANTATION GENETIC DIAGNOSIS. The genetic or genomic analysis of in vitro embryos to identify those that will not be transferred to the woman's uterus in the process of **in vitro fertilization**. *See also* ASSISTED REPRODUCTION; ASSISTED REPRODUCTIVE TECHNOLOGIES (ART).

PRENATAL DIAGNOSIS. This phrase names a wide range of techniques to evaluate the health status of a fetus. The **ethical justification** for prenatal diagnosis appeals to the **ethical principle of respect for autonomy**, because prenatal diagnosis provides information for the pregnant **patient** and her physician to consider in the **informed consent process** about the disposition of her pregnancy. The term *prenatal diagnosis* also refers to a set of invasive and noninvasive techniques for the evaluation of the fetus's clinical **condition**.

There are two invasive techniques. The first is **amniocentesis**, or obtaining amniotic fluid, which contains fetal cells, for genetic or genomic assessment of the fetus. The second is chorion villus sampling, which obtains tissue from the placenta for genetic or genomic assessment of the fetus. One advantage of chorion villus sampling is that it can be done earlier in pregnancy, which is **autonomy** enhancing. Both amniocentesis and chorion villus sampling permit genomic diagnosis and risk assessment (estimated probability for the onset of **disability** or **disease**) of the fetus.

There are three noninvasive techniques. The first is obstetric ultrasound, which can detect twin and higher order pregnancies and fetal structural anomalies as well as pathophysiology. The second is MRI, or magnetic resonance imaging, which permits more precise evaluation of fetal structures and physiology. The third is **noninvasive prenatal testing**, which should be called "noninvasive risk assessment," because it is not yet considered diagnostic. This technique, which can be performed very early in pregnancy, analyzes fetal cells circulating in maternal blood; the cells can be obtained by a blood draw on the pregnant woman, which poses no risk to the fetus. The results provide the pregnant patient with estimated risk of genetic anomalies, which are pertinent to her **decision making** with her physician about the disposition of her pregnancy.

Obstetric imaging, often using obstetric ultrasound and MRI, is used to refine fetal diagnoses that are candidates for fetal intervention. Like all diagnostic measures used to plan **clinical management** of the fetus's condition, the ethical justification for this use of imaging is **beneficence** based. The same is true of the use of other forms of prenatal diagnosis when the results are intended to be used to plan obstetric and neonatal clinical management. Before the development of **maternal-fetal surgery** and **maternal-fetal treatment** for fetal benefit, prenatal diagnosis was often criticized as enabling **induced abortion** because that was the only alternative to continuing a pregnancy complicated by a fetal anomaly. With the development of maternal-fetal surgery and maternal-fetal treatment for fetal benefit, this line of criticism has become unpersuasive. *See also* MATERNAL-FETAL SURGERY; OBSTETRIC ETHICS.

PRENATAL GENETIC DIAGNOSIS. The use of genetics or genomics in **prenatal diagnosis**.

PRESIDENTIAL COMMISSION. *See* PRESIDENTIAL COMMITTEE.

PRESIDENTIAL COMMITTEE. A group appointed by the president of the United States and charged to investigate specific topics in **bioethics** and **medical ethics** and report to the president. There have been presidential commissions, committees, or councils in the United States since the 1970s. Some commissions have been authorized and appointed by the United States Congress and report to the Congress. The U.S. National Commission for the Protection of Human Subjects of Biomedical and Behavioral Research (1974–1978) was the first such committee, which focused on the **ethics of human subjects research**. Its reports, including the ***Belmont Report***, became the basis of U.S. federal regulations of human subjects research (**45 CFR 46**). It is unusual for congressional commissions to have such lasting influence. Presidential committees have addressed the full range of topics in bioethics and medical ethics, with variable levels of influence. *See also* HEALTH POLICY; PUBLIC POLICY.

PRESIDENTIAL COUNCIL. *See* PRESIDENTIAL COMMITTEE.

PRESUMED CONSENT. The presumption that a **patient** has **consented** in clinical circumstances that do not permit time for the **informed consent process** or for **informed refusal** applies in **medical emergencies** unless there is valid refusal, for example, the patient has an **irreversible condition** or a **terminal condition** and has an applicable **advance directive** refusing **life-sustaining treatment**. From the perspective of the **ethical principle of respect for autonomy**, the application of this presumption confronts a very steep **burden of justification**.

PRESUMPTION OF DECISION-MAKING CAPACITY. All adult patients are presumed to have **decision-making capacity**. This means that the adult patient does not bear any **burden of justification** to establish that he or she has decision-making capacity. The burden of justification is on physicians and other healthcare professionals, who have clinically based concerns about the patient's decision-making capacity, to establish that the patient lacks decision-making capacity and that a **surrogate** is therefore needed to make decisions for the patient. This assessment should evaluate the components of decision-making capacity on the basis of **deliberative clinical judgment**. *See also* AUTONOMY; DECISION-MAKING CAPACITY; ETHICAL PRINCIPLE OF RESPECT FOR AUTONOMY.

PREVENTIVE ETHICS. An approach to **decision making** with patients based on the belief that it is better for **patients**, physicians, other healthcare team members, the patient's family members, and **organizational culture** to prevent **ethical conflict** about the **clinical management** of the patient's **condition, disability, disorder**, or **disease**. The tools of preventive ethics are modifications of the **informed consent process** and include making recommendations when they are justified in **deliberative clinical judgment** and **respectful persuasion**.

PRICE, RICHARD (1723–1791). Welsh Dissenter and philosopher. He is a founder of **moral realism**, the view that moral judgments are based on moral properties of things in the world that can be discovered reliably using the methods of observation elaborated by Francis Bacon (1561–1626). Price called the direct observation of moral properties **"intuition,"** by which he meant a direct, immediate, and therefore **bias**-free apprehension of moral properties. He wrote *A Review of the Principal Questions of Morals* (1787). Price's student, John Taylor (1694–1761), was one of **Thomas Percival**'s (1740–1804) teachers at the Warrington Academy in 1760 and 1761 and introduced Percival to Price's **moral philosophy**.

PRIMA FACIE ETHICAL OBLIGATION. An action that one should complete, except when in **ethical reasoning** another **ethical obligation** should be given priority. This higher-priority obligation limits the existing obligation. *See also* ABSOLUTE ETHICAL OBLIGATION.

PRIMA FACIE ETHICAL PRINCIPLE. An **ethical principle** that generates **ethical obligations** that have justified limits originating in other ethical principles and **professional virtues**. *See also* ETHICAL REASONING.

PRIMA FACIE NEGATIVE RIGHT. A **negative right** that creates an **ethical obligation** of noninterference that has **ethically justified** limits. A widely accepted justified limit is the **beneficence**-based **ethical obligation** to prevent impermissible harm to others, known as the **harm principle**. A prima facie negative **right** creates a **prima facie ethical obligation**. *See also* ABSOLUTE NEGATIVE RIGHT.

PRIMA FACIE POSITIVE RIGHT. A **positive right** that creates an **ethical obligation** with **ethically justified** limits to use one's resources to protect and promote the **interests** of the **rights**-bearer. A prima facie positive right creates a **prima facie ethical obligation**. *See also* ABSOLUTE POSITIVE RIGHT.

PRIMA FACIE RIGHT. A **right** that creates obligations with **ethically justified** limits. An adequate justification for a prima facie right will identify criteria to guide **judgment** about what those limits should be. *See also* ABSOLUTE RIGHT.

PRIMUM NON NOCERE. A Latinate version of **"First do no harm,"** attributed to **Worthington Hooker** (1806–1872). *See also* ETHICAL PRINCIPLE OF NONMALEFICENCE.

PRINCIPLE. Used as shorthand for **ethical principle.** In **David Hume's** (1711–1776) **moral** science, the term *principle* is used to refer to constitutive causal processes in animals and humans, their moral physiology, chief among which is **sympathy.** *See also* ETHICAL REASONING.

PRINCIPLE OF AUTONOMY. *See* ETHICAL PRINCIPLE OF RESPECT FOR AUTONOMY.

PRINCIPLE OF BENEFICENCE. *See* ETHICAL PRINCIPLE OF BENEFICENCE.

PRINCIPLE OF JUSTICE. *See* ETHICAL PRINCIPLE OF JUSTICE.

PRINCIPLE OF NONMALEFICENCE. *See* ETHICAL PRINCIPLE OF NONMALEFICENCE.

PRINCIPLE OF RESPECT FOR AUTONOMY. *See* ETHICAL PRINCIPLE OF RESPECT FOR AUTONOMY.

PRINCIPLE OF RESPECT FOR PERSONS. *See* ETHICAL PRINCIPLE OF RESPECT FOR PERSONS.

PRINCIPLES OF BIOMEDICAL ETHICS. The most commonly used textbook in courses on **bioethics** at the undergraduate, graduate, and medical school levels. Coauthored by philosopher Tom L. Beauchamp of Georgetown University and religious studies scholar James F. Childress of the University of Virginia, the first edition appeared in 1979 and has been followed by six editions. The current, seventh edition appeared in 2012 (Beauchamp and Childress 2012). The approach taken in this book treats ethical principles as originating in different sources, a **metaethics** that permits a pluralism of sources for ethical principles. The authors are insistent that no one of the four **ethical principles—beneficence, nonmaleficence, justice,** and **respect for autonomy**—has automatic priority in **ethical reasoning.** Instead, each ethical principle is a **prima facie ethical principle.** It is therefore a mistake to attribute to the authors, as some do, the view that the ethical principle of respect for autonomy is an **absolute ethical principle.** The authors are also insistent on deploying **virtues** in ethical reasoning. It is therefore a mistake to equate their approach as equivalent to the **"Georgetown Mantra"** or **principlism**, as some do. *See also* BIOMEDICAL ETHICS.

PRINCIPLES OF MEDICAL ETHICS OF THE AMERICAN MEDICAL ASSOCIATION. *See* AMERICAN MEDICAL ASSOCIATION *PRINCIPLES OF MEDICAL ETHICS.*

PRINCIPLISM. A neologism used in **bioethics**, **medical ethics**, and **professional medical ethics** to refer to a method of **ethical reasoning** based exclusively on **ethical principles** and thus omitting other ethically relevant considerations, especially **virtues**. *See also* VIRTUE ETHICS.

PRIVACY. The **negative right** of an individual to control access to information about himself or herself by other individuals, organizations, or the state. This **right** is asserted in response to the potentially predatory power of other individuals, organizations, or the state to use such information to harm the individual or to violate his or her other rights. Privacy is often taken in the literature of **bioethics** and **medical ethics** to be synonymous with **confidentiality**. This is a mistake, for two reasons. The physician's **ethical obligation** of confidentiality originates in **professional medical ethics** and applies to all patients, including patients who may not be rights-bearers, for example, fetal and neonatal patients. As a healthcare professional committed to protecting and promoting the patient's health-related **interests**, the physician is not a potential predator on those interests.

PROCEDURAL JUSTICE. A requirement of the **ethical principle of justice** that **decision making** about the allocation of resources and opportunities in a society take account of the **interests** and **rights** of all who will be affected by the outcome of decision making. There is **ethical controversy** about the best ways to do so. *See also* EGALITARIAN JUSTICE; HEALTHCARE JUSTICE; LIBERTARIAN JUSTICE; RAWLSIAN JUSTICE; UTILITARIAN JUSTICE.

PROCREATIVE FREEDOM. Ambiguous between freedom from noninterference (a **negative right**) and freedom of assistance (a **positive right**) to reproduce via sexual intercourse or **assisted reproduction**. Failure to specify the sense in which the phrase is used results in lack of **clarity** and **consistency**, which is impermissible in **ethical reasoning**. *See also* PROCREATIVE LIBERTY; PROCREATIVE RIGHT.

PROCREATIVE LIBERTY. Ambiguous between freedom from noninterference (a **negative right**) and freedom of assistance (a **positive right**) to reproduce via sexual intercourse or **assisted reproduction**. Failure to specify the sense in which the phrase is used results in lack of **clarity** and **consistency**, which is impermissible in **ethical reasoning**. *See also* PROCREATIVE FREEDOM; PROCREATIVE RIGHT.

PROCREATIVE RIGHT. Ambiguous between freedom from noninterference (a **negative right**) and freedom of assistance (a **positive right**) to reproduce via sexual intercourse or **assisted reproduction**. Failure to specify the sense in which the phrase is used results in lack of **clarity** and **consistency**, which is impermissible in **ethical reasoning**. *See also* PROCREATIVE FREEDOM; PROCREATIVE LIBERTY; RIGHT.

PROFESSION OF MEDICINE. *See* ETHICAL CONCEPT OF MEDICINE AS A PROFESSION.

PROFESSIONAL ASSOCIATIONS OF PHYSICIANS. There is a long history of professional associations of physicians, including general associations such as the **American Medical Association** and the **National Medical Association** and specialties societies in the United States, a pattern that is replicated in many other countries. Historically, these have been important instruments of self-regulation of the medical profession. These associations are important sources for **oaths** and **ethics statements** that provide guidance and sometimes establish norms for **clinical practice**, **research**, education, and **health policy**.

PROFESSIONAL COMMUNITY STANDARD. A standard for disclosure by the physician of information to the **patient** in the **informed consent process** that requires the physician to disclose information that any relevantly trained and experienced physician would disclose. This was once based on local practice but is increasingly based on national standards, as standards for **clinical practice** have become increasingly national. This standard is the legal standard in the minority of states in the United States. It is not regarded as an **ethically permissible** standard in **bioethics** and **medical ethics** because its inherent, systematic risk of underdisclosure is incompatible with the **ethical principle of respect for autonomy**. *See also* REASONABLE PERSON STANDARD; SUBJECTIVE STANDARD.

PROFESSIONAL CONSCIENCE. A fundamental set of beliefs and convictions about the commitments of **professional medical** ethics that apply to all physicians as a matter of **professional integrity**. Acting in ways inconsistent with the **ethical obligations** generated by professional conscience is not compatible with professional integrity and is therefore **ethically impermissible** for a physician. The **ethical justification** of **conscientious objection** sometimes appeals to professional conscience, for example, in **military medical ethics** when a physician makes the **judgment** that an order is unlawful because it violates professional conscience. *See also* CONSCIENCE; INDIVIDUAL CONSCIENCE.

PROFESSIONAL ETHICAL OBLIGATION. An **ethical obligation** originating in the social role of being a physician and **ethically justified** in **professional medical ethics**. *See also* PROFESSIONAL RESPONSIBILITY.

PROFESSIONAL ETHICS. **Ethical reasoning** about the **ethical obligations** of professionals that originate in **ethical principles** and **virtues** pertinent to a profession. The traditional professions are the law, medicine, the military, and the ministry. **Thomas Gisborne** (1758–1846) was one of the first to use the term *professional ethics*, while **Thomas Percival** (1740–1804) was perhaps the first to use the phrase to characterize **medical ethics**, this creating a **professional medical ethics**. Refer to the introduction and *see also* ETHICAL CONCEPT OF MEDICINE AS A PROFESSION.

PROFESSIONAL IDEAL. An **ideal** that is a component of **professional medical ethics**. Aspirational statements or ideals have long been such a component. *See also* MORAL NORM; NORM; PROFESSIONAL NORM.

PROFESSIONAL INTEGRITY. *See* PROFESSIONAL VIRTUE OF INTEGRITY.

PROFESSIONAL LIABILITY. The legal exposure to risk of litigation for malpractice. Physicians and healthcare organizations contract for insurance for the management of this risk. This is popularly known by the term *malpractice insurance*. Having such insurance is a matter of **legitimate self-interest**. Concern and especially fear of such litigation can incline physicians to base **clinical practice** on self-interest rather than on **deliberative clinical judgment**, introducing powerful and potentially uncontrollable **biases**. To the extent that physicians make such choices, which are almost always **voluntary**, they undermine the **ethical concept of medicine as a profession** by prioritizing **self-interest**.

PROFESSIONAL MEDICAL ETHICS. An ethics for **clinical practice, research**, education, and **health policy** based on the **ethical concept of medicine as profession**. Professional medical ethics differs from **bioethics** in its interpretation of the **ethical principle of beneficence, ethical principle of respect for autonomy, ethical principle of justice**, and **ethical principle of nonmaleficence** and in its emphasis on the **professional virtues**. Professional medical ethics was invented in the 18th century during the Scottish Enlightenment and the English Enlightenment. The coinventors of professional medical ethics were Scottish physician-ethicist **John Gregory** (1724–1773) and English physician-ethicist **Thomas Percival** (1740–1804). There is therefore no history of professional medical ethics dating to the ancient world, especially to the ethical writings of the **Hippocratic Corpus**. These texts are dominated by a contractual model of the relationship between practitioners and the sick (*aegrotus*; the word *patient* and therefore the ethical concept of being a patient do not appear in these texts) and the conception of medicine as a guild, where the primary concern is to protect and promote its trade secrets and thereby the interest of its members.

Professional medical ethics was intended by Gregory and Percival to be transnational, transreligious, and transcultural. More than two centuries later, it has taken on these characteristics. The history of this remarkable development has yet to be written. Such scholarship will, no doubt, identify multiple factors, for example, the role of colonialism in Africa, Asia, and Central and South America; the affinity of some schools of Islam for the sciences, as well as global war in the middle of the 20th century; and the long history of international trade. Refer to the introduction and *see also* MEDICAL ETHICS; PROFESSIONAL ETHICS.

PROFESSIONAL MILITARY MEDICAL ETHICS. Professional medical ethics for physicians who are officers in the military. In the United States, these physicians are members of the medical corps of the armed services: air force, army, coast guard, marines, and navy. These physician-officers have **professional responsibilities** as both physicians and military officers. As physicians, these physician-officers have **ethical obligations** to **patients** and **research subjects**. As officers, these physician-officers have taken an oath to defend the U.S. Constitution and to follow the *Uniform Code of Military Justice* (http://www.military.com/join-armed-forces/the-uniform-code-of-military-justice-ucmj.html, accessed 14 September 2017), which requires all military personnel to obey lawful orders. As officers, physician-officers have an ethical obligation to support military missions by providing **clinical management** that protects and promotes the health-related interests of military personnel and thus contributes to their fitness for combat.

Physician-officers are often said to have "dual loyalties" and, therefore, can face ethical challenges arising from **conflicts of commitment**. A physician-officer may be given an order that the physician judges to be unlawful because it is not compatible with ethical obligations created by professional medical ethics. A physician-officer will use **triage** to establish priorities for clinical management that limit patient **autonomy** and **decisional rights**. Some take the view that, in responsibly managing these and other conflicts of commitment, the default position should be fulfilling the ethical obligations of a physician. That is, the **burden of justification** should be on giving priority to ethical obligations of an officer. This is a matter of **ethical controversy**. *See also* PROFESSIONAL ETHICS; WAR.

PROFESSIONAL NORM. A standard of **clinical practice, clinical research**, scientific research, or medical education that is grounded in **deliberative clinical judgment, professional medical ethics,** or **scientific integrity**. *See also* IDEAL; NORM.

PROFESSIONAL OBLIGATION. An **ethical obligation** originating in the social role of being a physician and **ethically justified** in **professional medical ethics**. *See also* PROFESSIONAL ETHICAL OBLIGATION; PROFESSIONAL RESPONSIBILITY.

PROFESSIONAL RELATIONSHIP. The relationship between a member of one of the traditional professions (law, medicine, the military, and the ministry) and an individual subordinate to the **authority** and **power** of the professional. The member of the profession has an **ethical obligation** to adhere to **professional ethics** and **professional norms** in all aspects of his or her relationship with the individual. In a professional relationship, the professional has power over the individual and, therefore, has an ethical obligation, as the **fiduciary** of that individual, to protect the individual by adhering to the requirements of **professional integrity**, to protect the individual from the misuse of that power. A **contractual relationship** of free exchange between equals is conceptually inadequate to a professional relationship. A distinctive language is used to signal the professional relationship and its difference from a contractual relationship: attorneys serve clients; physicians serve **patients**; military officers serve their nation, subordinates, and enemy combatants; and clergy serve their congregants. No professional serves customers.

PROFESSIONAL RESPONSIBILITY. The **ethical obligations** generated by fulfilling the three commitments that define the **ethical concept of medicine as a profession**, specifically, the ethical obligations to **patients** and **research subjects** generated by the **professional virtues** of physicians and the **ethical principle of beneficence, ethical principle of nonmaleficence, ethical principle of respect for autonomy,** and **ethical principle of justice.** *See also* PROFESSIONAL MEDICAL ETHICS.

PROFESSIONAL SOCIETIES OF PHYSICIANS. Also known as "academies," "associations," and "colleges." Historically, these have been important instruments of self-regulation of the medical profession and production of **codes** and statements on topics in **professional medical ethics** and **health policy.** *See also* PROFESSIONAL ASSOCIATIONS OF PHYSICIANS.

PROFESSIONAL TRUST. The ability of patients to **trust** in their physicians to be professionals by adhering to the **ethical principle of medicine as a profession** and **professional medical ethics.** *See also* FIDUCIARY; PUBLIC TRUST.

PROFESSIONAL VIRTUE. A habit or trait of character required to fulfill the three commitments that constitute the **ethical concept of medicine as a profession.** The professional **virtues** include the **professional virtue of compassion,** the **professional virtue of integrity,** the **professional virtue of self-effacement,** and the **professional virtue of self-sacrifice.** *See also* CHARACTER; VICE.

PROFESSIONAL VIRTUE OF COMPASSION. The **virtue** or trait of character or habit that creates the **ethical obligations** of the physician to recognize when a **patient** is at risk of experiencing **distress, pain,** or **suffering** and acting to prevent them and to provide effective **clinical management** of distress, pain, and suffering when they occur. Fulfilling these ethical obligations is required by the second component of the **ethical concept of medicine as a profession.** *See also* PROFESSIONAL MEDICAL ETHICS.

PROFESSIONAL VIRTUE OF INTEGRITY. A bedrock **virtue** of **professional medical ethics** that creates an **ethical obligation** of the physician to adhere to standards of intellectual and moral excellence in medical education, **patient care,** and scientific **research** and the integration of a physician's life that results from sustained adherence to these standards of intellectual and moral excellence. Fulfilling this ethical obligation is required by the first component of the **ethical concept of medicine as a profession. Thomas Percival** (1740–1804) was probably the first to recognize that sustaining the professional virtue of integrity requires a supportive **organizational culture.** *See also* INTEGRITY.

PROFESSIONAL VIRTUE OF SELF-EFFACEMENT. The **virtue** or trait or habit of character that creates an **ethical obligation** of the physician to be aware of differences (country of origin, dress, first language, immigration status, race, religion, sex, gender, military uniform), when they are clinically irrelevant, between the physician and **patient** and not allowing these differences to bias **deliberative clinical judgment** or **patient care**. Fulfilling these ethical obligations is required by the second component of the **ethical concept of medicine as a profession**. *See also* PROFESSIONAL MEDICAL ETHICS.

PROFESSIONAL VIRTUE OF SELF-SACRIFICE. The **virtue** or habit or trait of character that creates an **ethical obligation** of the physician to take reasonable risks to the physician's convenience, family life, health, life, and time in **patient care** and **research**. Fulfilling these ethical obligations is required by the second component of the **ethical concept of medicine as a profession**. One of the most pressing ethical challenges is setting **ethically justified** limits on the ethical obligation to make self-sacrifices in patient care, research, and education. *See also* PROFESSIONAL MEDICAL ETHICS.

PROFESSIONALISM. *See* ETHICAL CONCEPT OF MEDICINE AS A PROFESSION.

PROXY. *See* SURROGATE.

PROXY DECISION MAKING. *See* SURROGATE DECISION MAKING.

PRUDENCE. A **virtue** that schools one in the discipline of identifying one's **legitimate self-interests**, distinguishing these from **mere self-interest**, and acting to protect and promote one's legitimate self-interests. This virtue plays a central role in the concept of *medicus politicus* or the "politic physician" in the *medicus politicus* literature, created by physician-ethicists such as **Rodrigo de Castro** (1550–1627) and **Friedrich Hoffmann** (1660–1738). Hoffmann made the major contribution of basing prudence on enlightened self-interest (i.e., defining the legitimate self-interests of the physician based on the patient's **interests**).

PSYCHOPHARMACOLOGY. The use of medications to provide **clinical management** for mental illnesses and disorders, for behavioral **disorders** of **patients**, and also for **behavioral control**. These medications often have side effects; some of these can be serious, far-reaching, and irreversible. In such clinical circumstances, **beneficence**-based **clinical judgment** approaches its limits, creating uncertainty about whether such medication is a **medically reasonable alternative**. This uncertainty is compounded by the intrinsic uncertainty of symptom-based or behavior-based diagnoses in mental health care. This synergistic uncertainty helps explain why psychopharmacology and its clinical limits can become an **ethical controversy** in itself and for **ethical reasoning** about **behavior control**. Pharmacogenomics may help reduce this uncertainty.

PUBLIC HEALTH. The prevention and management of a population's **conditions, diseases, disabilities, disorders**, or **injuries** based on **deliberative clinical judgment**. Public health measures should be based on reliable predictions of the outcomes of **clinical management**. When the outcomes of a public health measure cannot be reliably predicted, that public health measure becomes an **experiment**. Public health experiments should be conducted as **research**. *See also* FRANK, JOHANN PETER (1745–1821); HEALTH POLICY; PRECAUTIONARY PRINCIPLE; PUBLIC POLICY.

PUBLIC HEALTH ETHICS. Ethical reasoning about **public health**, in which the focus shifts from **beneficence**-based reasoning about one patient at a time to beneficence-based and **justice**-based ethical reasoning about the health of a population of patients. **Johann Peter Frank** (1745–1821) wrote one of the first public health ethics, based on the concept of **medical police**. *See also* HEALTH POLICY; PRECAUTIONARY PRINCIPLE; PUBLIC POLICY.

PUBLIC POLICY. Guidance from governments, nongovernmental organizations, and social organizations about acceptable behavior of individuals, organizations, businesses, and governments. In the federal system of the United States, public policy is made by city, county, state, and federal governments in the form of **common law, regulatory law**, and **statutory law**. As a general rule, what is not prohibited in health policy is permissible. **Ethical reasoning** about what public policy ought to be typically appeals to the **ethical principle of justice**. *See also* HEALTH POLICY.

PUBLIC TRUST. A phrase used by **Thomas Percival** (1740–1804) in his *Medical Ethics* (1803). The phrase is used to characterize the third component of the **ethical concept of medicine as a profession** and to explicitly reject the concept of medicine as a merchant guild (the guild's primary purpose is the protection and promotion of its members' economic and political **interests**), which had dominated **clinical practice** for centuries, except in faith communities, such as the infirmaries of the foundations of the Roman Catholic Church in Europe. *See also* FIDUCIARY; TRUST.

PVS. Ambiguous between **persistent vegetative state** and **permanent vegetative state**.

Q

QUACK. A derogatory term used by physicians to distinguish themselves from those practitioners who were considered "irregulars," in other words, not trained in the ways physicians were—by apprenticeship, by attending a university medical school, by having a license to practice—and therefore not possessing the knowledge and skills required to provide **patient care**. This term was almost always used out of **self-interest** in gaining and keeping market share among the few well-to-do individuals who could afford physicians' fees. The use of the term was on shaky grounds, inasmuch as the training of physicians varied widely, resulting in many physicians without the requisite knowledge and skill to provide patient care.

QUALITATIVE FUTILITY. This concept applies clinically when the outcome of **life-sustaining treatment** is the patient's survival, but the **patient** is either permanently unconscious or permanently dependent on such treatment (Schneiderman et al. 1996). *See also* FUTILITY; INTERACTIVE CAPACITY FUTILITY.

QUALITY. In **clinical practice**, the **professionally responsible** reduction of variation in the processes of **patient care** that improves outcomes and therefore should better manage costs. The first component of the **ethical concept of medicine as a profession** creates an **ethical obligation** of physicians and healthcare organizations to improve the quality of patient care by identifying uncontrolled variation in the processes of patient care, analyzing their causes, and eliminating or modifying the causes that contribute most to the observed variation following accepted methods of continuous quality improvement. *See also* EVIDENCE-BASED MEDICINE; PRECISION MEDICINE.

QUALITY OF LIFE. Engaging in valued life tasks and deriving satisfaction from doing so. The concept originated in the social sciences and came into **bioethics** in the 1970s. Which life tasks are worth valuing is a **judgment** that can be made reliably only by each individual for himself or herself. How much satisfaction from engaging in valued life tasks, even in a limited fashion, is acceptable is a judgment that can be make reliably only by each individual for himself or herself. To be morally **authoritative**, judgments by others about a patient's current or future quality of life must be made based on the patient's beliefs about valued life tasks and patient-oriented judgments about what level of satisfaction from engaging in valued life tasks would be acceptable to the patient. The concept of quality of life in **professional medical ethics** is therefore an **autonomy**-based concept. Predictions about future functional status, especially neurologic function, that are based in **deliberative clinical judgment** are relevant to judgments about the acceptability of predicted quality of life made by the patient or the patient's **surrogate** making decisions based on the **substituted judgment standard**. *See also* QUALITY-OF-LIFE FUTILITY.

QUALITY-OF-LIFE FUTILITY. There is no reasonable expectation that the predicted functional status of the patient will support a **quality of life** acceptable to the patient. The **ethical justification** for the application of this specification of **futility** appeals to the **ethical principle of respect for autonomy** that creates an **ethical obligation** of the care team to accept refusal to authorize clinical management as an outcome of the **informed consent process**. Respect for autonomy also creates an ethical obligation to accept the refusal of a **surrogate** to authorize clinical management when that refusal is reliably based on the patient's values and beliefs and therefore fulfills the **substituted judgment standard** of **surrogate decision making**. *See also* FUTILITY.

QUANTITATIVE FUTILITY. This concept applies clinically when in the past 100 attempts of an intervention it is "useless" (Schneiderman et al. 1996). *See also* FUTILITY.

QUARANTINE. The **voluntary** or **involuntary** confinement of a **patient** with a communicable disease that in **deliberative clinical judgment** is considered to pose a serious health risk to others. The confinement should be designed and implemented to prevent others from becoming infected. The **ethical justification** appeals to the **harm principle**, a beneficence-based **ethical principle** that creates an **ethical obligation** not to act in ways that are reliably predicted to harm innocent others. When the predicted harm is considered to be serious, far-reaching, and irreversible, the ethical obligation is considered strong enough to justify limits on an individual's **autonomy**, including involuntary confinement by order of **public health** authorities. This is a situation in which the **ethical principle of beneficence** overrides the **ethical principle of respect for autonomy**. Patients who are quarantined retain an important **autonomy**-based **prima facie negative right**, the **right to refuse treatment**, even if this creates the risk of serious, far-reaching, and irreversible harm to themselves, including **death**. *See also* HEALTH POLICY; PUBLIC POLICY.

QUICKENING. Used before the ability to detect heart sounds to describe fetal movement, usually in the second trimester. Now archaic. In 18th-century Europe, quickening was taken to signal the existence of a living fetus rather than not-yet-living fetus. When the fetus is alive, **induced abortion** after quickening became **ethically impermissible**, because quickening was taken to be a sign of **moral status**. As the ability to detect other signs of fetal life that occur sooner than quickening (e.g., detecting fetal heartbeat using auscultation) developed in the 19th century, using quickening as a cut-off for induced abortion being **ethically permissible** fell into disfavor (Baker and McCullough 2009d).

QUINLAN CASE. *See* ADVANCE DIRECTIVE.

R

RACISM. The false belief that one race is superior to another and therefore has the prerogative to organize social practices, organizations, and government with the privileged race always in the superior position, exercising **raw power** to oppress the race falsely believed to be inferior. Racism and racist practices are forms of **invidious discrimination**. As such, they are systematically incompatible with **ethical principles** and **virtues**, especially the **ethical principle of justice**, and are therefore **ethically impermissible**.

In **professional medical ethics**, racist practices in **patient care**, **research**, and education are incompatible with the commitment in the **ethical concept of medicine as a profession** to make the health-related **interests** of **patients** the physician's primary concern and motivation. Because they are based on false beliefs, the prerogatives claimed for themselves by racists are **mere self-interests** and, therefore, do not qualify as **legitimate self-interests**. Finally, racism and racist practice introduce unmanageable **bias** into **clinical judgment** and are therefore incompatible with the first commitment of the ethical concept of medicine as a profession, to scientific and clinical **competence** in patient care, research, and education.

RAMSEY, PAUL (1913–1988). American Methodist moral theologian who served for many years on the faculty of Princeton University and who was one of the founders of the field of **bioethics** in the United States. His *Patient as Person* (Ramsey 1973) was widely influential, explicating the concept of a person as embodied and fully human, not reducible to the abstraction of **autonomy** or **rights**. This became an important source for the **ethical principle of respect for persons** in the *Belmont Report* and therefore on the **ethics of human subjects research**. *See also* PATIENT AS PERSON.

RANDOMIZATION. A scientific **research** method used in randomized clinical trials (also known as **Phase III clinical trials**) to achieve populations of **research subjects** among which there will be no statistically significant differences in clinically relevant traits, such as age, **sex**, gender, race, and health status. Randomization means that subjects are not assigned to an arm of the clinical trial by the physician-investigators but on the basis of random assignment (usually generated by a computer). **Equipoise** is required as a necessary condition for randomization. It is essential in the **informed consent process** for **human subjects research** to make clear that assignment will be random and explain randomization to potential subjects, to prevent **therapeutic misconception**. *See also* CLINICAL TRIAL; RESEARCH.

RANDOMIZED CLINICAL TRIAL. *See* PHASE III CLINICAL TRIAL.

RATIONING. A tool for the **allocation of scarce medical resources**. There are several interpretations, based on **specifications** of the **ethical principle of justice**. One interpretation appeals to **libertarian justice** and allocates scarce medical resources by price and therefore ability to pay. This is an appeal to market solutions. That needs of some **patients** will go unmet is viewed as unfortunate but not unfair. Another interpretation appeals to **egalitarian justice**, which supports allocation by a lottery. A third interpretation appeals to **healthcare justice** and allocates according to medical need as defined in **deliberative clinical judgment**. A fourth interpretation appeals to outcomes that result in the greatest good for the greatest number, an appeal to **utilitarian justice**. The fifth appeals to **Rawlsian justice**, which gives preference to patients who are the least well off (i.e., patients with **conditions**, **disabilities**, or **diseases** that have serious, far-reaching, and irreversible consequences for patients and their family caregivers). When a specification of the ethical principle of justice allows for allocations that are not consistent with the **professional virtue of integrity**, that specification is not **ethically permissible** in **professional medical ethics**.

RAW POWER. Power that is exercised without **ethical justification**. In **professional medical ethics**, the exercise of raw power and an organizational culture based on raw power are both **ethically impermissible** because they are incompatible with the second and third components of the **ethical concept of medicine as a profession**.

RAWLSIAN JUSTICE. A **specification** of the **ethical principle of justice** that is a variant of **utilitarian justice** designed to prevent **exploitation** of those at the bottom end of the social, economic, and political ladders—the "least well off." This account of justice was developed by Harvard political philosopher John Rawls (1921–2002). He argued that the utilitarian imperative to maximize benefit is permissible but only when those least well off are also benefited. This is known as the maximin principle of justice. *See also* EGALITARIAN JUSTICE; HEALTHCARE JUSTICE; LIBERTARIAN JUSTICE.

REASONABLE PERSON STANDARD. A legal and ethical standard for disclosure of information to a **patient** or **surrogate** in the **informed consent process**. This is the majority legal standard in the United States and is the ethical standard. Courts have endorsed this standard because the **professional community standard** results in disclosure that is not adequate for making an informed **decision**. This standard requires the physician to disclose information about the patient's **condition**, diagnosis, treatment plan, and prognosis with and without treatment that any patient in the patient's condition needs to know.

This is a somewhat abstract standard because it does not mean what a particular patient needs to know at a particular time, which is known as the **subjective standard**. The reasonable person standard can be put into clinical practice by the physician identifying and disclosing clinically salient information (i.e., clinical information that shapes or should shape **deliberative clinical judgment**). Put more simply, if clinical information is or should be important to the physician it is important to the reasonable person. This implements the goal of the reasonable person standard: for the patient or surrogate to replicate for himself or herself the physician's deliberative clinical judgment and recommendations based on it. *See also* INFORMED CONSENT CASES; INFORMED REFUSAL; INFORMED REFUSAL CASE.

REC. Research Ethics Committee. The name in European and other countries for an **Institutional Review Board**. *See also* RESEARCH.

REED, WALTER (1851–1902). U.S. Army physician. During his time as an army physician, epidemics of yellow fever were common and incapacitated soldiers in camp and in the field. He supported the hypothesis that yellow fever is an infectious disease transmitted by mosquitos. His research to test this hypothesis was based on good science and required the **informed consent** of soldiers in writing to become **research subjects**. They received generous compensation. This **research** is considered a model for the conduct of research in military medicine and **military medical ethics**. *See also* ETHICS OF HUMAN SUBJECTS RESEARCH; HUMAN SUBJECTS RESEARCH.

REGENERATIVE MEDICINE. A set of biomedical technologies designed to repair or replace organs that have been damaged by **disease** or **injury**. These technologies include **embryonic stem cell research**, **reproductive cloning**, the use of adult stem cells that have been modified to be pluripotent stem cells, and scaffolding techniques in which cells are stripped from human or animal tissue and then repopulated with cells obtained from the **patient** with the goal of a diminished or absent immune response, a persistent clinical challenge of **transplantation**. Like all new biomedical technologies, the promise of regenerative medicine is sometimes oversold, resulting in **enthusiasm** followed by inevitable disappointment as **hopes** are not fulfilled (at all or only incompletely). This can be prevented by characterizing progress in ways that are disciplined by **deliberative clinical judgment**. *See also* STEM CELL RESEARCH.

REGULATORY LAW. Law in the form of regulations issued by the executive branch of government, following the provisions of **statutory law** for doing so. Regulatory law plays a major role in the prospective oversight of **animal subjects research** and **human subjects research**. *See also* ADMINISTRATIVE LAW; COMMON LAW.

RELIGIOUS BIOETHICS. Bioethics that draws on religious sources in a secular, non-doctrinal way, thus contributing to the pluralism of sources and methods in bioethics. *See also* MORAL THEOLOGY.

RELIGIOUS ETHICS. Ethical reasoning that draws on religious sources in a secular, non-doctrinal way. Religious ethics has made, and continues to make, contributions to **bioethics**. *See also* MORAL THEOLOGY.

RELIGIOUS MEDICAL ETHICS. Medical ethics that draws on religious sources in a secular, non-doctrinal way. The insights of religious ethics that can be expressed in **moral philosophy** can be incorporated into **professional medical ethics**.

REMMLINK REPORT (1990). In the Netherlands, this report documents cases of **euthanasia**—in the sense of **killing** of the **patient** by the physician—of patients who did not have **decision-making capacity**. This is **involuntary active euthanasia**, which is inconsistent with **professional integrity** and is therefore **ethically impermissible** in **professional medical ethics**. This practice was not consistent with the position of the Netherlands Supreme Court in the **Alkmaar Case**.

REN. A core concept in Chinese **medical ethics** based on the **moral philosophy** of **Confucius**. *Ren* is a **cluster concept** and includes altruism, **benevolence**, humaneness, humanity, and perfect virtue. *Ren* is the bridge that connects medicine to Confucian **ideals**, "thus elevating it to the art of humaneness" (Nie 2009, 338). For example, *ren* becomes the guiding concept for focusing on humane **clinical management** in **end-of-life care**.

REPRODUCTIVE CLONING. *See* CLONING.

REPRODUCTIVE TECHNOLOGY. *See* ASSISTED REPRODUCTION; ASSISTED REPRODUCTIVE TECHNOLOGIES (ART).

REPUTATION. The **judgments** of others about the behavior and **character** of an individual or the **organizational cultures** of healthcare organizations and governments. These judgments can be earned (i.e., have an evidence base) or unearned (i.e., result from sources that are influenced by **bias** or from **deception**). Reputation is one of the two bases for the *Hippocratic Oath* (the other is *techné*). The Hippocratic physician earns reputation as a good physician by following the prescriptions and proscriptions of the *Oath* and the other texts of the **Hippocratic Corpus.** A major risk of this approach to **medical ethics** is that a physician can have an unearned, good reputation.

RESEARCH. An **experiment** undertaken with a group of patients to create generalizable knowledge by adhering to the intellectual **norms** of scientific methods and the moral norms of **research ethics.** Research conducted with human subjects is **human subjects research.** Research conducted with non-human animal subjects, including nonhuman primates, is **animal subjects research.**

RESEARCH ETHICS. Ethical reasoning about **animal subjects research, human subjects research,** and biomedical research with cells and other biological materials. Ethical reasoning about animal subjects research dates to the ancient Western world, in which vivisection was practiced (Maehle 2009). Research with human subjects dates to the ancient Western world (Lederer 2009).

One of the earliest examples of ethical reasoning about such research is found in the **professional medical ethics** of **John Gregory** (1724–1773). He argued that experimental drugs should be administered only after all accepted remedies had been tried and failed to benefit the **patient** clinically. He also argued that physicians should not "sport" with patients, in other words, use patients to advance the physician's **self-interest** without regard for the patient's health and life, which is a form of **exploitation.** At that time, young physicians, ambitious to establish a name for themselves as what we would now call "cutting-edge" physicians, would declare patients incurable. The goal in doing so was not to abandon such patients, as had been accepted practice for centuries (a practice that Gregory rejected in his call for physicians to remain with dying patients and care for them), but to justify performing **experiments** on them. Gregory's admonition not to "sport" with patients was meant to condemn this self-serving, unprofessional practice. *See also* ETHICS OF ANIMAL SUBJECTS RESEARCH; ETHICS OF HUMAN SUBJECTS RESEARCH.

RESEARCH ETHICS COMMITTEE. The name in European and other countries for an **Institutional Review Board**. *See also* CLINICAL ETHICS COMMITTEE.

RESEARCH ETHICS CONSULTANT. An individual or team who provides **research ethics consultation** about research with **human subjects**. *See also* CLINICAL ETHICS CONSULTANT.

RESEARCH ETHICS CONSULTATION. The provision of **ethics consultation** about research with **human subjects**. The scope of such ethics consultation includes working with clinical investigators to identify and responsibly manage ethical challenges in research design, recruitment of subjects, the **informed consent process**, and the conduct of research. *See also* CLINICAL ETHICS CONSULTATION; CONSULTATION.

RESEARCH ON CHILDREN. Research with **pediatric patients**. The distinctive feature of **research ethics** includes **parental consent** and **pediatric assent** (the child must do more than not opt out but affirmatively agree to participate). Care must be taken in the **informed consent process** to ensure that the parents' **decision making** is **voluntary**, given the natural, very strong willingness of concerned parents to agree to any **clinical management** that might benefit a child, especially a child with a life-threatening **disease** or **injury**. Some **Institutional Review Boards** assess the projected risk/benefit ratio using the concept of **no more than minimal risk** (i.e., risk that is no greater than that experienced by a child in everyday life). The concept of minimal risk is invoked in the section of **45 CFR 46** about research with children. *See also* ETHICS OF HUMAN SUBJECTS RESEARCH.

RESEARCH ON EMBRYOS. *See* EMBRYO RESEARCH.

RESEARCH ON FETUSES. Research with fetuses, which necessarily also is research in pregnant women. **45 CFR 46** permits research on fetuses provided that the risk is minimized: among study designs that could answer the research question(s), the design that is least clinically risky to the fetus should be chosen. This is not the same as **no more than minimal risk** (i.e., risk that is no greater than that experienced by a child in everyday life). Currently, the **informed consent** of the father is required by 45 CFR 46. Care must be taken in the **informed consent process** to ensure that the pregnant woman's and father's **decision making** is **voluntary**, given the natural, very strong willingness of concerned, prospective parents to agree to any **clinical management** that might benefit their fetus and future child. The

ethical concept of the fetus as a patient has important implications for the ethics of research for fetal benefit. *See also* MATERNAL-FETAL SURGERY; MATERNAL-FETAL TREATMENT; OBSTETRIC ETHICS.

RESEARCH ON PRISONERS. Incarceration is an inherently **coercive** environment, calling into question whether any prisoner can engage in voluntary **decision making** about participating in **research**. There is **ethical controversy** about this matter. The regulation **45 CFR 46** requires safeguards to address this ethical challenge. *See also* ETHICS OF HUMAN SUBJECTS RESEARCH; VULNERABLE.

RESEARCH SUBJECT. A human being or animal used in scientific or clinical investigation. *See also* ETHICS OF ANIMAL SUBJECTS RESEARCH; ETHICS OF HUMAN SUBJECTS RESEARCH.

RESPECT. An attitude of due regard for the intrinsic worth and importance of an entity as well as behavior that expresses such due regard. This attitude is one of the components of **dignity**. The regard is "due" to the entity because it has **moral status**. This can be either **independent moral status** or **dependent moral status**. It is meaningless to speak of respect for an entity that does not have either form of moral status. *See also* ETHICAL PRINCIPLE OF RESPECT FOR AUTONOMY; ETHICAL PRINCIPLE OF RESPECT FOR PERSONS.

RESPECT FOR AUTONOMY. *See* ETHICAL PRINCIPLE OF RESPECT FOR AUTONOMY.

RESPECT FOR PERSONS. *See* ETHICAL PRINCIPLE OF RESPECT FOR PERSONS.

RESPECTFUL PERSUASION. A component of **preventive ethics** in response to refusal of offered or recommended **clinical management** by a **patient** or **surrogate**. The physician should assume that the patient or surrogate has good reason for refusing. The task is to identify those reasons and determine whether they support authorization of the clinical management. The physician can elicit information from the patient or surrogate by asking what is important for the patient to accomplish or avoid. (For surrogates, this approach implements the **substituted judgment standard**.) The responses will express the patient's **values**. When the patient's values support a **medically reasonable alternative** that has been offered or recommended, the physician should point this out and ask the patient or surrogate to reconsider. If this fails to result in authorization, **informed refusal** must be implemented by the physician. *See also* INFORMED CONSENT PROCESS.

RESPIRATOR. A machine that provides mechanical ventilation of **patients**. *See also* LIFE-SUSTAINING TREATMENT.

RHAZES (MOHAMMAD IBN ZAKARIYA AL-RAZI, 845–925). Persian physician and philosopher. His **medical ethics** emphasized obligations to both friends and enemies.

RIGHT. A justified claim of an individual against other individuals, organizations, or the state to be treated in a specified fashion. The **ethical justification** for a right is a set of reasons that explain the basis or foundation of the right. This justification should establish whether the right is an **absolute right** or a **prima facie right** (limited right). This justification should also make clear whether the right is a **negative right** or a **positive right**. There are no absolute positive rights. An adequate account of a right will clearly classify the right as either an **absolute negative right**, a **prima facie negative right**, or a **prima facie positive right**.

In the history of philosophy, various ethical justifications for rights have been proposed. One justification appeals to the concept of a **natural right**, a right that originates in our nature as human beings in a world created by the creator god and ordered to human good. This is known as **deism**. Because the state of nature precedes that of society and government, natural rights precede government, making government accountable to individuals. This is a frontal assault on the divine right of kings. John Locke (1632–1704), who provides a deistic account, enumerates four natural rights: life, liberty, health, and property. These are prima facie negative rights. The Declaration of Independence (1776) of the United States from the United Kingdom also appeals to a deistic account of natural rights and enumerates three: life, liberty, and the pursuit of happiness.

Another line of justification appeals to the **ethical principle of respect for autonomy** and **independent moral status** as the origin of rights. Like natural rights, these rights precede society and the state. They also precede the relationship between a physician and a patient and thus serve as a constraint on physician **paternalism**. Some in **bioethics** hold that autonomy-based rights are prima facie negative rights while others hold that autonomy-based rights are absolute negative rights.

A third line of justification appeals to **utilitarianism**. This line of justification holds that rights are essential for achieving the greatest good for the greatest number, correcting the erroneous claim that utilitarianism does not support rights and might even support slavery.

A fourth line of justification appeals to **dependent moral status** or rights that originate in social roles. This appeal uses the philosophical method of **pragmatism**. Rights exist because of a social role that is created for a purpose. This is the basis of **human rights** in the **United Nations Universal Declaration of Human Rights**. Human rights can be prima facie negative rights as well as prima facie positive rights.

RIGHT TO AN OPEN FUTURE. An imprecise concept that encompasses the **right** of a child to have one's future opportunities and choices remain as unrestricted as possible, to provide the widest possible range of choices. This right is **autonomy** based. This right creates an **ethical obligation** of parents to rear their child with this constraint in mind. There is **ethical controversy** about this right. It appears to make **ethically impermissible** raising a child in a faith community or with inherited family **values**, which ordinarily is considered to be **ethically permissible** in **moral philosophy** and is usually **ethically obligatory** in the **moral theology** of a faith community or by family tradition. This right appears also to create an ethical obligation to prevent the birth of children with **disabilities** that reduce cognitive, sensory, or motor functions. Invoking this right therefore bears the **burden of justification**. This requirement is not always recognized, especially in the literatures of **genethics** and **genomic ethics**. *See also* PARENTAL RESPONSIBILITY.

RIGHT TO CONFIDENTIALITY. A misnomer, inasmuch as the physician's **ethical obligation** to maintain **confidentiality** is based on **professional medical ethics**, independent of the **patient's rights**. The correct phrase is **right to privacy**.

RIGHT TO DIE. A phrase widely in use in the **bioethics** literature to refer to a **negative right** of a **patient** to refuse treatment that was causing an "unnatural" or "technological" prolongation of life that did not result in net clinical benefit for the **patient** and that undermined the patient's **quality of life**. In most cases, this was asserted as an **absolute negative right**. This phrase has been replaced by the **right to refuse treatment**. *See also* DEATH AND DYING; END-OF-LIFE CARE; EUTHANASIA; LETTING DIE.

RIGHT TO HEALTH. The **absolute negative right** or **prima facie negative right** not to have one's health damaged by another individual, organization, or the state. The philosopher and physician John Locke (1632–1704) included the right to health among the **natural rights** of human beings. Like all absolute negative rights, the absolute negative right to health bears the **burden of justification**. *See also* HEALTH POLICY; PUBLIC POLICY.

RIGHT TO HEALTHCARE. The **absolute positive right** or the **prima facie positive right** to the resources of others necessary to sustain one's health. This includes **access to healthcare** and the provision of healthcare based on **deliberative clinical judgment**. The right does not necessarily include clinical management based solely on the patient's preferences. The more broadly that the concept of health is understood, the more comprehensive the right to healthcare. Like all absolute positive rights, the absolute positive right to healthcare bears the **burden of justification**.

The right to healthcare was asserted as early as the 1790s, by the French revolutionary councils, which called for citizens of the new Republic of France to have a right to total, prompt, guaranteed, and free healthcare—a claim that could not realistically be satisfied at the time. The right to healthcare became an important component of the political agenda of the Progressives in late 19th- and early 20th-century America, with their calls for mandatory health insurance. *See also* HEALTH POLICY; PUBLIC POLICY.

RIGHT TO LIFE. There are four distinct meanings of this phrase: (1) an **absolute negative right** not to be **killed**; (2) a **prima facie negative right** not to be killed; (3) an **absolute positive right** to the resources of others necessary to remain alive; and (4) a **prima facie positive right** to the resources of others necessary to remain alive. Given that positive rights always come with limits, the concept of an absolute positive right to life is philosophically implausible. The prima facie positive right to life comes with limits; **ethical reasoning** concerns how those limits should be understood. This is also true for the prima facie negative right to life. Like all absolute negative rights, the absolute negative right to life bears the **burden of justification**. *See also* ABORTION; CAPITAL PUNISHMENT; INDUCED ABORTION; TERMINATION OF PREGNANCY.

RIGHT TO PRIVACY. *See* PRIVACY.

RIGHT TO REFUSE TREATMENT. The **absolute negative right** or the **prima facie negative right** not to authorize **clinical management**, including clinical management that in **deliberative clinical judgment** is expected to benefit the **patient** significantly. The **ethical justification** for this right appeals to the **ethical principle of respect for autonomy**. The right to refuse treatment is often treated as an absolute negative right. Indeed, it is often taken for granted that this is *the* meaning of the term *right to refuse treatment*. However, like all absolute negative rights, the absolute negative right to refuse treatment bears the **burden of justification**. One challenge to this view is that when a **patient** refuses to authorize clinical management but remains a patient, the patient in effect is exercising a **prima facie positive right** to alternative clinical management that may not be **medically reasonable** (Chervenak and McCullough 1991).

RIGHT TO TRY. The assertion of the **positive right** of a **patient** to have access to investigational drugs and devices, in the **hope** that the drug or device may have clinical benefit, if only to slow the process of **disease**. In the 1990s, this right was implemented to provide access to women with breast cancer to autologous bone marrow **transplantation**. The result for many women was shortening their lives and reducing their **quality of life**. This historical example serves as a cautionary tale for what can happen when **enthusiasm** replaces **deliberative clinical judgment** and false hope is not respectfully challenged by tempering the patient's beliefs to clinical reality. *See also* HEALTH POLICY; PUBLIC POLICY.

RISK ASSESSMENT. The estimation of the probability of a health outcome, including **morbidity** and **mortality**. Risk assessment for a **patient** can be based on a variety of factors, alone or usually in combination, including: a patient's history, including family history; physical examination; laboratory analysis; imaging; and genetic or genomic analysis. The concept of risk assessment does *not* mean that a patient is destined to experience an outcome or already has the **disease**. The disclosure of risk assessment information to the patient in the **informed consent process** should make this clear, as well as whether the risk can be modified. Risk assessment is a component of **clinical management**.

RO. One of the four key components in the concept of the life cycle in **medical ethics** in Japan, influenced by **Buddhism** and **Shintoism**. *Ro* "means aging, an inevitable phenomenon in our life cycle" (Kimura and Sakai 2009, 132). This concept plays a major role in **Kaibara Ekiken**'s (1630–1714) medical ethics. *See also BYO; SHI; SHO.*

ROE V. WADE (**410 U.S. 113 [1973]**). A case originating in Texas, decided by the United States Supreme Court in 1973, about the legal permissibility of **induced abortion**. *See also* ABORTION.

ROLE-RELATED ETHICAL OBLIGATION. An **ethical obligation** that is constitutive of a social role, such as being a physician. This way of thinking about ethical obligation has ancient roots in the history of Western philosophy, especially in the **moral philosophy** of the Roman moral philosopher **Cicero**. A core concept in Cicero's moral philosophy is *officium*, which is translated as **"office"** or "role." *See also* DEPENDENT MORAL STATUS.

ROMAN CATHOLIC BIOETHICS. Bioethics based on the **moral theology** of Roman Catholicism, drawing on such resources as the New Testament, Roman Catholic and other moral theologians, and the teachings of the Church, contributing to the pluralism of bioethics.

ROMAN CATHOLIC MEDICAL ETHICS. Medical ethics based on **Roman Catholic moral theology**, to guide Roman Catholic physicians, patients, and healthcare organizations. There is a long history of the contributions of Roman Catholic moral theologians to medical ethics, for example, **Alphonsus Liguori** (1696–1787), who made major contributions to **casuistry**, and Fathers **Charles Coppens, SJ** (1835–1920) and **Gerald Kelly, SJ** (1902–1964), who wrote books in the "manualist" tradition of providing reasoned, practical guidance for physicians. The **Ethical and Religious Directives for Catholic Health Care Services** provides a comprehensive guide, from the United States Conference of Catholic Bishops, to Roman Catholic **moral theology** pertaining to many topics in **bioethics** and medical ethics. Moral theology, because it is not secular, is not methodologically adequate to serve as the basis of **professional medical ethics**.

ROMAN CATHOLIC MORAL THEOLOGY. Moral theology based on sacred scripture, the teachings of the Fathers of the Church and the Doctors of the Church, the Magisterium (teaching authority that includes statements of Councils and Popes), philosophy, and other authoritative sources in the Roman Catholic faith community.

ROMANTIC RELATIONSHIPS WITH PATIENTS. *See* BOUNDARY ISSUES.

ROYAL INFIRMARY. Hospitals established in the United Kingdom and in its colonies, starting in the 18th century. These hospitals have charters from the monarch in London. They were established for the "worthy poor"—men, women, and children who worked on estates and in new industries such as coal fields, cotton mills, and shipyards, whose employers valued their skilled labor and rapid return to the workforce. The "unworthy" poor were not allowed admission for their own moral good. The employers paid an annual subscription to ensure free care for the hospital's *inmates*, the word used until the terms *the sick* and *patient* replaced it.

Royal Infirmaries became important for the careful study of the natural history of **diseases** and **injuries** and for **experiments**. In addition, for the first time, physicians and the hospital as an organization that controlled access to resources like drugs and wine in the formulary gained **power** over patients. There was, however, no ethics to guide and restrain this power, to prevent it from becoming **raw power**. The need for such ethics was among the motivations of **John Gregory** (1724–1773) and **Thomas Percival** (1740–1804), who wrote the first **professional medical ethics**.

RUSH, BENJAMIN (1746–1813). Physician and American patriot. He signed the Declaration of Independence for Pennsylvania and served as surgeon general of the Continental Army. Rush studied medicine at the University of Edinburgh and brought **John Gregory**'s **medical ethics** to North America in his *Observations on the Duties of a Physician, and the Methods of Improving Medicine. Accommodated to the Present State of Society and Manners in the United States* (1805). The duties or **ethical obligations** of a physician are based on the physician's **virtues**, especially humanity or **sympathy**, professional honor, and patriotism. Rush's medical ethics is strongly influenced by **Christian moral theology**. *See also* CHRISTIAN MEDICAL ETHICS.

RYAN, MICHAEL (1800–1840). Irish physician. He is the author of a text on **medical jurisprudence** that included what is regarded as the first **history of medical ethics**, *A Manual of Medical Jurisprudence, Compiled from the Best Medical and Legal Works* (1831). Ryan condemned **experiments** with dangerous medicine without the consent of the **patient**. He also argued that this practice should be replaced with investigation using animals in **animal research**.

S

SALICETO, GUGLIELMO DA (1220–1274). Italian physician. His surgical ethics describes the good physician, based on the concept of solemnity or solidity of character, especially when sharing bad news with the sick.

SANCTITY OF LIFE. A concept from **moral theology** that life is sacred, creating an **ethical obligation** to God not to violate that life. Some versions of the concept limit it to humans, others to all sentient creatures, and still others to all living things. Sanctity of life is a form of **dependent moral status**. The concept cannot be generalized beyond faith communities in which it has currency. *See also* DEISM; THEISM.

SCIENTIFIC INTEGRITY. A **virtue** that requires adherence to standards of intellectual and moral excellence in the design, execution, evaluation, and reporting of scientific investigation and the integration of the scientist's life that results from sustained adherence to standards of intellectual and moral excellence. *See also* PROFESSIONAL VIRTUE OF INTEGRITY; RESEARCH.

SCIENTIFIC RESEARCH. Investigations in the biological and physical sciences, mathematics, and quantitative social sciences following accepted methods for doing so. The scope of scientific research includes basic science and clinical science. A central concept of scientific research is **scientific integrity**. *See also* RESEARCH.

SCOTTISH ENLIGHTENMENT. One of the national enlightenments of the 18th century (Porter and Teich 1981) distinctive for its emphasis on **moral science**. Scottish moral science took the view that, of the two human faculties of reason and instinct, instinct was the stronger and drove moral **judgment** and behavior. This moral instinct is called **sympathy**, a constitutive causal process of human moral physiology that naturally engages us directly in the lived experiences of others, especially affective experience. **David Hume** (1711–1776) reports his scientific discovery of sympathy in his

Treatise of Human Nature (2000 [1739–1740]). Reason was the weaker and nothing more than a calculating machine for matching means to the ends, with the ends set by the workings of sympathy. Scottish moral science became a major source of influence for the **professional medical ethics** of **John Gregory** (1724–1773) and **Thomas Percival** (1740–1804). *See also* ENGLISH ENLIGHTENMENT.

SCREENING. This word is used ambiguously between: (a) testing a population of **patients** for the presence of **disease** as part of **public health**, to determine the prevalence of disease and advocate for resources to provide **clinical management**; and (b) evaluating patients for the purpose of **risk assessment**. The latter use of the word *screening* does not refer to diagnosing disease, while the former does. The two can become conflated when physicians use the phrase *screening test*.

SCRIBONIUS LARGUS (ca. 1–ca. 50). Roman court physician and ethicist. His *Compositiones*, a text on pharmacy, includes text on **medical ethics**, based on *humanitas*, or love of humanity, which creates the physician's obligation to care for all who present for care. This obligation is based on the **virtue** of **compassion**, which should move the physician to pity the plight of the sick and seek to alleviate human suffering.

SECURIS, JOHN (fl. 1550–1580). English physician. He argued that only learned physicians have the capability to heal and warned against commercialization of clinical practice. Learned physicians could be distinguished from the unlearned, **incompetent** physicians because the latter prescribe the same medication each time, practicing from rote rather than from recognition of the need to vary medication depending on the patient's **condition**. Drawing on the **Hippocratic Corpus**, Securis emphasizes the importance of having a good **reputation** and advises on how to achieve this goal.

SELECTIVE REDUCTION. *See* SELECTIVE TERMINATION.

SELECTIVE TERMINATION. Termination of pregnancy by **feticide** of one or more fetuses in a twin or higher-order pregnancy. This procedure is considered **ethically permissible** to reduce the increased risk of **mortality** and **morbidity** of triplet and higher pregnancy, with the pregnant **patient**'s **informed consent** or to prevent the birth of a fetus with a diagnosed anomaly. The use of feticide to reduce a twin to a singleton pregnancy when neither fetus has a diagnosed anomaly is **ethically controversial**. *See also* ABORTION.

SELF-CARE. Often the first response to the experience of illness is self-diagnosis and self-treatment, activities in which human beings have engaged since time immemorial. In the 18th century in Britain, this was called "self-physicking." Because of **disability**, including dementias, some **patients** may have impaired **decision-making capacity** (i.e., decisional autonomy) or **executive capacity** (i.e., **executive autonomy**) that results in lost capacity for self-care, creating the need for **long-term care**.

SELF-DETERMINATION. *See* AUTONOMY; ETHICAL PRINCIPLE OF RESPECT FOR AUTONOMY.

SELF-EFFACEMENT. *See* PROFESSIONAL VIRTUE OF SELF-EFFACEMENT.

SELF-EXPERIMENTATION. *See* AUTOEXPERIMENTATION.

SELF-INTEREST. An **interest** in one's stakes in the past, present, or future. In scientific **research** and **clinical practice**, self-interest is a source of **bias**, a problem identified by **Francis Bacon** (1561–1626) in his **philosophy of science** and **philosophy of medicine**. Preventing bias is responsibly managed by adhering to scientific method. Irresponsibly managed self-interest results in irresponsibly managed **conflicts of interest**.

SELF-REFERRAL. Self-referral names the practice of physicians who provide **clinical management** that the physician has offered or recommended to the **patient**. The physician then bills for these clinical services. By its very nature, self-referral is structured by a **conflict of interest**. It is assumed that patients understand that such a conflict of interest exists, given that this kind of conflict of interest pervades the practice of medicine. There is therefore no **ethical obligation** to disclose this conflict of interest to patients; the **informed consent process** is designed to provide information to patients that the physician cannot reasonably assume that the patient already has.

However, all conflicts of interest create the potential for **bias**. The antidote to this and all other forms of bias is adherence to the discipline of **deliberative clinical judgment** and the implications of the **professional virtue of integrity**. Doing so protects the patient from mistreatment, undertreatment, and overtreatment, all of which the **ethical principle of beneficence** makes **ethically impermissible**. The patient's trust that the physician is competent and committed to the primacy of the patient's health-related interests is therefore warranted.

SELF-SACRIFICE. *See* PROFESSIONAL VIRTUE OF SELF-SACRIFICE.

SEVERE FETAL ANOMALY. An anatomic or physiologic abnormality of the fetus that will result either in **in utero fetal demise**, stillbirth, live birth followed by a very high probability of death even with treatment, or live birth followed by survival with complete or near-complete and irreversible loss of cognitive developmental capacity (Chervenak and McCullough 2014). The **ethical obligation** to provide **aggressive obstetric management** or **neonatal critical care** is very limited. It is therefore **ethically permissible** to withhold or withdraw these forms of clinical management. *See also* PRENATAL DIAGNOSIS.

SEX. Biological classification based on reproductive role. The traditional, dimorphic view that all humans are either male or female has been replaced in the science and medicine of reproduction with the view that sex, like all human traits, ranges along a **biopsychosocial** continuum. This range is illustrated, for example, by **disorders of sexual development**. This variation also supports a wide variation in **gender**.

SEXUAL RELATIONSHIPS WITH PATIENTS. *See* BOUNDARY ISSUES.

"SHAM" SURGERY. An informal way to refer to a **placebo-controlled clinical trial** of a surgical procedure to assess its efficacy in achieving the outcomes for which it is performed. Like all placebo-controlled trials, placebo-controlled surgical trials bear the **burden of justification**.

SHARED DECISION MAKING. This phrase is used without fixed meaning. Some use it to characterize all **decision making** of physicians with **patients** with the goal of preventing **medical paternalism** and thus requiring physicians never to engage in **directive counseling**, because directive counseling is not compatible with the **ethical principle of respect for autonomy**. Some use this phrase to characterize all decision making with the goal of eliminating one-sided decision making and replacing it with the **ethical obligation** of physicians to elicit questions from patients, listen to their concerns, and address those concerns in the course of **clinical management**. Others use this phrase, not as a universal model, but in a restricted sense to characterize only clinical situations in which **non-directive counseling** should be adopted, in other words, when there are two or more **medically reasonable**

alternatives but, in **deliberative clinical judgment**, none is clinically superior. In such cases, the **patient**'s **values** and beliefs should be decisive. *See also* INFORMED CONSENT PROCESS.

SHI. One of four key components in the concept of the life cycle in **medical ethics** in Japan, influenced by **Buddhism** and **Shintoism**. *Shi* "means death and dying" (Kimura and Sakai 2009, 132). This concept plays a major role in **Kaibara Ekiken**'s (1630–1714) medical ethics. *See also BYO; RO; SHO.*

SHINTOISM. A religion in Japan defined by its rituals of worship on one's ancestors. The purpose of these rituals is to sustain living links with one's past and to drive away evil spirits. Shintoism is a source for four key concepts in Japanese **medical ethics**: *byo, ro, shi,* and *sho. See also* KAIBARA EKIKEN (1630–1714); MORAL THEOLOGY.

SHO. One of four key components in the concept of the life cycle in **medical ethics** in Japan, influenced by **Buddhism** and **Shintoism**. *Sho* "means both the life cycle and coming into existence in this world" (Kimura and Sakai 2009, 132). This concept plays a major role in **Kaibara Ekiken**'s (1630–1714) medical ethics. *See also BYO; RO; SHI.*

SIMON, MAXIMILIEN ISIDORE AMAND (1807–?; fl. 1845–1865). French physician. He wrote on the duties of physicians in his **Déontologie médicale** (Medical Deontology, 1845), in which he applies the "science of duties" of **Jeremy Bentham** to the **ethical obligations** and **rights** of physicians. For Simon, Jesus Christ is the moral exemplar whom physicians should emulate by caring for the poor. Simon also recognized that mental illnesses were real and required medical attention, if only to lessen their effects on **patients**.

SIMPLE CONSENT. Simple consent occurs when a **patient** or a **surrogate** either authorizes or refuses to authorize **clinical management**. Simple consent is **ethically permissible** when there is little risk to clinical management, for example, measuring blood pressure or drawing blood for laboratory analysis from a patient with no known bleeding **disorders** (Whitney et al. 2004). In **common law**, simple consent is taken to have been endorsed in a landmark **simple consent case** in 1914. See also INFORMED CONSENT; INFORMED CONSENT CASES; INFORMED CONSENT PROCESS.

SIMPLE CONSENT CASE. The landmark **common law** case of **simple consent** is *Schloendorff v. Society of New York Hospital* (105 N.E. 92, 93) of 1914 in the State of New York. The case originated in 1908 when it was alleged by the plaintiff that, while she agreed to physical examination, which discovered a large fibroid tumor, she refused surgery for the **clinical management** of this problem. The New York Court of Appeals (the highest **appellate court** for civil cases) opinion by Justice Benjamin Cardozo contains a frequently quoted sentence: "Every human being of adult years and sound mind has the right to determine what shall be done with his own body; and a surgeon who performs an operation without his patient's consent, commits an assault, for which he is liable in damages . . . except in cases of emergency where the patient is unconscious and where it is necessary to operate before consent can be obtained." This is taken to be a strong endorsement of simple consent.

Recent scholarship has shown that *Schloendorff* was not about consent but about the immunity from liability of a hospital as a charitable organization from what its professional staff does or fails to do (Lombardo 2005). Other scholars have examined the hospital record and documented that the patient did indeed authorize the surgery (Chervenak, McCullough, and Chervenak 2015). *See also* INFORMED CONSENT; INFORMED CONSENT CASES; INFORMED CONSENT PROCESS.

SIMS, J. MARION (1813–1883). American physician noted for his development of the surgical procedure to repair vesicovaginal fistula. He was a vocal opponent of the **American Medical Association** *Code of Medical Ethics* **of 1847** on the grounds that a physician's honor was sufficient foundation for good conduct in **patient care**. He is also well known, indeed infamous, for his use of "unanesthetized female slaves as involuntary **research subjects** to perfect his most famous gynecological operation, repair vesico-vaginal fistula" (Baker 2009, 454). *See also* EXPERIMENT; INFORMED CONSENT.

SINGLE-BLINDED CLINICAL TRIAL. A **clinical trial** using **blinding** in which the **research subjects** do not know what treatment they are receiving. This method is used to prevent **bias** in self-reporting by subjects of symptoms and other outcomes that are end points of the trial. The **informed consent process** must disclose and explain the nature and purpose of such blinding.

SOCIAL CONTRACT. The agreement of individuals to create a government and delineate its **powers**. This is usually thought in political philosophy to be a hypothetical contract, a source of limitations of the concept. Perhaps the most well-known conception of the social contract appears in the political philosophy of John Rawls (1921–2002) and is the basis for **Rawlsian justice**.

SOCIALIZED MEDICINE. Used colloquially in political discourse in the United States to mean the unacceptable involvement of the federal government in the delivery of healthcare, either as a payer or provider. More precisely, socialized medicine means that the government (local, regional, state, or federal) owns healthcare facilities and pays the physicians and other professional staff for **patient care**. In this meaning, Veterans Health Affairs, the medical corps of the armed services, the Indian Health Service, and the Public Health Service are all forms of federal socialized medicine. County and city hospitals and clinics are regional and local forms of socialized medicine. **Medicare** and **Medicaid**, which pay for patient care, are not forms of socialized medicine. Socialized medicine was common in the Union of Soviet Socialist Republics, from after World War II until its collapse in 1991. See also ZEMSKAYA MEDICINE; ZEMSKIE PHYSICIANS.

SOLIDARITY. A core **value** in **bioethics** in Europe, but not in bioethics in the United States, that reflects the complex webs of interdependency in contemporary societies and the vulnerability to the **power** of others, especially large organizations such as corporations and the state. The most effective response to this vulnerability is to stand with others. The more people who stand together, the greater the capacity to protect oneself in one's vulnerability to power.

This concept originates in the devastation of World War II in Europe and the recognition that transnational ties of cooperation can help to prevent war from recurring, especially in an era of nuclear weapons. The American experience of the war was different, which may explain the absence of the concept of solidarity from the discourses of politics and bioethics in the United States. In social discourse in the United States, there is the colloquial saying "We are all in this together and together we are stronger," which can be read as an expression of the concept of solidarity. See also COMMUNITARIAN ETHICS; EGALITARIAN JUSTICE; RAWLSIAN JUSTICE.

SOMATIC CELL GENETIC/GENOMIC ENGINEERING. The use of techniques to alter the portions of the genome that are thought to cause a **patient**'s **condition**. Somatic cell engineering has the potential to reduce the **biopsychosocial** burden of **disability, disease, disorder**, or **injury** for an individual patient. Ethical concerns about this form of genetic engineering include unknown short-term and long-term risk resulting from genetic material being inserted in the wrong place or functioning incorrectly. When in **deliberative clinical judgment** such intervention is expected to result in net clinical benefit, it becomes a **medically reasonable alternative** that should be offered to the patient in the **informed consent process**. Somatic cell engineering undertaken as **innovation** or **research** may be offered only after it has been prospectively reviewed and approved by an **Institutional Review Board** for its scientific and clinical **justification**, an acceptable level of risk, and its informed consent process. *See also* GERM LINE GENETIC/GE-NOMIC ENGINEERING.

SONG, GUOBIN (1893–1952). Chinese physician and ethicist. He wrote *Professional Ethics in Medicine* (1933), the first **professional medical ethics** in China in the 20th century, integrating Western **medical ethics** into Chinese **clinical practice**.

SPECIFICATION. The process in **ethical reasoning** of adapting general action guides such as **ethical principles** to specific circumstances, such as **clinical practice** or **clinical research** (Richardson 1997). For example, there are multiple specifications of the **ethical principle of justice** and the concept of **futility**.

SPERRY, WILLIAM (1882–1954). American Protestant theologian and dean of Harvard University Divinity School. He wrote *The Ethical Basis for Medical Practice* (1950), emphasizing the importance of **codes of ethics**. *See also* MEDICAL ETHICS.

SPONTANEOUS ABORTION. The evacuation of the contents of the uterus before **fetal viability** as a result of **disease** or **injury** during pregnancy. This is also called a miscarriage. There is little or no **ethical controversy** about spontaneous abortion. Spontaneous abortion has clinical ethical significance because of the need to identify its causes by means of a postmortem examination. This information can be used to calculate recurrence risk and plan preventive approaches to a subsequent pregnancy; both of these figure prominently in counseling women who have experienced spontaneous abortion. The **professional virtue** of **compassion** creates an **ethical obligation** to provide counseling and psychosocial support for women who have experienced spontaneous abortion. *See also* ABORTION; INDUCED ABORTION.

SPORTS MEDICINE. **Patient care** for athletes and **research** to improve patient care for athletes. Physicians providing **patient** care for teams sponsored by schools, colleges, and universities as well professional teams confront both **conflicts of commitment** and **conflicts of interest**. These physicians have conflicts of commitment between their **professional responsibility** to patient-athletes and their role-related **ethical obligation** to athlete-patients and their sponsors and fans who help field teams. These physicians also have conflicts of interest because if they prioritize their professional responsibility to patient-athletes, as they should, they risk being dismissed from their positions.

"STARK LAW". Federal **statutory** law and **regulatory law** based on the statute and named for Representative Fourtney Hilman "Pete" Stark, a Democrat who represented the 13th Congressional District of California in the United States House of Representatives from 1993 to 2013 and who authored the legislation. This statute prohibits physicians from referring **Medicaid** or **Medicare** beneficiaries to facilities providing "designated health services" and in which the physician or an immediate family member of the physician has an ownership **interest**, which creates a **conflict of interest**. The Stark Law manages this conflict of interest by eliminating it. There is evidence that physicians with an ownership interest in imaging facilities refer patients as much as three times as often as justified by criteria established by the American Academy of Radiology. Failure to follow these criteria can unnecessarily increases the risk of exposure to radiation, especially cumulative dosing, which is **ethically impermissible** in **professional medical ethics**.

STATUTORY LAW. Law made by legislatures at the local, state, and federal levels. In the federal system of self-government in the United States, the states regulate the practice of medicine based on statutory law. An important example for the ethics of **end-of-life care** are state **Advance Directives Acts**. *See also* ADMINISTRATIVE LAW; COMMON LAW; REGULATORY LAW.

STEADINESS. In the **professional medical ethics** of **John Gregory** (1724–1773), one of the two **virtues** that regulate **sympathy**, the other being **tenderness**. "Women of learning and virtue" were Gregory's exemplars of both virtues. Steadiness allows the physician to enter directly into the experience of the **patient** by maintaining self-mastery (an element of **Stoicism** in Gregory's professional medical ethics). For Gregory, the moral exemplars of the virtue of steadiness were "women of learned and virtue," which makes steadiness a virtue in **feminine medical ethics**. Steadiness differs from both **empathy** (the distancing of the physician from the patient's lived experience by creating a non-affective idea of that experience) and *aequanimitas* (an affective imperturbability). Steadiness is also one of the four virtues that form the basis for **Thomas Percival**'s (1740–1804) professional medical ethics, along with **tenderness**, **authority**, and **condescension**.

STEM CELL RESEARCH. Research using stem cells, **valued** for their potency to become different cells in the body, to improve **regenerative medicine**. Research using stem cells engineered from **patients** is not **ethically controversial**. By contrast, **embryonic stem cell research** is ethically controversial.

STERILIZATION. A surgical or medical procedure to eliminate a **patient**'s reproductive capacity. There is a long history in the United States and other countries of **involuntary sterilization** (i.e., sterilization without the **informed consent** of patients) both in patients who had **decision-making capacity** and patients who did not. Women from racial and ethnic minorities, lower socioeconomic status, and with intellectual disabilities especially have been subject to involuntary sterilization. This practice is considered **ethically impermissible**. Because of this history of abuse, **informed consent** is **ethically obligatory**. Many states have imposed waiting periods, to protect women from manipulation who may later withdraw their authorization, and on the ability of **surrogates** to consent to sterilization of patients who do not have decision-making capacity. *See also* CONTRACEPTION.

STOIC. An adherent of **Stoicism**. Reflecting the nature of Stoicism, the word is also used to characterize **patients** who are willing to endure **pain**, especially pain that is resistant to complete relief by analgesia. Physicians may be challenged on the basis of the **professional virtue of compassion** to accept a patient's willingness to endure considerable pain.

STOICISM. A philosophy and way of life created in ancient Athens that accepts the limits and frailty of human nature and creates an **ethics** based on accepting the natural order and cultivating the **virtues** required for doing so, such as **courage**, humility (not calling attention to one's plight), and **self-sacrifice**. The Stoic also carries himself or herself with style, a habitual insouciance, in response to aging, loss (loss of loved ones to disease and the perils of childbirth for women and of comrades in battle was constant in the ancient world), infirmity, and **death**. The Stoic uses contemplation in this lifelong work, especially in *ars moriendi*, preparing for a death with **dignity**. The lifelong commitment to and achievement of self-mastery becomes the central task of the Stoic. *See also* AURELIUS, MARCUS (121–180); CICERO, MARCUS TULLIUS (106–43 BCE).

STRIKES. Organized work actions, with or without unionization, to stop work, as a bargaining tool with owners and leaders of healthcare organizations. To prevent a group-level **conflict of interest**, physicians have the **professional responsibility** to prioritize **patient care**. This means that, during strikes, there is a **beneficence**-based **ethical obligation** to prevent the risk of serious, far-reaching, and irreversible harm to **patients**. This obligation is fulfilled by preventing denial of urgently **clinical management**. There is **ethical controversy** about strikes that do not meet this condition.

SUBJECTIVE STANDARD. An ethical standard for disclosure of information to a **patient** or **surrogate** in the **informed consent process**. This standard requires the physician to disclose information about the **patient**'s **condition**, diagnosis, treatment plan, and prognosis with and without treatment that a particular patient in the patient's particular condition needs to know at the time. Because it is not reliably enforceable (the patient could retrospectively add to his or her informational needs, which is not fair to the physician), the subjective standard has not been widely adopted as a legal standard. In a very small number of jurisdictions in the United States, the subjective standard has been adopted explicitly or implicitly in the **common law**. The **ethical justification** for the application of the subjective standard to dying patients appeals to the profound nature of the **biopsychosocial** needs of such patients, which includes, for patients who express an interest in it, more information than the **reasonable person standard** or **professional community standard** would support.

SUBSTANTIVE JUSTICE. *See* DISTRIBUTIVE JUSTICE.

SUBSTITUTED JUDGMENT STANDARD. The priority, **autonomy**-based ethical standard for **surrogate decision making** that requires the **surrogate** to make decisions for an adult patient based on a reliable understanding the patient's **values** and beliefs. This standard does not require 100 percent accuracy of such understanding. In some jurisdictions, this ethical standard is the applicable legal standard. Some jurisdictions have adopted the preponderance of evidence standard (i.e., the understanding of the patient's values and beliefs by the surrogate is more likely than not to be accurate). Some jurisdictions have adopted the clear and convincing standard (i.e., the understanding of the patient's values and beliefs by the surrogate is highly probable to be accurate). When the substituted judgment standard cannot be reliably met, the surrogate should follow the **best interests standard**. *See also* CRUZAN CASE.

SUFFERING. The experience of unwelcome limits on one's aims, intentions, plans, or **hopes** for the future accompanied by a negative affect. **Pain** can cause suffering, but suffering can occur in the absence of pain, for example, the suffering of grief upon the death of a loved one. **Distress** can cause suffering, especially prolonged distress, but suffering can occur in the absence of distress. *Suffering* is therefore not synonymous with the term *distress*. The phrase *mental pain* is imprecise and sometimes has the same meaning as *distress* or *suffering*. When this is the case, *suffering* should be used. In **professional medical ethics**, there is an **ethical obligation** to prevent suffering and to manage suffering effectively when it occurs. This obligation, which has been recognized in the history of professional medical ethics since **John Gregory** (1724–1773) and later the emergence of psychiatry as a specialty, is based on the **ethical principle** of **beneficence** and the **professional virtue of compassion**.

SUICIDE. Self-killing. In many **moral theologies**, suicide is **ethically impermissible**, inasmuch as life is a gift from God and is therefore not something that a human being is free to destroy. In **moral philosophy**, there is **ethical controversy** about whether suicide is **ethically permissible**. As a consequence, **physician-assisted suicide** is ethically controversial. The prohibition in the ***Hippocratic Oath*** against giving poisons is often cited by opponents of physician-assisted suicide. However, the *Oath* provides no **justification** for this position, which means that there is no textual evidence for this appeal. *See also* AUTONOMY; RIGHT TO DIE.

SUPREME COURT ABORTION CASES. *See* ABORTION.

SURGICAL ETHICS. Ethical reasoning about **patient care, research**, and education in surgery and the surgery-related specialties such as obstetrics and gynecology.

SURROGATE. The individual(s) designated by applicable law to make decisions for a patient who is a legal minor or who is an adult who has been reliably determined not to have **decision-making capacity**. Parents or guardians are the surrogates for legal minors who are patients. For adult patients, applicable law tends to favor family members in a priority order, starting with the spouse (including a common law spouse), adult child or children, parents, and siblings. If the patient has a completed **durable power of attorney for healthcare** or a **medical power of attorney**, the individual named as surrogate usually has priority over family members, as may the individual(s) named as surrogates in a patient's **living will** or **directive to physicians**. The decisions of surrogates are guided by two ethical (and often legal) standards, in priority order: **substituted judgment standard** or **best interests standard**. In some jurisdictions, the word *proxy* is used instead of *surrogate*. *See also* SURROGATE DECISION MAKING.

SURROGATE DECISION MAKING. Making decisions by a **surrogate** for a patient who lacks **decision-making capacity**. The surrogate decision maker should base decisions for the patient on one of two standards, in the following priority order: the **substituted judgment standard** and the **best interests standard**. In some jurisdictions, these are also the legal standards for surrogate decision making under the substituted judgment standard. Some states accept the standard of preponderance of the evidence: it is more likely true than false that the surrogate is reliably representing the patient's **values** and beliefs. Some states have a more demanding standard, the clear and convincing standard or 75 percent probability false that the surrogate is reliably representing the patient's values and beliefs. *See also* CRUZAN CASE.

SURROGATE MOTHERHOOD. *See* ASSISTED REPRODUCTION; SURROGATE PREGNANCY.

SURROGATE PREGNANCY. A pregnancy undertaken by a woman who contractually agrees, in the case of live birth, to give her child to a couple. This is a component of **assisted reproduction** when the female **patient** is not able to become pregnant or to become pregnant safely (i.e., without putting her life in jeopardy or her health at risk for serious, far-reaching, and irreversible damage). Sometimes the embryos are created with the couple's gametes and sometimes with donor gametes. This is an **ethically controversial** practice because of its ethical challenges, including protecting the **right** of the pregnant woman to make decisions about the **clinical management** and disposition of her pregnancy; blurred parenthood—the child will have a gestational mother, biological mother, and rearing father with, in some cases, the biological mother not being the rearing mother or the biological father not being the rearing father; enforcement of legal contracts; and refusal of the commissioning couple to accept the baby. The **biopsychosocial** risks are obviously complex and potentially unmanageable to the satisfaction of all parties, calling this practice into question on the grounds of the **virtue** of **prudence**. *See also* ASSISTED REPRODUCTIVE TECHNOLOGIES (ART).

SYMPATHY. The capacity to enter directly into the lived experience of others, especially affective experience. In his *Treatise of Human Nature* (2000 [1739–1740]), **David Hume** (1711–1776) reports his scientific discovery of the **principle** of sympathy, using the methods of **moral science**. *Principle* in Scottish moral science means a constitutive, causal process of human nature. Sympathy becomes a key **ethical concept** in the **professional medical ethics** of **John Gregory** (1724–1773). *See also* EMPATHY; STEADINESS; TENDERNESS.

SYSTEM OF MEDICAL ETHICS. The title given to statements and **codes of ethics** by the colonial and state medical societies in British North America in the 18th century and by the United States in the 19th century. The New York State Medical Society adopted its *System of Medical Ethics* in 1823 (State Medical Society of New York 1823). It "comprises all the moral principles and regulations which should govern physicians and surgeons in the exercise of their professional avocation with the public in general, in private and confidential cases, as well as in their intercourse with other medical men, and before magistrates and courts of justice" (State Medical Society of New York 1823, 6). The foundation of this **professional medical ethics** is the physician's character. Its acknowledged sourses include the professional medical ethics of **John Gregory** (1724–1773) and **Thomas Percival** (1740–1804). *Systems of Medical Police* played an important role in the formation of a **profession of medicine** in the United States and set the stage for the **American Medical Association** *Code of Medical Ethics* of **1847**. *See also* PROFESSIONAL ASSOCIATIONS OF PHYSICIANS.

T

TECHNÉ. Used in the **Hippocratic Corpus**, especially in the *Hippocratic Oath*, to mean the unchanging and unchangeable body of scientific and clinical knowledge and skill set of a physician. This is why it has to be kept "pure" according the *Oath*. The concept of *techné* is incompatible with the concept of modern science—which is both changing and changeable owing to the sustained application of the scientific method. This stark contrast between *techné* and the first commitment of physicians, to scientific and clinical competence, of the **ethical concept of medicine as a profession** makes the *Oath* unacceptable as a basis for **professional medical ethics**. *Techné* is commonly translated as "art," which has encouraged the interpretation that *techné* names the prerogative of a physician to alter clinical practice on an individualized basis. This is an incorrect interpretation because *techné* names what Hippocratic physicians took to be the unchanging body of knowledge that was applied to *patterns* of signs and symptoms, which are not unique but common to patients sharing a diagnosis.

TECHNOLOGICAL IMPERATIVE. The belief that the adoption of new biomedical technology into **clinical practice** has a momentum of its own, originating the very natures of technology and medicine. The result will be **clinical management** based on **enthusiasm** that will blind physicians to the inevitable limits of new technology and cause overtreatment in violation of the **ethical principle of beneficence** and the **professional virtue of integrity** in **professional medical ethics**. To prevent the technological imperative, it has been argued that new technologies should be introduced only as **clinical research** before they are adopted into routine **clinical care**.

TEMPERANCE. A **virtue** that obligates the physician not to imbibe spirit beverages or to do so only in small quantities. This admonition appears in the **medical ethics** literature of the 18th and 19th centuries in the United Kingdom and the United States because it was common for a physician calling on private **patients** in their homes to be offered a "cordial" or spirit beverage (in a time before potable water was routinely available). In the course of a day, a physician who accepted could become inebriated and thus be at high risk of defective **clinical judgment**. Today, the temperance pertains to **ethical reasoning** about whether it is **ethically permissible** for a physician who is on call to imbibe even a small amount of spirit beverages during the time he or she is on call and therefore could be called by telephone about a patient's care or required to go in to the hospital to care for a patient.

TENDERNESS. In the **professional medical ethics** of **John Gregory** (1724–1773), one of the two **virtues** that regulates **sympathy**, the other being **steadiness**. Tenderness allows the physician to enter directly into the experience of the **patient** while maintaining self-mastery (an element of **Stoicism** in Gregory's professional medical ethics) by adhering to steadiness. For Gregory, the moral exemplars of the virtue of tenderness were "women of learning and virtue," which makes tenderness a virtue in **feminine medical ethics**. Tenderness differs sharply from both **empathy** (the distancing of the physician from the patient's lived experience by creating a non-affective idea of that experience) and *aequanimitas* (an affective imperturbability). Tenderness is also one of the four virtues that form the basis for **Thomas Percival**'s (1740–1804) professional medical ethics, along with **steadiness**, **authority**, and **condescension**.

TERMINAL CONDITION. A condition that is defined in applicable **advance directive** legislation and, when it has been diagnosed by the patient's attending physician, creates a legal permission to discontinue **life-sustaining treatment**. Typically, a terminal condition is defined in advance directive legislation as a condition expected to result in the patient's death in six months, even if life-sustaining treatment is continued. A terminal condition differs from an **irreversible condition** in that a patient with an irreversible condition is not expected to die in the near future. The invocation of this concept in **clinical ethical reasoning** rejects **vitalism**. *See also* END-OF-LIFE CARE.

TERMINAL SEDATION. For a **patient** with a **terminal condition** or an **irreversible condition**, whose **distress, pain**, or **suffering** has become unacceptable from the patient's perspective, the use of high doses of sedating drugs to induce loss of awareness but not high enough doses to kill the patient. Terminal sedation is therefore not a form of **killing** or **suicide**. This is followed by withholding or discontinuing the administration of artificial hydration and nutrition, forms of **life-sustaining treatment** that are **ethically permissible** and legally permissible to **withhold** or **withdraw** from such patients under the provision of the applicable **Advance Directives Act**. The patient's **death** then ensues in a short period of time. The **ethical justifica-**

tion for this clinical practice appeals to the **ethical principle of beneficence**, the **professional virtue of compassion**, and the principle of **double effect**. *See also* END-OF-LIFE CARE; PALLIATIVE CARE.

TERMINATION OF PREGNANCY. The end of a pregnancy. This can occur as a result of **spontaneous abortion, induced abortion, feticide, in utero fetal demise,** or delivery resulting in either stillbirth or live birth. The phrase *termination of pregnancy* is therefore not synonymous with *abortion, induced abortion,* or *feticide*. Some forms of termination of pregnancy are ethically uncontroversial, such as spontaneous abortion and in utero fetal demise. Other forms of termination of pregnancy are **ethically controversial**, especially induced abortion and feticide. The ethics of termination of pregnancy is therefore indeterminate.

"TEST-TUBE BABY". A phrase used in the 1970s and 1980s to refer to babies conceived and born by **in vitro fertilization**. *See also* ASSISTED REPRODUCTION; ASSISTED REPRODUCTIVE TECHNOLOGIES (ART).

THEISM. The belief in a creator God in the religion of faith communities. Theistic accounts of creation and nature originate in specific faith communities and have no or only very limited application in other faith communities. These theistic accounts will have no application for individuals and communities that reject the existence of God. Theistic accounts of the concept of **natural rights** therefore will differ from nontheistic accounts, especially accounts based on **deism**.

THERAPEUTIC CLONING. *See* CLONING.

THERAPEUTIC EXCEPTION. *See* THERAPEUTIC PRIVILEGE.

THERAPEUTIC MISCONCEPTION. Originally meant the lack of understanding of a **research subject** or a potential research subject that some aspects of a **clinical trial** have been chosen based on scientific design rather than clinical benefit, which differs from **clinical practice** (Appelbaum et al. 1982). Examples include increased dosing in a **Phase I clinical trial** and **randomization** and **blinding** in a **Phase III clinical trial**. This concept has come to have a very broad meaning: the lack of understanding that a **patient** is participating in clinical research. The antidote to this lack of understanding is an **informed consent process** that makes it clear to a potential research subject or **surrogate** that **clinical research** will be conducted and that some aspects of the study design have been chosen for **scientific reasons** and would therefore ordinarily not be part of clinical practice. *See also* PATIENT CARE; RESEARCH.

THERAPEUTIC/NONTHERAPEUTIC RESEARCH DISTINCTION. There is **ethical controversy** about whether therapeutic **research**—research that benefits current and future **patients**—can be reliably distinguished from nontherapeutic research—research that does not benefit current or future patients. For example, a **Phase I** safety and efficacy trial of a new drug may not benefit those enrolled early but may benefit those enrolled later because of higher doses of the study medication (Brody 1998).

THERAPEUTIC PRIVILEGE. The freedom of a physician to withhold information from the **patient** about the patient's **condition**, diagnosis, treatment plan, and prognosis with and without treatment on the **beneficence**-based ground that providing such information would be seriously **biopsychosocially** harmful to the patient. Inasmuch as the risk of such harm is most commonly created by how the physician makes the disclosure rather than the content of the disclosure, the invocation of therapeutic privilege bears a very steep **burden of justification**. It is therefore **ethically permissible** only very rarely. Some take the view that it is never ethically permissible. The invocation of therapeutic privilege to protect the physician from the (understandable) **distress** of giving the patient bad news is never acceptable as an **ethical justification**. *See also* HONESTY; TRUTH-TELLING.

THOMAS, DYLAN (1914–1953). Welsh writer and internationally renowned poet. Two of his poems are cited in the literature of **bioethics**, **medical ethics**, and **professional medical ethics**—"**Do Not Go Gentle into That Good Night**" and "And Death Shall Have No Dominion" (Thomas 2003)—for taking a stance in favor of not accepting **death**, usually accompanied by a critique of Thomas's stance.

TIPPING. An informal but expected practice in many of the countries that were under the control of Soviet Russia and that were officially socialist societies. **Patients** would make off-the-books cash payments for "goods and services [that] could only be obtained by tips in many countries that were nothing but bribes" (Blasszauer 2009, 624). These had a systemic effect on the **physician-patient relationship** and helped to undermine the official socialist policy of free healthcare. Given the low compensation rates by the state, this source of revenue was valued by physicians. *See also* CONFLICT OF INTEREST; PROFESSIONAL MEDICAL ETHICS.

TORTURE. The United Nations defines torture in the following manner:

> For the purposes of this Convention, the term "torture" means any act by
> which severe pain or suffering, whether physical or mental, is intentional-
> ly inflicted on a person for such purposes as obtaining from him or a third
> person information or a confession, punishing him for an act he or a third
> person has committed or is suspected of having committed, or intimidat-
> ing or coercing him or a third person, or for any reason based on discrimi-
> nation of any kind, when such pain or suffering is inflicted by or at the
> instigation of or with the consent or acquiescence of a public official or
> other person acting in an official capacity. It does not include pain or
> suffering arising only from, inherent in or incidental to lawful sanctions.
> (United Nations Office of the High Commissioner 1984)

Thus understood, torture violates the **ethical principle of beneficence**, the
ethical principle of justice, the **ethical principle of nonmaleficence**, the
ethical principle of respect for autonomy, the **ethical principle of respect
for persons**, the **professional virtue of compassion**, the **professional virtue
of integrity**, and the **professional virtue of self-effacement**. It is therefore
impossible to provide an **ethical justification** of torture in **professional
medical ethics**. There is therefore an **absolute ethical obligation** of physicians never to participate in any way in torture, including especially physicians in the medical corps of the armed services of the United States or in
government intelligence and national security agencies. This conclusion is
rare in professional medical ethics, a distinctive feature of the ethics of torture. *See also* PROFESSIONAL MILITARY MEDICAL ETHICS.

TRANSSEXUALITY. The experience of discordance between one's **gender** identity and one's **sex**. One form of **clinical management** is the combination of medication and surgery to support a **patient**'s transition to the
gender with which the patient identifies. The **informed consent process** for
such clinical management should be led by a multidisciplinary team to address the **biopsychosocial** issues with care and attention to the needs of the
patient. The informed consent process with adolescents is more complex,
inasmuch as the discordance may not be durable, a challenging **clinical judgment** to make. **Confidentiality** and its limits with adolescent patients also
needs to be addressed, for example, parents may have to authorize release of
records for insurance payment or may see claims for their child's care. The
parents' role in, and especially support for, their child's care may be key to
the success of that care. *See also* DISORDERS OF SEXUAL DEVELOP-
MENT.

TRANSPLANTATION. The surgical removal of organs or tissues from a cadaver (the "dead donor") or **patient** (the "living donor") that are then surgically placed into a patient, to replace organs and tissues that have been lost to **disease** or **injury** (the "recipient"). The **ethics** of transplantation comprise **ethical reasoning** about **organ allocation**, **organ donation**, and **organ procurement**. In the United States, the **United Network for Organ Sharing**, a nongovernmental organization supported by the transplantation community, promulgates **ethically justified** guidelines about organ allocation, organ donation, and organ procurement. There is **ethical controversy** about some aspects of transplantation, for example, procurement of a partial liver from a living donor and whether the **dead donor rule** should be reconsidered or even abandoned.

TRIAL COURT. A court of law in a state or in the federal system that hears a civil or criminal case. Sometimes also known as the court of original jurisdiction. Verdicts of guilty in criminal cases and all verdicts in civil cases can be appealed to higher courts, known as **appellate courts**. The results of trial courts in civil cases have no or extremely limited value as precedents or **paradigm cases** in the **casuistry** of the **common law**, if only because results are sometimes unreported, unlike appellate cases.

TRIAGE. A system for making **deliberative clinical judgment** about which **patients** should receive priority for **clinical management** when the number of patients exceeds the available resources to treat all of them in a timely way. Patients are prioritized by medical need, an approach invented by Baron Dominique-Jean Larrey (1766–1842) in the 1790s. This means that some patients may die and other patients survive but with increased risk of **disability** and **disease**. Triage is also used in emergency medicine and is a component for the response to mass casualty events, for example, mass shootings or a bioterrorism attack.

The **World Medical Association** has proposed the following priority list: "patients who can be saved but whose lives are in immediate danger"; "patients whose lives are not in immediate danger and who are in need of urgent but not immediate medical care"; "injured persons requiring only minor treatment"; "psychologically traumatized individuals who do not require treatment for bodily harm but might need reassurance or sedation if acutely disturbed"; "patients whose condition exceeds the available therapeutic resources, who suffer from extremely severe injuries such as irradiation or burns to such an extent and degree that they cannot be saved in the specific circumstances of time and place, or complex surgical cases requiring a particularly delicate operation which would take too long, thereby obliging the physician to make a choice between them and other patients" (World Medical Association 2006a). This priority list is based on the **ethical principle of beneficence**. The **ethical principle of respect for autonomy** plays no role in the **ethical justification** of triage in **professional medical ethics**, which is a distinctive feature of triage. *See also* ALLOCATION OF SCARCE MEDICAL RESOURCES.

TRUST. The term *trust* has two meanings.

In its first meaning, *trust* names a stance of confidence of an individual in the **judgment, decision making**, and behavior of another individual, organization, or government. Trust is earned when another individual, organization, or government is **competent** in the scope of its expertise, uses that competence primarily for the benefit of others, is transparent, and is accountable. Trust means that one can act with confidence that these beliefs are true. When another individual, organization, or government fails in one or more of these respects, trust is lost: one can no longer believe what they say or base behavior on what they say or do. When the consequences of the inability to act on what an individual, organization, or government official or agency says or does are serious, far-reaching, and irreversible, it is very difficult to re-earn trust once trust has been lost. The three commitments of physicians in the **ethical concept of medicine as a profession** were framed by the concept's inventors, **John Gregory** (1724–1773) and **Thomas Percival** (1740–1804), to earn the trust of the sick and transform them into **patients**.

In its second meaning, a *trust* is a social institution that holds and protects things of **value**, for example, an estate created by an individual's last will and testament, for the beneficiaries of them. That institution has a **fiduciary** responsibility to prevent its **self-interest** from **biasing** its decisions about the management of these things of value. Percival coined the phrase *public trust* to conceptualize medicine as a profession: it holds and protects biomedical science and its clinical application for the benefit of current *and* future patients, physicians, and trainees. Percival thereby sharply distinguished medicine as a profession from what it had been for centuries, a merchant guild that acted primarily to protect and promote its own interests in its social, economic, and political **power**, as well as social and political status. The history of **medical ethics** pivots on this conceptual shift.

TRUTH-TELLING. The **ethical obligation** to communicate in a factually correct fashion with the **patient** about the patient's **condition**, diagnosis, treatment plan, and prognosis with and without treatment. This rules out as **ethically impermissible** all **lies** and **deceptions**. The main **ethical justification** appeals to the **ethical principle of respect for autonomy**, which supports the patient's right to be informed and thus be able to participate in the **informed consent process**. The ethical justification also appeals to the **ethi-**

cal principle of beneficence in that it is biopsychosocially better for the patient to be informed than it is for the patient to speculate or worry in the absence of truthful communication or to find out clinical information inadvertently and therefore without the psychosocial support of the physician and team in the informed consent process.

It is commonly stated in the literature of bioethics and medical ethics that the ethical norm in the history of medical ethics was for physicians not to be truthful with patients, a form of medical paternalism. This has been shown not to be accurate (McCullough 2011). Reluctance was expressed about fulfilling the ethical obligation to be truthful, but on the grounds that fulfilling this obligation was distressing for the physician (Gregory 1772). Not being truthful with a patient for self-protecting motives is not paternalism because the resulting restriction of the patient's autonomy (the first criterion for the application of the concept of paternalism) is not done to protect the patient (the second, beneficence-based criterion for the application of the concept of paternalism) but to protect the physician (i.e., from [understandable] self-interest). See also HONESTY; INFORMED CONSENT PROCESS; THERAPEUTIC PRIVILEGE.

"TUBE-FEEDING". A misnomer for provision of artificial nutrition. The use of the term tube-feeding is misleading because artificial nutrition is processed food not food, and therefore should not be used. See also END-OF-LIFE CARE; LIFE-SUSTAINING TREATMENT.

TUSKEGEE SYPHILIS EXPERIMENT. A study of the natural history of syphilis among African American men, conducted by the United States Public Health Service starting in 1931 in Macon County, Georgia. The study's name is taken from the Tuskegee Institute, the hospital that collaborated in the study. The study was kept secret until it became public in 1972 and was shut down later that year. At the time the study was started, there was no safe, effective treatment for syphilis, a sexually transmitted disease that, in its later stages, affects many organ systems and causes disability or death. Its natural history was not well understood. The study was designed as what Francis Bacon (1561–1626) called a "natural experiment," also known as an "experiment in nature," a study design that is ethically permissible when there is no effective treatment for a disease.

Subjects were enrolled in a deceptive consent process. Potential subjects were told that they had "bad blood." This phrase then had a wide range of meanings, which include benign conditions but also diagnoses such as syphilis but not limited to syphilis. The goal was to have potential subjects think that their condition was benign, thus creating a false belief (Jones 2003 [1993]). Penicillin, an antibiotic that is safe and effective for the treatment of syphilis, became available in 1945 and became the drug of choice for syphilis in 1947. However, the study's policy was not to inform subjects about this curative treatment or provide it. This should have been done immediately to fulfill the **beneficence**-based **professional responsibility** to informed **research subjects** about such treatment and provide it to them. It was no longer **ethically justified** to continue a natural history study, and so it should have been stopped in 1947. This underscores the **ethical obligation** of investigators and oversight groups such as **data and safety monitoring boards** to stop a clinical trial when it is no longer **ethically permissible** to continue it. However, the study continued until it became public and was shut down 25 years after it should have been.

The exposure of the Tuskegee Syphilis Experiment influenced the creation of the National Commission for the Protection of Human Subjects of Research that produced the ***Belmont Report*** (Jonsen 1998). On 16 May 1997, at a White House ceremony, President William Jefferson Clinton (term of office: 1993–2001) issued a formal apology for wrongs done in the Tuskegee Syphilis Experiment.

TWIN-TWIN TRANSFUSION SYNDROME. "Twin-twin transfusion syndrome (TTTS) is a serious condition that occurs in approximately 10 to 15 percent of pregnancies with identical twins that share one placenta (monochorionic). Abnormal blood vessel connections cause the fetuses to share blood supply, and the smaller (donor) twin pumps blood to the larger (recipient) twin. Because it has more blood, the recipient twin makes too much urine, which may enlarge the bladder, produce too much amniotic fluid and cause heart failure. The donor twin has lower levels of blood, amniotic fluid and urine, and a smaller bladder" (http://women.texaschildrens.org/program/texas-childrens-fetal-center/twin-twin-transfusion-syndrome-ttts?gclid= EAIaIQobChMIibXIoo7L1QIVRWp-Ch260AKxEAAYAyAAEgLzufD_ BwE, accessed 14 September 2017). Treatment aims at reducing the number of abnormal connections, with the goal of preventing **death** in both fetuses. When **fetal demise** does occur, it is accepted in **ethical reasoning** using the principle of **double effect**, because the death of one of the two fetuses is not the cause of preventing death in the other fetus. *See also* MATERNAL-FETAL TREATMENT.

U

ULYSSES CONTRACT. Takes its name from the episode in the *Odyssey* in which Ulysses and his crew were sailing close to the island of the Sirens, whose lovely song drove men mad and resulted in their sailing toward the island and coming to grief by running aground on the island's deadly reefs. In a Ulysses contract, a **patient** with a mental illness or disorder instructs his or her psychiatrist to ignore his or her refusal of treatment in the clinical circumstance in which the patient's **condition** deteriorates to the point that the patient has lost **decision-making capacity** and provide treatment. The contract, in effect, authorizes **surrogate decision making** by the physician based on the **substituted judgment standard**. *See also* MENTAL HEALTH DIRECTIVE.

UNACCEPTABLE OPPORTUNITY COST. *See* OPPORTUNITY COST.

UNETHICAL. Characterizes actions as **ethically impermissible**. *See also* ETHICAL; IMMORAL; MORAL.

UNIT 731. One of the biological warfare groups established by the Imperial Japanese Army between 1932 and 1945 in China and other locations (Nie, Tsuchiya, and Li 2009). Their mission was to create biological weapons, and they engaged in what one group of scholars has called "murderous experiments," including deliberately infecting people followed by **vivisection** and subjecting people to bomb blasts (Nie, Tsuchiya, and Li 2009). Other such groups included Units 100, 1644, 1885, and 9420 in various locations in East Asia. Leaders of these groups were not brought to trial after the unconditional surrender of the Empire of Japan to the Allied powers concluded World War II, unlike the prosecution of the Nazi doctors. *See also* NAZI MEDICAL WAR CRIMES.

UNITED NETWORK FOR ORGAN SHARING (UNOS). A nongovernmental organization in the United States supported by the **organ transplantation** community that promulgates **ethically justified** guidelines about **organ allocation**, **organ donation**, and **organ procurement** (https://www.unos.org/, accessed 14 September 2017). The goal in creating UNOS was to replace competitive, uncoordinated practices that were not consistent with **egalitarian justice**, **healthcare justice**, and perhaps **utilitarian justice** with an **ethics of cooperation**.

UNIVERSAL DECLARATION OF HUMAN RIGHTS. Adopted by the United Nations, December 10, 1948, in response to the violation of **human rights** during World War II, especially by Nazi Germany and Imperial Japan (http://www.un.org/en/universal-declaration-human-rights/, accessed 14 September 2017). The Declaration appeals for its **ethical justification** to human **dignity** and inalienable **rights** (i.e., rights that cannot be taken away by the state or waived by an individual). The Declaration does not appeal to **natural rights**, a strategic decision aimed at achieving transnational and transcultural support (McKeon 1948). The Declaration asserts a wide range of rights, including civil, economic, political, and social rights, expressed as both **negative rights** and **positive rights**. The Declaration has become an important source for **medical ethics** and **bioethics** based on human rights.

UNIVERSAL DECLARATION OF HUMAN RIGHTS AND BIOETHICS. Published by the United Nations Educational, Scientific and Cultural Organization (better known as UNESCO) in 2005 (United Nations Educational, Scientific and Cultural Organization 2005). Based on the **Universal Declaration of Human Rights**, this document deals with "ethical issues related to medicine, life sciences and associated technologies as applied to human beings, taking into account their social, legal and environmental dimensions" on the basis of **human rights** and **dignity**.

UNJUST. A behavior, **health policy**, **public policy**, or practice that is incompatible with the **ethical principle of justice** in all of its **specifications**. *See also* JUST.

UNLIMITED RIGHT. An **absolute right**, either an **absolute negative right** or an **absolute positive right**.

UNOS. *See* UNITED NETWORK FOR ORGAN SHARING (UNOS).

UNREPRESENTED PATIENT. A **patient** who has lost **decision-making capacity** but who has no one on the legally designated list of **surrogates** who is a family member or (where allowed by **advance directive** law) a close friend. Most states make provisions for a nonfamily surrogate, for example, the patient's physician and one other physician not previously involved in the patient's care. For such patients, the application of the **substituted judgment standard** of **surrogate decision making** is unlikely to be possible, requiring decision making based on the **best interests standard**. *See also* ADVANCE DIRECTIVES ACT.

UTILITARIAN JUSTICE. A **specification** of the **ethical principle of justice** that creates an **ethical obligation** to act in such a way as to result in the greatest good for the greatest number. *See also* UTILITARIANISM.

UTILITARIANISM. An approach to **ethical reasoning** first articulated by British philosopher **Jeremy Bentham** (1748–1832) that holds that an action or policy is **ethically justified** if it results in the greatest good for the greatest number. Deploying utilitarianism requires one to clearly state the meaning of the terms *good*, *greatest good*, and *greatest number*, and to clearly define the time period in which consequences will be identified. There is considerable variation in how these tasks are to be accomplished, which means that utilitarianism is an abstract ethical theory that requires **specification**. It is also important that completion of these tasks prevents an ethical theory that justifies **exploitation**. Prevention of the risk of exploitation is intrinsic to utilitarian ethical theory. Utilitarianism is classified as a variant of **consequentialism**. *See also* UTILITARIAN JUSTICE.

V

VALUE. A standard used to assess the worth of people, events, and things in multiple domains, including the moral domain. One purpose of **ethics** is to critically appraise values that people assert to make a **judgment** about whether the value in question should be asserted and accepted by others to guide and assess their thought, speech, and behavior. *See also* IDEAL; NORM.

VEGETATIVE STATE. A clinical condition in which the **patient** has lost awareness and exhibits sleep-wake cycles. Such patients can appear to family members as aware, a false belief that should be addressed sensitively and respectfully. The determination that a vegetative state exists is a function of **clinical judgment**. A vegetative state may be considered potentially reversible, in which case it is classified as a **persistent vegetative state**. A vegetative state that is considered irreversible is classified as a **permanent vegetative state**. These classifications are based on the length of time that a vegetative state has existed, using criteria established by the American Academy of Neurology (https://www.aan.com/Guidelines/Home/GetGuidelineContent/83, accessed 14 September 2017). Because the determination that a patient is in a vegetative state is a function of clinical judgment, the boundaries between that state and a **minimally conscious state** may be unclear, but this is not surprising about any clinical judgment made in the absence of confirming findings from serological analysis or imaging.

The use of the word *vegetative* comes from the Aristotelian hierarchy of life forms, with rational animals or **persons** at the top, then other animals, then plants or vegetation. Rational animals, human beings, and other animals are individuals, but vegetation is not individuated. Metaphysically, vegetation is of a different and lower order of reality and therefore of **moral status** than rational animals. In this metaphysical context, the use of the word *vegetative* signals uncertainty about the moral status of a human being who, because awareness has been lost, is not a rational animal.

VENTILATOR. A machine that oxygenates the lungs of a **patient** who is not able to breathe on his or her own. Ethical challenges arise about setting **ethically justified** limits on this **life-sustaining treatment**.

VIABILITY. The ability to stay alive, given the available level of clinical care. The concept of viability, therefore, has both a biological and a biomedical component. In obstetrics, viability means the ability of a fetus to survive *ex utero* albeit with the full technological support of **neonatal critical care**. In high-income countries, which provide access to neonatal critical care, fetal viability occurs at approximately 24 completed weeks of gestation. There is scientific, clinical, and **ethical controversy** about whether fetuses at 23 completed weeks of gestation should be considered viable. Low-income countries may not be able to provide neonatal critical care. Fetal viability in such countries may therefore occur at a later gestational age. This is not a problem when one recalls that the concept of viability includes biomedical components. Some philosophers hold that the concept of viability is a solely biological concept, which is clinically inadequate and, therefore, should not be used in **bioethics**, **medical ethics**, or **professional medical ethics**. *See also* FETAL VIABILITY.

VICE. A disvalued trait or habit of **character** that originates in **self-interest** and that inclines an individual to disregard the **interests** of others and **ethical obligations** to them. Vices are therefore antithetical to good character and **ethically impermissible** to develop. For physicians, vices give primacy to self-interest and thus undermine the second commitment of the **ethical concept of medicine as a profession**, which means that, in **professional medical ethics**, vices are ethically impermissible to develop. *See also* VIRTUE.

VIRTUE. A **valued** trait or habit of character that creates **ethical obligations** and thereby blunts **self-interest** as one's primary concern and motivation. For physicians, the **professional virtues** are essential for fulfilling the three commitments of the **ethical concept of medicine as a profession**. *See also* PROFESSIONAL VIRTUE OF COMPASSION; PROFESSIONAL VIRTUE OF INTEGRITY; PROFESSIONAL VIRTUE OF SELF-EFFACEMENT; PROFESSIONAL VIRTUE OF SELF-SACRIFICE; VICE; VIRTUE ETHICS.

VIRTUE ETHICS. An approach to **ethical reasoning** based on appeals to **virtues**. Such an approach needs to identify and provide an **ethical justification** for the virtues to which appeal is made. Some take the view that virtue ethics is an antidote to **principlism** in **bioethics** and **medical ethics**, while others take the view that virtue ethics and principlism exhibit **complementarity**: neither is adequate for ethical reasoning and thus must be deployed together so that limitations of each are addressed by the other.

A major risk of virtue ethics arises in the limits of reasoning from good behavior to good character (i.e., distinguishing behavior that expresses a virtue and behavior that expresses **self-interest**). The Scottish physician-ethicist **John Gregory** (1724–1773) was aware of and addressed this risk in his **professional medical ethics**. The true physician treats patients the same, regardless of their social class and source of payment, and never calls attention to himself or herself, no matter the level of **self-sacrifice** required by **patient care**, **research**, or an organizational leadership position. *See also* METAETHICS.

VITALISM. The view that there is an **absolute ethical obligation** to preserve the life of the **patient**, irrespective of the patient's diminished functional status and the resultant **quality of life**. Vitalism has never been endorsed in the global history of medical ethics or in **codes of ethics** of professional associations of physicians. Vitalism is endorsed by some faith communities, for example, Orthodox Judaism and some schools of Islam. *See also* END-OF-LIFE CARE; MORAL THEOLOGY.

VIVISECTION. A form of **animal subjects research** or **human subjects research** in which the subject is surgically dissected and anatomy and physiology observed, with or without anesthesia, for the purposes of scientific investigation and not **clinical care**. While both practices were undertaken in the past, there came to be **ethical controversy** about both. It is now accepted that both forms of vivisection are **ethically impermissible**. *See also* UNIT 731.

VOLUNTARY. A decision or implementation of a decision is voluntary when it is free of internal controlling influences, such as extreme **pain** or unreasoning fear, or external controlling influences, such as **coercion**. *See also* AUTONOMY; INVOLUNTARY.

VOLUNTARY ACTIVE EUTHANASIA. **Killing** a **patient** with the patient's authorization in the **informed consent process**. When the patient authorizes the physician to prescribe a life-taking medication and the patient ingests that medication, this is known as **physician-assisted suicide**. *See also* EUTHANASIA.

VOLUNTARY CONSENT. The **consent** of a **patient** that is free from controlling influence by both internal and external factors. *See also* DECISIONAL AUTONOMY; INVOLUNTARY.

VOLUNTARY EUTHANASIA. Euthanasia undertaken with the authorization of the **patient** in the **informed consent process.** When this is done by **killing** the patient, this is known as **voluntary active euthanasia.** When this is done by **letting the patient die,** this is known as **voluntary passive euthanasia.** *See also* INVOLUNTARY EUTHANASIA.

VOLUNTARY PASSIVE EUTHANASIA. Discontinuing **life-sustaining treatment** of a **patient** with a **terminal condition** or an **irreversible condition,** or **letting die,** with the authorization of the patient in the **informed consent process.** This is **ethically permissible** when it implements the **voluntary, informed decision** of a patient with **decision-making capacity.** This is also ethically permissible when a patient with a terminal condition or an irreversible condition lacks **decision-making capacity** but has completed a **directive to physicians** or **living will** under applicable **advance directives** law. This is also ethically permissible when a patient with a terminal condition or an irreversible condition lacks decision-making capacity but has completed a directive to physicians or living will under applicable advance directives law, when the patient's legally designated **surrogate** authorizes discontinuation of life-sustaining treatment. *See also* EUTHANASIA.

VULNERABLE. Used to characterize **patients** with reduced capacity to engage in **decision making** that is informed and **voluntary.** The risk is that such patients cannot protect themselves and thus are at risk for **exploitation.** There are two different contexts in which the concept of vulnerability applies. Patients with cognitive impairments may not be capable of **informed consent.** Patients subject to **coercion** by others or who are in an intrinsically coercive organizational setting such as a prison may not be capable of voluntary decision making. *See also* AUTONOMY.

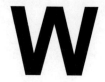

W

WAR. Armed conflict between or among nations or between nations and nonstate actors such as terrorists. From a historical perspective, war has been and continues to be one of the most influential behaviors of human beings. The **biopsychosocial** effects of war can last for decades or even centuries. **Ethical reasoning** about warfare is governed by **just** war ethical theory, which addresses *jus ad bellum* (the rightness of going to war) and *jus in bello* (the rightness of the conduct of war). Just war theory addresses both. Ethical reasoning about *jus ad bellum* appeals to such concepts as the **right** of a nation to continue to exist, proportionate means, and avoiding civilian casualties (sometimes invoking the principle of **double effect**). Ethical reasoning about *jus in bello* appeals to such concepts as the minimization of force needed to achieve the goal of battle: to close with and destroy the enemy's capacity and will to fight with a minimum of casualties on both sides. The latter condition is thought essential for winning the peace at the conclusion of armed conflict.

A core concept of **professional military ethics** is that officers should issue only lawful orders and their subordinates should obey only lawful orders. As double professionals, military physicians (who are commissioned officers) may appeal to **professional medical ethics** as the basis for **judging** whether an order is lawful or unlawful. This will create a **conflict of commitment**.

WARNOCK COMMITTEE. The Committee of Inquiry into Human Fertilisation and Embryology, established by the British government and chaired from 1982 to 1984 by Dame Helen Mary Warnock, an English philosopher with a distinguished record as a public intellectual and of public service. This report of the committee, known as the Warnock Report, resulted in the Human Fertilisation and Embryology Act enacted by Parliament in 1990 that provides for the regulation of **assisted reproductive technologies** in the United Kingdom. *See also* HEALTH POLICY; PRESIDENTIAL COMMITTEE; PUBLIC POLICY.

WHOLE EXOME SEQUENCING. Sequencing of the active coding regions of the genome. *See* GENOME SEQUENCING.

WHOLE GENOME SEQUENCING. Sequencing of the entire genome. *See* GENOME SEQUENCING.

WILLOWBROOK SCHOOL CASE. This case concerned the clinical investigation of hepatitis in a state school for cognitively impaired or disabled children (the phrase then in use was *mentally retarded*, now no longer acceptable) in which hepatitis was common from unsanitary living conditions about which nothing was done (Lederer 2009). This study, once it was revealed publicly in the 1960s by Senator Edward M. Kennedy (1932–2009; term of office: 1962–2009), Democrat of Massachusetts, was considered **ethically impermissible** in the **bioethics** literature, and still is, for a variety of reasons, including giving uninfected children live hepatitis to ingest and observing the results, the **exploitation** of a **vulnerable** population, and lack of **informed consent** by **surrogates**. It is a considered a **paradigm case** of the abuse of **research subjects**. *See also* ETHICS OF HUMAN SUBJECTS RESEARCH; RESEARCH ON CHILDREN.

WITHDRAWING TREATMENT. Discontinuing treatment after it has been initiated, including **life-sustaining treatment**. There are two **ethical justifications** that make discontinuing treatment **ethically permissible**: (1) in **deliberative clinical judgment** there is no reasonable expectation of clinical benefit for the patient from continuing treatment, which means that discontinuing treatment does not violate **beneficence**-based **ethical obligations** to the patient; or (2) a patient with **decision-making capacity** has refused to authorize continuation of treatment in the **informed consent process**, which means that discontinuing treatment does not violate **autonomy**-based ethical obligations to the patient. *See also* WITHDRAWING/WITHHOLDING DISTINCTION; WITHHOLDING TREATMENT.

WITHDRAWING/WITHHOLDING DISTINCTION. Some take the view that the distinction between **withdrawing treatment** and **withholding treatment** is not ethically significant. This view has become so commonplace that it is often invoked with no explanation. The explanation is that the **ethical justification** for withholding treatment is the same as the ethical justification for withdrawing treatment. Those who maintain the distinction hold that, while there was an **ethical obligation** to initiate treatment, including **life-sustaining treatment**, it can become the case, as clinical circumstances of the patient change for the worse, that there is no longer an ethical obligation to continue treatment. For example, for a life-threatening condition, initiating life-sustaining treatment is **ethically justified**, but later there may no longer exist either a **beneficence**-based ethical obligation or an **autonomy**-based ethical obligation to continue treatment when the patient's **disease** or **injury** becomes life-taking despite the provision of treatment. That is, the absence of a distinction between withdrawing and withholding treatment is invoked to claim, correctly, that initiating treatment does not, by itself, create an ethical obligation in all cases to continue treatment. *See also* KILLING/LETTING DIE DISTINCTION.

WITHHOLDING TREATMENT. Not initiating treatment, including **life-sustaining treatment**. There are two **ethical justifications** that make not initiating treatment **ethically permissible**: (1) in **deliberative clinical judgment** there is no reasonable expectation of clinical benefit for the patient from initiating treatment, which means that not initiating treatment does not violate **beneficence**-based **ethical obligations** to the patient; or (2) a patient with **decision-making capacity** has refused to authorize initiation of treatment in the **informed consent process**, which means that not initiating treatment does not violate **autonomy**-based ethical obligations to the patient. *See also* WITHDRAWING TREATMENT; WITHDRAWING/WITHHOLDING DISTINCTION.

WMA. *See* WORLD MEDICAL ASSOCIATION.

WOMEN'S RIGHTS. The **rights** of women, including female **patients**, and the primary focus of **feminist ethics, feminist bioethics,** and **feminist medical ethics**.

WORLD MEDICAL ASSOCIATION. An international association of national professional associations of physicians (https://www.wma.net/, accessed 14 September 2017). Its *Oath of Physicians* is important for **bioethics, medical ethics,** and **professional medical ethics**. Its **Declaration of Helsinki** is important for **research ethics**. *See also* PROFESSIONAL ASSOCIATIONS OF PHYSICIANS.

X

XENOGRAFTS. The **transplantation** of organs or tissue from nonhuman animals into **patients**. The safety and efficacy of this practice is well established, for example, the use of pig valves in heart-valve replacement. Baby Fae became the first recipient of a nonhuman primate heart in **innovation** of **xenotransplantation** for the **clinical management** of hypoplastic left heart syndrome in 1984, before current surgical techniques that have reduced mortality from this cardiac anomaly were available. This was considered an **ethical controversy** at the time, for reasons of safety (e.g., cross-species infection, massive immune response) and because of disagreement about **organ procurement** from nonhuman primates that caused death. Moreover, this is a form of **vivisection** on a nonhuman animal. *See also* RESEARCH.

XENOTRANSPLANTATION. Transplantation of a nonhuman organ into a **patient**. *See also* XENOGRAFTS.

Y

***YELLOW EMPEROR'S CLASSIC OF MEDICINE (HUANGDI NEIJ-ING)* (SECOND TO FIRST CENTURIES BCE).** Author unknown. The work has the status in the history of Chinese medicine that the **Hippocratic Corpus** has in the history of Western medicine. This text calls for physicians to follow the *Dao* or way of medicine and describes medicine as the ultimate **virtue**. Students for the study of medicine should be selected based on their character.

"YUCK FACTOR". A **gut feeling** of revulsion invoked to justify character-izing **clinical practice** or **research** as **ethically impermissible**. Despite its attraction for some, appeal to the "yuck factor," like all appeals to gut feel-ings, is not a form of **argument** and therefore produces only **mere opinion**.

Z

ZACCHIAS, PAULUS (1584–1659). Italian physician, medical educator, and papal physician. He wrote a comprehensive **medical ethics** that also incorporated legal reasoning. His *Questiones Medico-Legales (Medical-Legal Questions)* was published from 1621 to 1625. He argued against using medicines with the poor that they could not afford, thus addressing the impact on **patient care** of reduced ability to self-pay, which remains an ethical challenge in the current era of high deductibles and co-payments in many health insurance plans. He also recognized that the sick have a limited **ethical obligation** to follow the physician's care plan when it entails medicines with iatrogenic effects that are so harsh that a sick individual is reasonable to want to avoid them.

ZEMSKAYA MEDICINE. A form of medical care in late 19th-century Russia that was based on providing free medical care that was accessible and included preventive medicine. This was a "prototype for socialized health care in Russia" (Lichterman and Yarovinsky 2009, 440). *See also* SOCIALIZED MEDICINE.

ZEMSKIE PHYSICIANS. Physicians in Tsarist Russia in the 19th century who practiced **Zemskaya medicine**. With the advent of medical specialists in the early 20th century, Zemskie physicians could not be specialists in all diseases and they began to shrink in numbers. *See also* SOCIALIZED MEDICINE.

ZERBI, GABRIELE (1445–1505). Italian physician and ethicist. In the *de cautelis* tradition, he wrote *De Cautelis Medicorum*, emphasizing the fidelity of the physician to the sick. The physician should always continue to learn, especially through rigorous, retrospective self-evaluation, always looking for ways to improve **quality**. While he cites the ***Hippocratic Oath***, he differs somewhat from the **Hippocratic Corpus** by calling for the physician to remain with those who are seriously ill but accepts the Hippocratic injunction to abandon the **dying**.

Bibliography

CONTENTS

INTRODUCTION

The literature of medical ethics includes thousands of articles each year in scientific and medical journals, as well as in journals of moral philosophy, religious ethics, moral theology, and the medical humanities. As a field of inquiry to which the disciplines of the humanities contribute, the field of medical ethics is also a book culture. This is important for medical student, resident, fellow, academic, and practicing physician users of this dictionary to appreciate, because, it is fair to say, medicine is not the book culture it once was.

The defining feature of the dictionary is its historical perspective on medical ethics. The disciplines of history—history of medicine, history of ideas, history of moral philosophy, history of moral theology, history of religious ethics—are very much book cultures. The bibliography in the dictionary, therefore, draws mainly from books—authored and edited—that contain original research.

REFERENCE WORKS ON MEDICAL ETHICS AND BIOETHICS

The single, most reliable reference work to which to turn for a concise, scholarly, and well-referenced introduction to topics of interest has been and remains the *Encyclopedia of Bioethics*. The first edition, in four volumes, both consolidated the nascent field of bioethics and provided the impetus for subsequent scholarship. There are four editions:

Reich, Warren T., ed. *Encyclopedia of Bioethics*. New York: Macmillan, 1978.

Reich, Warren T., ed. *Encyclopedia of Bioethics*. 2nd ed. New York: Macmillan, 1995.

Post, Stephen Garrard, ed. *The Encyclopedia of Bioethics*. 3rd ed. New York: Gale Group, 2004.

The *Encyclopedia* in its fourth edition has been renamed, simply, *Bioethics*:

Jennings, Bruce, ed. *Bioethics*. 4th ed. Farmington Hills, MI: Gale Cengage Learning, 2014.

The 1978 and 1995 editions of the *Encyclopedia* each contain a long section, "Medical Ethics, History of," providing a remarkably comprehensive history of medical ethics and signaling that the history of medical ethics is part of bioethics and medical ethics. Modern scholarship on the history of medical ethics was launched, it is reasonable to claim, in the first edition of the *Encyclopedia of Bioethics*. The third edition of the *Encyclopedia* reformatted material on and related to the history of medical ethics in an appendix titled "Historical Perspectives on Medicine, Ethics, and Health Care," focusing mainly on the history of Western medical ethics. The fourth edition takes a more global perspective.

Entries in the *Encyclopedia of Bioethics* often include a historical perspective on the topic under consideration. In addition, readers can gain a historical perspective on the historiography of scholarship on topics in the *Encyclopedia of Bioethics* over the past four decades by reading, in sequence, entries on a specific topic, for example, abortion or informed consent.

There is an *Encyclopedia* devoted to Jewish medical ethics:

Steinberg, Avram. *The Encyclopedia of Jewish Medical Ethics*. Translated by Fred Rosner. Jerusalem: Feldheim Publishers, 2003.

There is also a global encyclopedia of bioethics:

ten Have, Henk. *Encyclopedia of Global Bioethics*. Cham, Switzerland: Springer International Publishing, 2016.

Readers may find more general reference works to be of use:

Becker, Lawrence C., and Charlotte Becker, eds. *Encyclopedia of Ethics*. 3rd ed. New York: Routledge, 2013.

Callahan, Dan, and Peter Singer, eds. *Encyclopedia of Applied Ethics*. Cambridge, MA: Academic Press, 2011.

Zalta, Edward N. *Stanford Encyclopedia of Philosophy*. Available at https://plato.stanford.edu/ [accessed 14 September 2017].

The following edited collections serve as introductions to topics in medical ethics:

Alora, Angeles Tan, and Josephine M. Lumitao, eds. *Beyond a Western Bioethics: Voices from the Developing World.* Washington, DC: Georgetown University Press, 2001.

Chadwick, Ruth F., Eric M. Meslin, and Henk ten Have, eds. *The Sage Handbook of Health Care Ethics.* London: Sage Publications, 2011.

Guinn, David E., ed. *Handbook of Bioethics and Religion.* New York: Oxford University Press, 2006.

Kuhse, Helga, and Peter Singer, eds. *A Companion to Bioethics.* Chichester, Sussex, United Kingdom: Wiley-Blackwell, 2009.

Steinbock, Bonnie, ed. *The Oxford Handbook of Bioethics.* New York: Oxford University Press, 2007.

ten Have, Henk A .M. J., and Bert Gordijn, eds. *Handbook of Global Bioethics.* Cham, Switzerland: Springer International Publishing, 2013.

In a 13-year effort, funded by the National Endowment for the Humanities, the Milbank Memorial Funds, and the Earhart and Littauer Foundations, my academic partner in the history of medical ethics, Robert B. Baker, the William D. Williams Professor of Philosophy at Union College (Schenectady, New York), and I led 55 scholars from 27 countries to provide a global, comprehensive history of medical ethics from the ancient world to the dawn of the 21st century:

Baker, Robert B., and Laurence B. McCullough, eds. *The Cambridge World History of Medical Ethics.* New York: Cambridge University Press, 2009.

Professor Baker has also provided a concise history of medical ethics in a leading reference work for the history of medicine:

Baker, Robert B. "The History of Medical Ethics." In *Companion Encyclopedia of the History of Medicine*, edited by William F. Bynum and Roy Porter, 852–87. London: Routledge, 1993.

Albert Jonsen, one of the founders of the field of bioethics, has provided a "short history" of bioethics, in the tradition of books in philosophy on the "short history" of topics in philosophy:

Jonsen, Albert R. *A Short History of Medical Ethics.* New York: Oxford University Press, 2000.

The book culture of the history of medical ethics grows ever more robust, with books on a wide range of topics. Professor Baker worked with colleagues at the Wellcome Institute for the History of Medicine in London on two conferences on the history of medical ethics that were unique and remarkable for bringing historians of medicine, historians of medical ethics, and medical ethicists together for the first time. The result was two books in the Philosophy and Medicine book series published by Kluwer, now absorbed into Springer:

Baker, Robert B., ed. *Codification of Medical Morality: Historical and Philosophical Studies of the Formalization of Western Medical Morality in the Eighteenth and Nineteenth Centuries: Anglo-American Medical Ethics and Jurisprudence in the Nineteenth Century*. Dordrecht, Netherlands: Kluwer Academic Publishers, 1995.
Baker, Robert B., Dorothy Porter, and Roy Porter, eds. *Codification of Medical Morality: Historical and Philosophical Studies of the Formalization of Western Medical Morality in the Eighteenth and Nineteenth Centuries: Medical Ethics and Etiquette in the Eighteenth Century*. Dordrecht, Netherlands: Kluwer Academic Publishers, 1993.

Professor Baker has also contributed two books on the history of American medical ethics before the emergence of bioethics in the 1960s and 1970s:

Baker, Robert B. *Before Bioethics: A History of American Medical Ethics from the Colonial Period to the Bioethics Revolution*. New York: Oxford University Press, 2013.
Baker, Robert B., Arthur L. Caplan, Linda L. Emanuel, and Stephen R. Latham, eds. *The American Medical Ethics Revolution: How the AMA Code of Ethics Has Transformed Physicians' Relationship to Patients, Professionals, and Society*. Baltimore, MD: Johns Hopkins University Press, 1999.

Other scholars have produced, written, or edited volumes on other periods in the history of medical ethics:

Burns, Chester R., ed. *Legacies in Ethics and Medicine*. New York: Science History Publications, 1977.
Carrick, Paul. *Medical Ethics in the Ancient World*. Washington, DC: Georgetown University Press, 2001.
Edelstein, Ludwig. *Ancient Medicine: Selected Papers of Ludwig Edelstein*. Edited by Owsei Temkin and Lilian Temkin. Baltimore, MD: Johns Hopkins University Press, 1967.

Fissell, Mary E. *Patients, Power, and the Poor in Eighteenth-Century Bristol.* Cambridge: Cambridge University Press, 1991.

Haakonssen, Lisbeth. *Medicine and Morals in the Enlightenment: John Gregory, Thomas Percival, and Benjamin Rush.* Amsterdam: Editions Rodopi, 1997.

Jacobovitz, Immanuel. *A Comparative and Historical Study of the Jewish Religious Attitude to Medicine and Its Practice.* New York: Bloch Publishing Company, 1959.

Konold, Donald. *A History of American Medical Ethics: 1847–1922.* Madison: State Historical Society of Wisconsin, University of Wisconsin, 1962.

Lederer, Susan E. *Subjected to Science: Human Experimentation in America before the Second World War.* Baltimore, MD: Johns Hopkins University Press, 1995.

Maehle, Andreas-Holger, and Johanna Geyer-Kordesch, eds. *Historical and Philosophical Perspectives on Biomedical Ethics.* Aldershot, United Kingdom: Ashgate, 2003.

McCullough, Laurence B. *John Gregory and the Invention of Professional Medical Ethics and the Profession of Medicine.* Dordrecht, Netherlands: Springer (originally Kluwer Academic Publishers), 1998.

Miles, Steven H. *The Hippocratic Oath and the Ethics of Medicine.* New York: Oxford University Press, 2004.

Nie, Jing-Bao. *Medical Ethics in China: A Transcultural Interpretation.* London: Routledge, 2011.

Numbers, Ronald L., and Darrell W. Amundsen, eds. *Caring and Curing: Health and Medicine in Western Religious Traditions.* New York: Macmillan, 1986. Reprinted Baltimore, MD: Johns Hopkins University Press, 1998.

Reiser, Stanley Joel, Arthur J. Dyck, and William Curran, eds. *Ethics in Medicine: Historical Perspectives and Contemporary Concerns.* Cambridge, MA: MIT Press, 1977. (This was the first anthology for teaching medical ethics that included extensive historical materials.)

Schleiner, Winfried. *Medical Ethics in the Renaissance.* Washington, DC: Georgetown University Press, 2007.

Schmidt, Ulf. *Karl Brandt, the Nazi Doctor: Medicine, and Power in the Third Reich.* London: Hambleton Continuum, 2007.

Unschuld, Paul. *Medical Ethics in Imperial China: A Study of Historical Anthropology.* Berkeley: University of California Press, 1979.

Veatch, Robert M. *Disrupted Dialogue: Medical Ethics and the Collapse of Physician-Humanist Communication, 1770–1980.* New York: Oxford University Press, 2004.

Wear, Andrew, Johanna Geyer-Kordesch, and Roger French, eds. *Doctors and Ethics: The Earlier Historical Setting of Professional Ethics.* Amsterdam: Editions Rodopi, 1993.

There are several histories of bioethics:

Jonsen, Albert R. *The Birth of Bioethics*. New York: Oxford University Press, 1998.
Rothman, David J. *Strangers at the Bedside: A History of How Law and Bioethics Have Transformed Medical Decision Making*. New York: Basic Books, 1991.
Stevens, M. L. Tina. *Bioethics in America: Origins and Cultural Politics*. Baltimore, MD: Johns Hopkins University Press, 2000.

WORKS CITED

American Academy of Pediatrics. "Informed Consent, Parental Permission, and Assent in Pediatric Practice." Committee on Bioethics. *Pediatrics* 95, no. 2 (February 1995): 314–17.
———. "Informed Consent in Decision Making in Pediatric Practice." *Pediatrics* 138, no. 2 (August 2016): e20161484.
American Medical Association. "Code of Ethics." 1847. In *The American Medical Ethics Revolution: How the AMA's Code of Ethics Has Transformed Physicians' Relationships to Patients, Professionals, and Society*, edited by Robert B. Baker, Arthur L. Caplan, Linda L. Emanuel, and Stephen R. Latham, 324–34. Baltimore, MD: Johns Hopkins University Press, 1999.
———. *Principles of Medical Ethics*. Chicago, IL: American Medical Association, 1903. In *The American Medical Ethics Revolution: How the AMA's Code of Ethics Has Transformed Physicians' Relationships to Patients, Professionals, and Society*, edited by Robert B. Baker, Arthur L. Caplan, Linda L. Emanuel, and Stephen R. Latham, 335–45. Baltimore, MD: Johns Hopkins University Press, 1999.
———. *Principles of Medical Ethics*. Chicago, IL: American Medical Association, 1912. In *The American Medical Ethics Revolution: How the AMA's Code of Ethics Has Transformed Physicians' Relationships to Patients, Professionals, and Society*, edited by Robert B. Baker, Arthur L. Caplan, Linda L. Emanuel, and Stephen R. Latham. Baltimore, MD: Johns Hopkins University Press, 1999: 346–54.
———. *Principles of Medical Ethics*. Chicago, IL: American Medical Association, 1957. In *The American Medical Ethics Revolution: How the AMA's Code of Ethics Has Transformed Physicians' Relationships to Pa-*

tients, Professionals, and Society, edited by Robert B. Baker, Arthur L. Caplan, Linda L. Emanuel, and Stephen R. Latham, 355–37. Baltimore, MD: Johns Hopkins University Press, 1999.

———. *Principles of Medical Ethics*. Chicago, IL: American Medical Association, 1980. In *The American Medical Ethics Revolution: How the AMA's Code of Ethics Has Transformed Physicians' Relationships to Patients, Professionals, and Society*, edited by Robert B. Baker, Arthur L. Caplan, Linda L. Emanuel, and Stephen R. Latham, 358–59. Baltimore, MD: Johns Hopkins University Press, 1999.

———. *Principles of Medical Ethics*. Chicago, IL: American Medical Association, 2001. Available at https://www.ama-assn.org/sites/default/files/media-browser/principles-of-medical-ethics.pdf [accessed 14 September 2017].

———. *AMA Code of Medical Ethics*. Chicago, IL: American Medical Association, 2016. Available at https://www.ama-assn.org/delivering-care/ama-code-medical-ethics [accessed 14 September 2017].

Amundsen, Darrell W. "The Discourses of Early Christian Medical Ethics." In *The Cambridge World History of Medical Ethics*, edited by Robert B. Baker and Laurence B. McCullough, 202–10. New York: Cambridge University Press, 2009a.

———. "The Discourses of Roman Catholic Medical Ethics." In *The Cambridge World History of Medical Ethics*, edited by Robert B. Baker and Laurence B. McCullough, 218–24. New York: Cambridge University Press, 2009b.

Appelbaum, Paul S., Loren H. Roth, and Charles Lidz. "The Therapeutic Misconception: Informed Consent in Psychiatric Research." *International Journal of Law and Psychiatry* 5, nos. 3–4 (1982): 319–29.

Audi, Robert. "Intuition and Its Place in Ethics." *Journal of the American Philosophical Association* 1, no. 1 (April 2015): 57–77.

Aurelius, Marcus. *The Communings with Himself of Marcus Aurelius Emperor of Rome*. Translated by C. R. Haines. Cambridge, MA: Harvard University Press, 1937. Composed ca. 171–175.

Bacon, Francis. *De Augmentis Scientiarum* [*On the Dignity and Advancement of Learning*]. In *The Works of Francis Bacon*, edited by J. Spedding. Reprinted by Cambridge University Press. Cambridge: Cambridge University Press, 2000. Originally published in 1623.

Baker, Robert B. "Bioethics and History." *Journal of Medicine and Philosophy* 27, no. 4 (August 2002): 447–74.

———. "The Discourses of Practitioners in Nineteenth- and Twentieth-Century Britain and the United States." In *The Cambridge World History of Medical Ethics*, edited by Robert B. Baker and Laurence B. McCullough, 446–64. New York: Cambridge University Press, 2009.

———. *Before Bioethics: A History of American Medical Ethics from the Colonial Period to the Bioethics Revolution*. New York: Oxford University Press, 2013.

Baker, Robert B., Arthur L. Caplan, Linda L. Emanuel, and Stephen R. Latham, eds. *The American Medical Ethics Revolution: How the AMA's Code of Ethics Has Transformed Physicians' Relationships to Patients, Professionals, and Society*. Baltimore, MD: Johns Hopkins University Press, 1999.

Baker, Robert B., and Laurence B. McCullough, eds. *The Cambridge World History of Medical Ethics*. New York: Cambridge University Press, 2009a.

———. "What Is the History of Medical Ethics?" In *The Cambridge World History of Medical Ethics*, edited by Robert B. Baker and Laurence B. McCullough, 3–15. New York: Cambridge University Press, 2009b.

———. "The Discourses of Philosophical Medical Ethics." In *The Cambridge World History of Medical Ethics*, edited by Robert B. Baker and Laurence B. McCullough, 281–309. New York: Cambridge University Press, 2009c.

———. "Medical Ethics through the Life Cycle in Europe and the Americas." In *The Cambridge World History of Medical Ethics*, edited by Robert B. Baker and Laurence B. McCullough, 137–62. New York: Cambridge University Press, 2009d.

Beauchamp, Tom L., and James F. Childress. *Principles of Biomedical Ethics*. New York: Oxford University Press, 1979.

———. *Principles of Biomedical Ethics*. 7th ed. New York: Oxford University Press, 2013.

Beck, Theodoric Romeyn. *Elements of Medical Jurisprudence*. Albany, NY: Webster and Skinner, 1823.

Bell, John. "Introduction to the Code of Medical Ethics." *Minutes of the Proceedings of the National Medical Convention held in the City of Philadelphia, in May 1847*, 83–92. In *The American Medical Ethics Revolution: How the AMA's Code of Ethics Has Transformed Physicians' Relationships to Patients, Professionals, and Society*, edited by Robert B. Baker, Arthur L. Caplan, Linda L. Emanuel, and Stephen R. Latham, 317–23. Baltimore, MD: Johns Hopkins University Press, 1999.

Bernard, Claude. *Introduction à l'étude de la medicine expérimentale* [*Introduction to the Study of Experimental Medicine*]. Paris: J. B. Bailliére, 1865.

Biffl, W. L., D. A. Spain, A. M. Reitsma, R. M. Minter, et al. Society of University Surgeons Innovations Project Team. "Responsible Development and Application of Surgical Innovations: A Position Statement of the Society of University Surgeons." *Journal of the American College of Surgeons* 2006, no. 6 (June 2008): 1204–9.

Binding, Karl, and Alfred Hoche. *Die Freigabe der Vernichtung lebensunwerten Lebens: Ihr Mass und ihre Form* [*The Release and Destruction of Life Devoid of Value: Its Measure and Form*]. Leipzig, Germany: Verlag von Felix Meiner, 1920.

Blasszauer, Bela. "Medical Ethics and Communism in Eastern Europe." In *The Cambridge World History of Medical Ethics*, edited by Robert B. Baker and Laurence B. McCullough, 617–24. New York: Cambridge University Press, 2009.

Blumenthal-Barby, J. S., and Hadley Burroughs. "Seeking Better Health Care Outcomes: The Ethics of Using the 'Nudge.'" *American Journal of Bioethics* 12, no. 2 (February 2012): 1–10.

Braun, Ursula K., Aanand D. Naik, and Laurence B. McCullough. "Reconceptualizing the Experience of Surrogate Decision Making: Reports vs. Making Decisions." *Annals of Family Medicine* 7, no. 3 (May/June 2009): 249–53.

Brody, Baruch A. *The Ethics of Biomedical Research: An International Perspective*. New York: Oxford University Press, 1998.

——. *Taking Issue: Pluralism and Casuistry in Bioethics*. Washington, DC: Georgetown University Press, 2003.

Campbell, Alastair V. "My Country 'Tis of Thee—the Myopia of American Bioethics." *Medicine, Health Care and Philosophy* 3, no. 2 (May 2000): 195–98.

Castro, Rodrigo de. *Medicus Politicus; sive, De officiis medico-politicis tractatus, quatuor libris* [*The Politic Physician; or, On Medico-Politic Duties, Treated in Four Volumes*]. Hamburg: Frobenianus, 1614.

Chervenak, Frank A., and Laurence B. McCullough. "Justified Limits on Refusing Treatment." *Hastings Center Report* 21, no. 2 (April 1991): 12–18.

——. "The Diagnosis and Management of Progressive Dysfunction of Health Care Organizations." *Obstetrics and Gynecology* 105, no. 4 (April 2005): 882–87.

——. *The Professional Responsibility Model of Perinatal Ethics*. Berlin: Walter de Gruyter, 2014.

Chervenak, Frank A., Laurence B. McCullough, Amos Grünebaum, Birgit Arabin, Malcolm I. Levene, and Robert L. Brent. "Planned Home Birth: A Violation of the Best Interests of the Child Standard?" *Pediatrics* 132, no. 5 (November 2013): 921–23.

Chervenak, Judith, Laurence B. McCullough, and Frank A. Chervenak. "Surgery without Consent or Miscommunication: A New Look at a Landmark Legal Case." *American Journal of Obstetrics and Gynecology* 212, no. 5 (May 2015): 586–90.

Clouser, K. Danner. "Bioethics." In *Encyclopedia of Bioethics*, edited by Warren T. Reich, 115–27. New York: Macmillan, 1978.

"Consensus Statement of the Society of Critical Care Medicine's Ethics Committee Regarding Futile Care and Other Possibly Inadvisable Treatments." *Critical Care Medicine* 25, no. 5 (May 1997): 887–91.

Coppens, Charles, SJ. *Moral Principles and Medical Practice: The Basis of Medical Jurisprudence*. New York: Benziger Brothers, 1897.

Coverdale, John H., Laurence B. McCullough, and Frank A. Chervenak. "Enhanced Decision-Making by Depressed Pregnant Patients." *Journal of Perinatal Medicine* 30, no. 4 (April 2002): 349–51.

"A Definition of Irreversible Coma: A Report of the *Ad Hoc* Committee of the Harvard Medical School to Examine the Definition of Brain Death." *Journal of the American Medical Association* 205, no. 6 (5 August 1968): 337–40.

Engel, George. "The Need for a New Medical Model: A Challenge for Biomedicine." *Science* 196, no. 4286 (8 April 1977): 129–36.

Engelhardt, H. Tristram, Jr. *The Foundations of Bioethics*. 2nd ed. New York: Oxford University Press, 1996.

———. "The Discourses of Orthodox Christian Medical Ethics." In *The Cambridge World History of Medical Ethics*, edited by Robert B. Baker and Laurence B. McCullough, 211–17. New York: Cambridge University Press, 2009.

Fan, Ruiping. "The Discourses of Confucian Medical Ethics." In *The Cambridge World History of Medical Ethics*, edited by Robert B. Baker and Laurence B. McCullough, 195–201. New York: Cambridge University Press, 2009.

Ferngren, Gary B. "The Discourses of Protestant Medical Ethics." In *The Cambridge World History of Medical Ethics*, edited by Robert B. Baker and Laurence B. McCullough, 255–63. New York: Cambridge University Press, 2009.

Fletcher, Joseph. *Morals and Medicine*. Boston, MA: Beacon Press, 1954.

Flint, Austin. *Medical Ethics and Medical Etiquette: The Code of Ethics Adopted by the American Medical Association with Commentaries by Austin Flint, M.D.* New York: Appleton and Company, 1882.

Frank, Johann Peter. *System einer vollständigen medicinischen Polizei [A System of Complete Medical Police]*. Mannheim, Germany: C. F. Schwann, 1779.

Gãlvao-Sobrinho, C. R. "Hippocratic Ideals, Medical Ethics, and the Practice of Medicine in the Early Middle Ages: The Legacy of the Hippocratic Oath." *Journal of the History of Medicine and Allied Health Sciences* 51, no. 4 (October 1996): 438–55.

Gefanis, Eugenius. "The Discourses of Bioethics in Post-Communist Eastern Europe." In *The Cambridge World History of Medical Ethics*, ed. Robert B. Baker and Laurence B. McCullough. New York: Cambridge University Press, 2009: 495–500.

Gisborne, Thomas. *An Enquiry into the Duties of Men in the Higher and Middle Classes of Society in Great Britain Resulting from Their Respective Stations, Professions and Employment.* London: B. & J. White, 1794.

Gracia, Diego. "The Discourses of Practitioners in Nineteenth- and Twentieth-Century Spain." In *The Cambridge World History of Medical Ethics*, edited by Robert B. Baker and Laurence B. McCullough, 427–31. New York: Cambridge University Press, 2009.

———. "Philosophy: Ancient and Contemporary Approaches." In *Methods in Medical Ethics*, 2nd ed., edited by Jeremy Sugarman and Daniel P. Sulmasy, 55–72. Washington, DC: Georgetown University Press, 2010.

Gracia, Jorge. *Introduction to the Problem of Individuation in the Early Middle Ages.* 2nd ed. Munich, Germany: Philosophia Verlag, 1988.

Anonymous [John Gregory]. *Observations on the Duties and Offices of a Physician, and on the Method of Prosecuting Enquiries in Philosophy.* London: W. Strahan and T. Cadell, 1770. In *John Gregory's Writings on Medical Ethics and Philosophy of Medicine*, edited by Laurence B. McCullough, 93–159. Dordrecht, Netherlands: Springer (formerly Kluwer Academic Publishers), 1998.

Gregory, John. *Lectures on the Duties and Qualifications of a Physician.* London: W. Strahan and T. Cadell, 1772. In *John Gregory's Writings on Medical Ethics and Philosophy of Medicine*, edited by Laurence B. McCullough, 161–248. Dordrecht, Netherlands: Springer (formerly Kluwer Academic Publishers), 1998.

———. *Lectures on the Duties and Qualifications of a Physician.* London: W. Strahan and T. Cadell, 1772. Translated anonymously into German as *Vorlesungen über die Pflichten und Eigenschaften eines Artzes: Aus dem Englischen nach der neuen und verbesserten Ausgabe.* Leipzig, Germany: Caspar Fritsch, 1778.

———. *Lectures on the Duties and Qualifications of a Physician.* London: W. Strahan and T. Cadell, 1772. Translated into Italian by F. F. Padovano as *Lexioni Sopra I Doveri e la Qualita di un medico.* Florence: Gaetano Cambiagi, 1789.

———. *Lectures on the Duties and Qualifications of a Physician.* London: W. Strahan and T. Cadell, 1772. Translated into French by B. Verlac as *Discours sur les dévoirs, les qualités et les connaissances du médicin, avec un cour d'études.* Paris: Crapart & Briands, 1797.

———. *Lectures on the Duties and Qualifications of a Physician.* Philadelphia: M. Carey and Son, 1817.

Gregory, Juan. *Discurso sobre los deberes, qualidades y conocimientos del medico, con el método des sus estudios.* Madrid: Imprenta Real, 1803.

Grünebaum, Amos, Laurence B. McCullough, Kate J. Sapra, Robert L. Brent, Malcolm I. Levene, Birgit Arabin, and Frank A. Chervenak. "Apgar Score of Zero at Five Minutes and Neonatal Seizures or Serious Neurologic Dysfunction in Relation to Birth Setting." *American Journal of Obstetrics and Gynecology* 209, no. 4 (October 2013): 323.e1–323.e6.

Hippocrates. *The Art.* Translated by W. H. S. Jones. In *Hippocrates,* vol. 2, with an English translation by W. H. S. Jones, 185–217. Cambridge, MA: Harvard University Press, 1923a.

———. *The Sacred Disease.* Translated by W. H. S. Jones. In *Hippocrates,* vol. 2, with an English translation by W. H. S. Jones, 127–83. Cambridge, MA: Harvard University Press, 1923b.

Hoffmann, Friedrich. *Medicus Politicus; sive, Regulae Prudentiae secundum quas Medicus Juvenis Studia sua & Vitae Rationem Dirigere Debet [The Politic Doctor; or, Rules of Prudence according to which a Young Physician Should Direct His Studies and Reason of Life].* Leiden, Netherlands: Philip Bonk, 1738.

Hooker, Worthington. *Physician and Patient; or, A Practical View of the Mutual Duties, Relations and Interests of the Medical Profession and Community.* New York: Baker and Scribner, 1849.

Hufeland, Christian. *Enchiridion medicum order Anleitung zur medizinische Praxis: Vermächtnis funfzigjäbrigen Erfahrung [Manual of the Practice of Medicine: The Results of Fifty Years' Experience].* 2nd ed. Berlin: Jonas Verlagsbuchhandlung, 1836.

Hume, David. *A Treatise of Human Nature.* Edited by David Fate Norton and Mary J. Norton. New York: Oxford University Press, 2000. Originally published 1739–1740.

Ilkilic, Ilhan. "The Discourses of Islamic Medical Ethics." In *The Cambridge World History of Medical Ethics,* edited by Robert B. Baker and Laurence B. McCullough, 270–77. New York: Cambridge University Press, 2009.

Jacobovitz, Immanuel. *A Comparative and Historical Study of the Jewish Religious Attitude to Medicine and Its Practice.* New York: Bloch Publishing Company, 1959.

Jennings, Bruce, ed. *Bioethics.* 4th ed. of *Encyclopedia of Bioethics.* Farmington Hills, MI: Gale Cengage Learning, 2014.

Jones, James H. *Bad Blood: The Tuskegee Syphilis Experiment.* 2nd ed. New York: Free Press, 2003. First edition published in 1993.

Jones, James W., Laurence B. McCullough, and Bruce W. Richman. "A Comprehensive Primer on Surgical Informed Consent." *Surgical Clinics of North America* 87, no. 4 (August 2007): 903–18, viii.

Jonsen, Albert R. *The Birth of Bioethics.* New York: Oxford University Press, 1998.

———. *A Short History of Medical Ethics.* New York: Oxford University Press, 2000.

———. "The Discourses of Bioethics in the United States." In *The Cambridge World History of Medical Ethics*, edited by Robert B. Baker and Laurence B. McCullough, 477–85. New York: Cambridge University Press, 2009.

Jonsen, Albert R., Mark Siegler, and William J. Winslade. *Clinical Ethics: A Practical Approach to Ethical Decisions in Clinical Medicine*. 7th ed. New York: McGraw-Hill, 2010.

Jouanna, Jacques. *Hippocrates*. Translated by M. B. DeBevoise. Baltimore, MD: Johns Hopkins University Press, 1999.

Kant, Immanuel. *Groundwork of the Metaphysics of Morals*. Translated by H. J. Paton. New York: Harper Torchbooks, 1964.

Kappa Lambda Society. *Extracts from the Medical Ethics of Dr. Percival*. Philadelphia: Kappa Lambda Society, 1823. Privately published.

Kelly, Gerald. *Medico-Moral Problems*. 5 parts. St. Louis, MO: Catholic Hospital Association of the United States, 1949–1954.

Kimura, Rihito, and Shizu Sakai. "Medical Ethics through the Life Cycle in Japan." In *The Cambridge World History of Medical Ethics*, edited by Robert B. Baker and Laurence B. McCullough, 132–36. New York: Cambridge University Press, 2009.

Landau, Sidney L. *Dictionaries: The Art and Craft of Lexicography*. 2nd ed. Cambridge: Cambridge University Press, 2001.

Leake, Chauncey, ed. *Percival's Medical Ethics*. Baltimore, MD: Williams and Wilkins, 1927.

Lederer, Susan E. "The Ethics of Experimenting on Human Subjects." In *The Cambridge World History of Medical Ethics*, edited by Robert B. Baker and Laurence B. McCullough, 558–65. New York: Cambridge University Press, 2009.

Lichterman, Boleslaw L., and Mikhail Yarovinsky. "The Discourses of Practitioners in Eighteenth- to Twentieth-Century Russia." In *The Cambridge World History of Medical Ethics*, edited by Robert B. Baker and Laurence B. McCullough, 439–45. New York: Cambridge University Press, 2009.

Lombardo, Paul A. "Phantom Tumors and Hysterical Women: Revising Our View of the Schloendorff Case." *Journal of Law, Medicine, and Ethics* 33, no. 4 (Winter 2005): 791–801.

Maehle, Andres-Holger. "The Ethics of Experimenting on Animal Subjects." In *The Cambridge World History of Medical Ethics*, edited by Robert B. Baker and Laurence B. McCullough, 552–57. New York: Cambridge University Press, 2009.

Mainetti, José Maria. "The Discourses of Medical Ethics in Latin America." In *The Cambridge World History of Medical Ethics*, edited by Robert B. Baker and Laurence B. McCullough, 501–4. New York: Cambridge University Press, 2009.

Marx, Karl Friedrich Heinrich. *Ärtzlicher Katechismus: Über die Anforderungen an die Ärtze* [*Medical Catechism: On the Requirements on Physicians*]. Stuttgart, Germany: Verlag von F. Enke, 1876.

McCormick, Richard. *Ambiguity in Moral Choice*. Milwaukee, WI: Marquette University Press, 1977.

McCullough, Laurence B. *John Gregory and the Invention of Professional Medical Ethics and the Profession of Medicine*. Dordrecht, Netherlands: Springer (originally Kluwer Academic Publishers), 1998.

———. "The Ethical Concept of Medicine as a Profession: Its Origins in Modern Medical Ethics and Implications for Physicians." In *Lost Virtue: Professional Character Development in Medical Education*, edited by Nuala Kenny and Wayne Shelton, 17–27. New York: Elsevier, 2006.

———. "Was Bioethics Founded on Historical and Conceptual Mistakes about Medical Paternalism?" *Bioethics* 25, no. 2 (February 2011): 66–74.

McCullough, Laurence B., John H. Coverdale, and Frank A. Chervenak. "Argument-Based Medical Ethics: A Formal Tool for Critically Appraising the Normative Medical Ethics Literature." *American Journal of Obstetrics and Gynecology* 191, no. 4 (October 2014): 1097–102.

McKeon, Richard. "The Philosophical Basis and Material Circumstances of the Rights of Man." *Ethics* 58, no. 3 (April 1948): 180–87.

Menikoff, Jerry, Julie Kaneshiro, and Ivor Pritchard. "The Common Rule, Updated." *New England Journal of Medicine* 376, no. 7 (16 February 2017): 613–15.

Miles, Steven H. *The Hippocratic Oath and the Ethics of Medicine*. New York: Oxford University Press, 2004.

Moll, Albert. *Ärtzliche Ethik: Die Pflichten des Artzes in allen Bezeihungen seiner Thätighiet* [*Doctor's Ethics: The Duties of the Doctor with Regard to All His Activities*]. Stuttgart, Germany: Verlag von F. Enke, 1902.

Moreno, Jonathan. *Deciding Together: Bioethics and Moral Consensus*. New York: Oxford University Press, 1995.

Nie, Jing-Bao. "The Discourses of Practitioners in China." In *The Cambridge World History of Medical Ethics*, edited by Robert B. Baker and Laurence B. McCullough, 335–44. New York: Cambridge University Press, 2009.

Nie, Jung-Bao, Takashi Tsuchiya, and Lun Li. "Japanese Doctors' Experimentation, 1932–1945, and Medical Ethics." In *The Cambridge World History of Medical Ethics*, edited by Robert B. Baker and Laurence B. McCullough, 589–94. New York: Cambridge University Press, 2009.

Nutton, Vivian. The "Discourses of European Practitioners in the Tradition of the Hippocratic Texts." In *The Cambridge World History of Medical Ethics*, edited by Robert B. Baker and Laurence B. McCullough, 359–62. New York: Cambridge University Press, 2009.

Nye, Robert A. "The Discourses of Practitioners in Nineteenth- and Twentieth Century France." In *The Cambridge World History of Medical Ethics*, edited by Robert B. Baker and Laurence B. McCullough, 418–26. New York: Cambridge University Press, 2009.

Osler, William. *Aequanimitas: Valedictory Remarks to the Graduates in Medicine of the University of Pennsylvania, May 1, 1889*. Philadelphia: W. F. Fell and Company, 1889.

Percival, Thomas. *Medical Jurisprudence; or, A Code of Ethics and Institutes, Adapted to the Professions of Physic and Surgery*. Manchester, England: privately published, 1794.

———. *Medical Ethics; or, A Code of Institutes and Precepts, Adapted to the Professional Conduct of Physicians and Surgeons*. London: Johnson & Bickerstaff, 1803.

Pilcher, Lewis. "Codes of Medical Ethics." In *An Ethical Symposium: Being a Series of Papers Concerning Medical Ethics and Etiquette from a Liberal Standpoint*, edited by Albert C. Post et al., 42–43, 52–53. New York: G. P. Putnam, 1883.

Placencia, Frank X., and Laurence B. McCullough. "The History of Ethical Decision Making in Neonatal Intensive Care." *Journal of Intensive Care Medicine* 26, no. 6 (November–December 2011): 368–84.

Porter, Dorothy, and Roy Porter. *Patient's Progress: Doctors and Doctoring in Eighteenth-Century England*. Stanford, CA: Stanford University Press, 1989.

Porter, Roy, and Mikuláš Teich, eds. *The Enlightenment in National Context*. Cambridge: Cambridge University Press, 1981.

Rachels, James. "Active and Passive Euthanasia." *New England Journal of Medicine* 292, no. 2 (9 January 1975): 78–80.

Ramsey, Paul. *The Patient as Person: Explorations on Medical Ethics*. New Haven, CT: Yale University Press, 1973.

Rawls, John. *A Theory of Justice: Revised Edition*. Cambridge, MA: Harvard University Press, 1999. Revision of 1971 edition.

Reich, Warren T., ed. *Encyclopedia of Bioethics*. New York: Macmillan, 1978.

Richardson, Henry S. *Practical Reasoning about Final Ends*. Cambridge: Cambridge University Press, 1997.

Rush, Benjamin. *Observations on the Duties of a Physician, and the Methods of Improving Medicine. Accommodated to the Present State of Society and Manners in the United States*. In *Medical Inquiries and Observations*, 2nd ed., vol. 1, edited by B. Rush, 345–408. Philadelphia: J. Conrad & Co., 1805.

Ryan, Michael. *A Manual of Medical Jurisprudence, Compiled from the Best Medical and Legal Works: Comprising an Account of: I. The Ethics of the Medical Association, II. The Charter and Status Relating to the Faculty, and III. All Medico-Legal Questions, with the Latest Discussions. Being an Analysis of a Course of Lectures on Forensic Medicine Annually Delivered in London and Intended as a Compendium for the Use of Barristers, Solicitors, Magistrates, and Medical Practitioners.* London: Rensaw and Rush, 1831.

Schneiderman, Lawrence J., Nancy S. Jecker, and Albert R. Jonsen. "Medical Futility: Response to Critiques." *Annals of Internal Medicine* 125, no. 8 (15 October 1996): 669–74.

Scribonius Largus. *Compositiones.* Available as *De compositione medicamentorum liber.* Basileae: Cratandrus, 1529. Originally published ca. 47.

Shem, Samuel (pseud.). *The House of God.* New York: R. Marek Publishers, 1978.

Shestack, Jerome T. "The Philosophical Foundations of Human Rights." *Human Rights Quarterly* 20, no. 2 (May 1998): 201–34.

Simon, Maximilien Isidore Amand . Déontologie médicale; ou, Les devoirs et les droits des médicins dans l'état actuel de la civilisation [Medical Deontology; or, The Duties and Rights of Physicians in the Current State of Civilization]. Paris: Ballière, 1845.

Snyder, Lois, for the American College of Physicians Ethics, Professionalism, and Human Rights Committee. "American College of Physicians Ethics Manual, Sixth Edition." Annals of Internal Medicine 156, no. 1, pt. 2 (3 January 2012): 73 –104.

Song, Guobin. *Yiye Lunlixue* [*Professional Ethics in Medicine*]. Shanghai: Guoguang Bookstore, 1933.

Sperry, Willard. *The Ethical Basis for Medical Practice.* New York: P. B. Hoeber, 1950.

State Medical Society of New York. *A System of Medical Ethics, Published by the Order of the State Medical Society of New York.* New York: printed by William Grattan, 1823.

Steinberg, Avram. *The Encyclopedia of Jewish Medical Ethics.* Translated by Fred Rosner. Jerusalem: Feldheim Publishers, 2003.

Strawson, Peter F. *Individuals: An Essay in Descriptive Metaphysics.* Garden City, NJ: Anchor Books, 1963.

Thaler, Richard H., and Cass R. Sunstein. *Nudge: Improving Decisions about Health, Wealth, and Happiness.* New York: Penguin Books, 2009.

Thomas, Dylan. *The Poems of Dylan Thomas,* edited and notes by Daniel Jones with a preface by Dylan Thomas. New York: New Directions Books, 2003.

Thomas, Tessy A., and Laurence B. McCullough. "A Philosophical Taxonomy of Ethically Significant Moral Distress." *Journal of Medicine and Philosophy* 14, no. 1 (February 2015): 102–20.

Tong, Rosemary. *Feminine and Feminist Ethics.* Belmont, CA: Wadsworth, 1993.

Tooley, Michael. *Abortion and Infanticide*. New York: Macmillan, 1981.

United Nations Educational, Scientific and Cultural Organization. "Universal Declaration of Human Rights and Bioethics." Paris: United Nations Educational, Scientific and Cultural Organization, 2005. Available at http://unesdoc.unesco.org/images/0014/001461/146180E.pdf [accessed 14 September 2017].

United Nations Office of the High Commissioner. "Convention against Torture and Other Cruel, Inhuman or Degrading Treatment or Punishment." Adopted and opened for signature, ratification, and accession by General Assembly resolution 39/46 of 10 December 1984, entry into force 26 June 1987, in accordance with article 27 (1). Available at http://www.ohchr.org/EN/ProfessionalInterest/Pages/CAT.aspx [accessed 14 September 2017].

U.S. National Commission for the Protection of Human Subjects of Biomedical and Behavioral Research. *The Belmont Report*. Washington, DC: United States Government Printing Office, 1979. Available at https://www.hhs.gov/ohrp/regulations-and-policy/belmont-report/index.html [accessed 14 September 2017].

Veatch, Robert M. *The Basics of Bioethics: A Balanced and Systematic Ethical Framework*. 3rd ed. New York: Pearson Education, 2012.

Verhagen, Eduard, and Pietter J. J. Sauer. "The Groningen Protocol—Euthanasia in Severely Ill Newborns." *New England Journal of Medicine* 352, no. 10 (10 March 2005): 959–62.

von Staden, Heinrich. "In a Pure and Holy Way: Personal and Professional Conduct in the Hippocratic Oath." *Journal of the History of Medicine and Allied Health Sciences* 51, no. 4 (October 1996): 404–37.

———. "The Discourses of Practitioners in Ancient Europe." In *The Cambridge World History of Medical Ethics*, edited by Robert B. Baker and Laurence B. McCullough, 352–58. New York: Cambridge University Press, 2009.

Watterberg, Kristi L., on behalf of the Committee on Fetus and Newborn, American Academy of Pediatrics. "Policy Statement on Planned Home Birth: Upholding the Best Interests of Children and Families." *Pediatrics* 132, no. 5 (November 2013): 924–26.

Whitney, Simon N., Amy L. McGuire, and Laurence B. McCullough. "A Typology of Shared Decision Making, Informed Consent, and Simple Consent." *Annals of Internal Medicine* 140, no. 1 (6 January 2004): 54–59.

Wijdicks, E. F., P. N. Vareles, G. S. Gronseth, and D. M. Greer. "Evidence-Based Guideline Update: Determining Brain Death in Adults: Report of the Quality Standards Subcommittee of the American Academy of Neurology." *Neurology* 74, no. 23 (8 June 2010): 1911–18.

World Health Organization. "Constitution of WHO: Principles." Appended to bottom of text: The Constitution was adopted by the International Health Conference held in New York from 19 June to 22 July 1946, signed on 22 July 1946 by the representatives of 61 States and entered into force on 7 April 1948. Later amendments are incorporated into this text. Available at http://www.who.int/about/mission/en/ [accessed 14 September 2017].

World Medical Association. "International Code of Medical Ethics." Adopted 1949, last revised 2006a. Available at https://www.wma.net/policies-post/wma-international-code-of-medical-ethics/ [accessed 14 September 2017].

———. "Declaration of Geneva: Physician's Oath." Adopted 1946, last revised 2006b. Available at https://www.wma.net/policies-post/wma-declaration-of-geneva/ [accessed 14 September 2017].

———. "Statement on Medical Ethics in the Event of Disasters." Adopted 1994, revised 2006c. Available at https://www.wma.net/policies-post/wma-statement-on-medical-ethics-in-the-event-of-disasters/ [accessed 14 September 2017].

———. "Declaration of Helsinki: Ethical Principles for Research with Human Subjects." Adopted 1964, last revised 2013. Available at https://www.wma.net/policies-post/wma-declaration-of-helsinki-ethical-principles-for-medical-research-involving-human-subjects/ [accessed 14 September 2017].

Young, Katherine K. "The Discourses of Practitioners in India." In *The Cambridge World History of Medical Ethics*, edited by Robert B. Baker and Laurence B. McCullough, 324–34. New York: Cambridge University Press, 2009a.

———. "Medical Ethics through the Life Cycle in Buddhist India." In *The Cambridge World History of Medical Ethics*, edited by Robert B. Baker and Laurence B. McCullough, 113–25. New York: Cambridge University Press, 2009b.

———. "Medical Ethics through the Life Cycle in Hindu India." In *The Cambridge World History of Medical Ethics*, edited by Robert B. Baker and Laurence B. McCullough, 101–12. New York: Cambridge University Press, 2009c.

Zohar, Noam J. "The Discourses of Jewish Medical Ethics." In *The Cambridge World History of Medical Ethics*, edited by Robert B. Baker and Laurence B. McCullough, 264–69. New York: Cambridge University Press, 2009.

About the Author

Laurence B. McCullough is adjunct professor of ethics in obstetrics and gynecology and of medical ethics in medicine at the Weill Medical College of Cornell University in New York City. He is also distinguished emeritus professor at the Center for Medical Ethics and Health Policy of Baylor College of Medicine in Houston, Texas. He received his A.B., cum laude with honors, in art history from Williams College in 1969 and his Ph.D. in philosophy from the University of Texas at Austin in 1975. He was a research associate and predoctoral fellow at the Institute for the Medical Humanities of the University of Texas Medical Branch at Galveston (1975–1976) and a postdoctoral fellow at the Hastings Center, 1975–1976, which was funded by the National Endowment for the Humanities. He was elected a fellow of the Hastings Center in 2003.

McCullough has made his academic career for more than 40 years as a philosopher and medical educator. He has held his adjunct appointment at Weill Cornell since 1987, and he and his fellow scholar Frank A. Chervenak have published more than 250 papers in the peer-reviewed literature and two books, including *The Professional Responsibility Model of Perinatal Ethics* (2014). He was professor of medicine and family medicine at Baylor College of Medicine from 1988 to 2016, where he was also the Dalton Tomlin chair in medical ethics and health policy (2008–2016). While in Houston, he served as adjunct professor of philosophy at Rice University (2001–2016) and taught medical students, residents, and fellows at Baylor (Texas Children's Hospital and the Michael E. DeBakey Veterans Affairs Medical Center) and mentored 140 medical students in Baylor's national award-winning ethics track. He received Baylor's Barbara and Corbin J. Robertson Presidential Award for Excellence in medical education in 2013, the college's highest teaching award.

McCullough's research interests include ethics in obstetrics and gynecology, the history of medical ethics, ethics in pediatrics (including ethics in pediatric cancer genomics), teaching medical ethics to medical students and residents, and the philosophy of Gottfried Wilhelm Leibniz (1646–1716). His research in the history of medical ethics has been funded by an American Council of Learned Societies fellowship (1995–1996) and by the National Endowment of the Humanities, the Milbank Memorial Fund, and the Earhart and Littauer foundations (1999–2002). He collaborated at Baylor with colleagues on multidisciplinary research projects funded by the National Institutes of Health on conflicts of interest in scientific research, ethical challenges in research under an emergency waiver, and the ethics of introducing whole exome sequencing into the clinical care of children with cancer. This is his 15th book.